SACRED PLANTS
HUMAN VOICES

SACRED PLANTS HUMAN VOICES

Nancy Herrick, P.A.

◆

PROVINGS
OF SEVEN
NEW PLANT
REMEDIES

Hahnemann Clinic Publishing

Other books from Hahnemann Clinic Publishing:

- *Animal Mind, Human Voices* by Nancy Herrick P.A.
- *Desktop Guide To Keynotes and Confirmatory Symptoms* by Roger Morrison M.D.
- *Desktop Companion To Physical Pathology* by Roger Morrison M.D.

Lectures from Hahnemann College of Homeopathy:

HOME STUDY VIDEO SERIES:

- *Foundations of Acute Prescribing*
- *Foundations of Materia Medica I – Polycrests*
- *Foundations of Materia Medica II – Polycrests*
- *Foundations of Homeopathic Theory I*
- *Foundations of Homeopathic Theory II*

www.hahnemanncollege.com

Hahnemann Clinic Publishing
13974 Glenn Pines
Grass Valley, CA 95945
Telephone and facsimile: 530-477-7397
E-mail Address: jaffemarks@yahoo.com

Copyright © 2003 Nancy Herrick, P.A.

All rights reserved (including all translations into foreign languages). No part of this publication may be reproduced, stored in a retrieval system, or transmitted in any form or by any means, electronic, mechanical, photocopying, recording or otherwise, without the prior written permission of the copyright holder.

The quotation by Jalaluddin Rumi on page xxi is from *The Essential Rumi*. Translated by Coleman Barks with John Moyne, A. J. Arberry, Reynold Nicholson. The poem title is *Being a Lover: The Sunrise Ruby*. Copyright © 1995 by Coleman Barks Harper/Sanfrancisco

Book and cover design by Lubosh Cech *okodesignstudio.com*
Illustrations by Ana Capitain

1 2 3 4 5 6 7 8 9

ISBN 0-9635368-3-4

Printed in the United States of America

For Naomi,

My daughter,

Whom

I

Love

Rapturously.

CONTENTS

Foreword *ix*
Introduction *xi*
Acknowledgments *xix*

LOTUS *1*
Themes *11*
Rubrics *31*
Provers' Journals *43*

GINSENG *109*
Themes *121*
Rubrics *137*
Provers' Journals *145*

MANDRAGORA *175*
Themes *183*
Rubrics *223*
Provers' Journals *237*

ROSA GALLICA *291*
Themes *299*
Rubrics *319*
Provers' Journals *329*

ROSA ST. FRANCIS *373*
Themes *383*
Rubrics *407*
Provers' Journals *421*

AYAHUASCA *459*
Themes *469*
Rubrics *479*
Provers' Journals *487*

ANHALONIUM *511*
Themes *519*
Physical States *539*

Bibliography *543*
Resources *551*
Ordering Information *553*

FOREWORD

The fundamental contributions of homeopathy to medicine begin and end with its peculiar conception of medicines. They are more than simply weapons against this or that disease or symptom, they are unique totalities or ensembles of symptom-responses that must be studied for their own sake and understood as a whole. Aided by genius and a touch of uncommonly good luck, Hahnemann began giving remedies to himself and his students, and eventually completed his investigation of over ninety of them in his own lifetime. His method of proving them on healthy volunteers still remains the core of the homeopathic enterprise, the supreme test of how medicines are to be known and used.

Doubtless because of their quasi-canonical status in our movement, new provings tend to be minutely scrutinized for the slightest hint of revision of or deviation from Hahnemann's two-hundred-year-old method. This is especially true at times like the present, when important new teachings are being presented and the homeopathic community is riven by serious disagreement about their legitimacy and value.

The present volume is the second series of provings conducted by the noted homeopath Nancy Herrick, whose *Animal Mind, Human Voices* broke new ground when it was published several years ago, and aroused a storm of protest as well. No doubt partly in response to these criticisms, she has been even more scrupulous than before in following both the letter and the spirit of Hahnemann's instructions, with one notable exception.

What is missing from the literature of provings, and what students are least likely to understand or appreciate without actually participating in one of them, is the crucial inter-mediate step between compiling the detailed symptomatology of the individual subjects, the "raw data" of the proving, and its end point of making specific additions to the Repertory. This is the same mysterious but indispensable process by which students learn to grasp the whole or "essence" of each remedy from the sum of its parts. It is this pivotal issue around which every Materia Medica runs the risk of saying either too much, and losing the forest for the trees, or too little, by reducing remedies to pat formulae and ignoring the details on which their meaning is built. Such tricky navigation is at the heart of what we do, and is seldom easy or free from ambiguity.

Like her previous book, Nancy Herrick's latest volume offers homeopathic students and practitioners alike a new kind of compass to guide them through these virtually uncharted waters. From the raw data of the proving, she extracts the additions she can cast in Repertory language, as is customary, but takes the further step of identifying a series of underlying and hopefully important themes that tie them together. To safeguard the objectivity and reliability of her findings, she discovers these themes by a novel process of group discussions that continue until a consensus is reached, based solely on the subjects' reported symptoms and their own feelings about them. Although her results will require years of clinical experience to verify, they offer the prospect of a deeper understanding and more skillful use of these remedies as their estimable reward.

As with her first book of animal remedies, her title *Sacred Plants, Human Voices* implies a sort of criterion for selecting these seven particular plants to be proved, which also made me ask her what she meant by the loaded word "sacred." In a very pragmatic way, she told me that:

1) She chose only "new" remedies, i. e., unproved or imperfectly proved, and thus left out such candidates as Agaricus, Cannabis, Coca, or Opium, that are already familiar to us from past investigations; and

2) She uses the word "sacred" in a much wider sense, to include not only psycho-active plants used in shamanic rituals (peyote, ayahuasca), but also some with broad and even universal powers of healing and/or poisoning and black magic, encompassing the physical, spiritual, religious, and mythical realms, like ginseng, mandrake, lotus, and, most interestingly, two different species of rose.

In short, her list is simply representative of a much larger number that might have been included, just as *Animal Mind, Human Voices* represents tantalizing excerpts rather than a synopsis of the animal kingdom as a whole.

Once again, the homeopathic community is indebted to Nancy Herrick not only for her pioneering investigations of new remedies that deserve to be better known, but above all for her courage in daring to try, in a serious, principled fashion, what nobody else will touch with a ten-foot pole, namely, to seek the bioenergetic "essence" of each proving, and thus to provide a basis for students, colleagues, and future generations to establish or improve upon.

—Richard Moskowitz, M.D.

INTRODUCTION

All who commit themselves to the practice of classical homeopathy know that it is a rigorous discipline. A thorough understanding of materia medica is at the center of this discipline. But what is materia medica? Is it merely a list of symptoms? Or is it something deeper and more inclusive? Something that pulls together all of the disparate pieces into one grand and truly "whole" picture?

As most agree, Kent was the master of providing a perspective on materia medica that coalesced symptoms into a meaningful and memorable totality. Following that tradition, I have always tried to read every proving, review every patient's symptoms, and teach every remedy as an expression of a greater whole. With the number of new provings dramatically increasing (over 600 in the past ten years), the wealth of new information has become increasingly difficult to synthesize. Even with a determined intent to study, prescribe, and teach new remedies, the amount of information is daunting. With the advance of computer technology, we have easier access to the symptoms expressed in a proving, but the core expressions of the remedy often remain elusive.

My very first provings were a labor of love in which I did all the typing, making of rubrics, etc. This proved fortuitous because in reviewing the provers' words many times over I began to notice certain ideas and phrases being repeated in more than one prover. For example, in the proving of Lac leoninum, Prover #3 has a dream where his wife is accused of theft. Prover #6 has the actual experience of a strong and completely unusual impulse to steal perfume as she walks through a department store. She also has a dream of someone stealing a part of her sewing machine. Then I noted that Prover #4 dreams of a child being kidnapped. It struck me as rather remarkable that out of seven provers, three would have such distinctly similar dreams and experiences. I concluded that any symptom repeatedly reflected in the proving journals, was likely to be an excellent clue for the prescription of the remedy. I called these repeated elements "Themes" and made a list of them for each of the remedies I proved.

In some of these remedies, the themes were obviously related in some way to the animal from which the remedy was taken. For example, in the proving of Lac leoninum there is the theme of **CATS/CATLIKE**. A number of provers had dreams about cats, in one of them the prover's boyfriend is sitting on the ground, he is very hairy, licking his leg and rubbing his face on it. Could this be merely coincidence? Returning to the theme of **THEFT** found in the same proving, I did not see how this theme, which was so strong in the proving journals, could be related to Lion. Only much later as I studied their behavior did I realize that much of the lion's life is about "stealing." This is most evident in the lion's symbiotic link with hyenas. The hyenas will make a kill and the lion consistently steals the hyena's food. Sometimes if a lion is alone and makes a kill, the hyenas, will attack as a group, stealing the food from the lion. Basically, the lion although capable of hunting, often uses his strength to overpower and take food from other animals. I also learned that within the pride, the king of the jungle holds his throne only briefly. Younger males are constantly challenging the king, attempting to "take" his territory and his family. Theft, it turns out, is a major theme in the life of the lion. The hypothesis seemed confirmed: The themes often directly relate to the remedy's source.

When I began to take the idea of "uncovering" themes seriously I saw that every remedy elicited symptoms which fell into a number of thematic categories. Consistently these thematic categories expressed the fundamental nature of the remedy's source. Again, only by deep analysis and consideration did that revelation occur. Taking into consideration this deeper understanding of the source of the remedy even tentatively, became an invaluable tool in prescribing and subsequently in teaching these remedies. In preparing my first book, *Animal Mind, Human Voices*, I felt I had to provide more than a list of symptoms for my fellow homeopaths to ponder. A complete presentation had to include the observations of the consistent themes that emerged after serious study of all the individual symptoms.

From the very beginning it was clear that a standardized proving protocol and analytical process for developing themes must be developed. The themes needed to be extracted directly from the proving material and never be based on subjective impressions or "intuition." Slowly, a procedure for extracting themes emerged that could be taught and replicated.

Over the years this process has become more sophisticated. The following procedures have been developed over time, greatly aided by the work of James Tyler Kent, Rajan Sankaran, and Jeremy Sherr. May they be a guide for your own work and a helpful insight into the provings which follow.

Pre-proving
- Choose ten to twenty provers.
- Each prover is provided with a set of instructions, a date for starting the proving, a journal (listing the mental and body systems to reflect on each day), and a proving supervisor.
- Provers are required to sign a release form indicating that they are fully aware of

what a proving is and that uncomfortable symptoms can and often will occur and occasionally may continue past the proving experience.
- The provers are given a contact person who will follow their symptoms should they develop a serious problem.

Proving
- All provings are done blind; only two people know the source of the remedy, the pharmacist and the proving master.
- On a pre-set date, the provers take an initial dose.
- If no significant symptoms occur, provers are instructed to consult with the proving master or supervisors, and re-dose up to two more times (maximum).
- For three to four weeks, all provers keep a daily journal, noting any uncharacteristic experiences, thoughts, or sensations.
- If a prover is comfortable with having a proving supervisor available for consultation and to serve as an outside observer of the prover's state, one is provided. (Optional)

Proving Meeting
- At the end of three to four weeks a proving meeting takes place with the proving master, proving supervisors and provers. This meeting requires three to four hours. Ideally it is videotaped for future reference.
- Each prover reads their journal aloud to the group. A transcript is made of the meeting.
- The source of the unlabeled remedy is revealed to them at the end of the meeting.

Proving Journals
- The proving journals are typed. Any elaboration on symptoms, dreams, and/or events that occur during the proving meeting is incorporated into the final version of the proving journals. *Note: No comments or notes are included once the name of the remedy is revealed to the group.*
- Any content that represents a "pre-proving state" is deleted from the proving journal material.
- Limited editing is done, to ensure that the journals remain true to the exact words and writing style of the provers.

Development of Themes
- Two to five homeopaths or students of homeopathy are chosen to work on themes with the proving master. Sometimes the provers or proving supervisors are part of this group. After an initial meeting, each person independently studies

the completed proving journals, noting repetitive themes, words, or main points for every line of the proving. A list of possible themes and supportive quotes is developed by each person (often 20–30+ themes long).
♦ The list of possible themes and their quotes is reviewed as a group and individually, pooling (together) similar themes under single headings, and eliminating those which do not meet the specified criteria (see below). This process requires four to six meetings.

Theme criteria
♦ Each theme must be confirmed by proving entries from at least *three* different provers. Entries from one or two provers cannot make a theme no matter how strong their experience. *Note: Many of the themes are confirmed by many or most of the provers.*
♦ The themes come exclusively from the words of the provers. *Note: In the case of Ayahuasca, some journal excerpts from material dose experiences were used to elucidate corresponding themes but were not used in the development of those themes.*
♦ No theme developed is based on a study of the substance or any known aspect of the substance.
♦ A theme is considered very strong if it has confirmation from: 1) emotional/mental states, 2) events, 3) dreams, and 4) physical sensations. For example:

BLOOD/LACERATIONS (*theme from Rosa St. Francis*)

#6 Woke up at 6 a.m. with a pleasant sensation of internal heat; diffused in bones, around the mouth, on my head. It was as if the blood in the veins were warmer.
#6 Dream: . . . I was lying on a bed and a nurse was putting a needle in my right arm for phleboclysis. . . . Then there were some problems with a patient that a doctor, dirty with blood, carried away with a white sheet. . . .
#1 Lots of mosquito bites, large red welts . . . I scratch 'til the skin breaks.
#1 I did an inordinate amount of suturing (in the ER) – complicated lacerations (fingertips, face, kids). I don't know what it means but it caught my attention.
#3 Dream: . . . ends with a dog (bloodhound) attacking me – I see little cuts on (the palm of) my hands, very minor, like scratches, and two of my cousins are there (one of whom is trying to give me a tetanus shot (!?) . . .
#4 Dream: . . . A phlebotomist arrives and is upset . . .
#5 . . . Saw stars when I blew my nose, some blood in discharge. . . .

Rubrics
♦ Each symptom of the proving is given a rubric.
♦ Intense effort is made to see that very few new rubrics are added to the repertory.

Already existing rubrics or sub-rubrics are used whenever possible. As a result there are usually only a few new rubrics made for each proving.

An example of a new rubric from Ayahuasca:

MIND: CONFRONTATIONAL

Examples of new sub-rubrics from Ginseng:

MIND; AVERSION;
    newspaper or television news, to
    small talk, to

- The only exception to the above rule is in the case of dreams, which by necessity, are often represented by new rubrics. Every attempt is made to express the main feeling or idea of a dream in as few rubrics as possible.
- Rubrics are reviewed repeatedly to minimize or eliminate mistakes and duplications.
- Rubrics are italicized if more than two provers had the symptom. They are bolded if more than two provers had the symptom and it has been cured in at least one confirmed case. (This is based on Kent's system of analyzing rubric strength.)

Write-up (after the themes are developed)
- Each substance is researched. Its physical properties, broad natural and cultural history, and its impact on human consciousness is explored.
- Outside sources provide a broad perspective of each substance proved and are cited in text.
- When research on a substance illustrates a theme from the proving material, that theme is parenthetically inserted into the body of the text. For example, in Ayahuasca where death is a theme we found an excerpt from *Visionary Vine* by Peter Stafford which reads:

> . . . In some places, natives refer to Banisteriopsis as "the vine of death" – meaning that it causes one to "die," and then be "born anew." *(354)* (**DEATH**)

In our work on the sacred plant provings, it was again remarkable to see the relationship between the impact of the remedy on the provers and the impact of the substance on our collective consciousness. The connection was predictable and corroborative in the Rosa gallica and Rosa St. Francis proving when many provers commented numerous times on gardens. **GARDENS** emerged as a strong theme in both provings and another satisfying confirmation that blind provings can indeed reflect the deep inner nature of a substance. In the Lotus proving, a jarring and unexpected theme of **KILLING** and **VIOLENCE** appeared, an image that is not in the popular culture surrounding this flower. But extensive research of the substance showed a strong undercurrent of this theme in the plant's history and mythology. The Mandragora and Ginseng provings had strong themes around the color **RED**. These plants both have large and powerful roots but otherwise do not have any biological connection that would account for this strange similarity.

Additionally, the impact of a plant's genetic structure on a remedy and its themes was also observed. For example: Rosa gallica's proving has the strong themes of **OLD LOVERS, GARDENS, LOVING FEELINGS/COMPASSION, REBELLING AGAINST AUTHORITY**, and **FOOD/HUNGER**. This series of themes was not reflected in any of my other sixteen provings . . . except one: Rosa St. Francis, Rosa Gallica's botanical cousin. It was amazing to observe this congruence of symptoms – which were developed by independent teams and without my realizing their similarity until many months later!

The plant remedies in general proved to be more elusive and subtle in their thematic content than were the animals. They required much more in-depth study and analysis. This analysis proved to be deeply satisfying as the plants slowly revealed their mysteries.

I would also like to address the question some pose as to whether new remedies are needed at all. Hahnemann gave us a blueprint for creating remedies; he used common medicines, poisonings, and folk remedies particular to his own era in order to heal the illnesses common to his age. We would best follow Hahnemann's lead by doing the same, that is, to look in our own environment for remedies appropriate to the illnesses of our own time.

I believe deep thematic analysis of these new remedies is essential. Without it, these provings are far less accessible to the busy practitioner. And since the proving synthesis requires of the proving master and assistants such deep familiarity with the details of the proving, it is incumbent upon us to offer this level of analysis with the raw material.

The process of analyzing a proving to this extent is both rigorous and time consuming. However, the results have proven to be invaluable. Not only because they provide insight into the provings themselves, but when the "picture" of a new remedy is clarified it becomes readily available to the average prescriber and a benefit to all.

I sincerely hope you will find these provings useful in your practice. This book is for you, the sincere and dedicated practitioner. The goal of this effort is to expand our materia medica with well-proven and analyzed remedies to cure the patient.

I do not expect the research and themes that I've done to be exhaustive nor do I expect it to take the place of direct study of the proving itself. I offer these as a starting point, leaving you the task of further enlightening our understanding of each remedy through your own study and cured cases. As I have mentioned in my previous book, I personally, and the homeopathic community at large, welcome any additions or revisions derived from clinical experience. I would deeply appreciate hearing cases where you have found these remedies curative or even useful. As always, I believe that with the use of these remedies, more insights, themes, symptoms, and rubrics will emerge. They will grow as we as homeopaths grow.

—Nancy Herrick

ACKNOWLEDGMENTS

*F*irst and foremost, I wish to extend my deepest gratitude to all the wonderful unnamed provers who, for the sake of ameliorating the suffering of humanity, have been willing to dedicate many weeks and, sometimes months, of their precious time to doing a proving. Of course this book would not exist without their ceaseless dedication, hard work, and sometimes, intense physical or mental pain.

Next come the very special students and graduates of Hahnemann College of Homeopathy who worked on these provings with me; sifting, sorting, analyzing, and pouring over the words of the provers for as much as two years for each proving. Out of their hard work we get the benefit of the themes, the exact quotes from each prover to support the themes, and of course, the all-important rubrics.

For Rosa gallica, I wish to thank Jessica Jackson, LAC who worked unstintingly on themes and rubrics and Lynn Snow who carefully typed the words of each prover, going over video tapes and difficult-to-read transcripts, to get the job done perfectly.

For Ayahuasca, I also wish to thank Jessica Jackson for her special efforts with working on themes. We had a lot of fun with this unusual proving.

For Mandragora, the most enormous proving of them all, I wish to thank Andrew Bonner, N.D., Becky Reese, M.D., and Doug Brown, P.A. We met for almost two years and struggled unceasingly with an almost overwhelming amount of material. Finally, to our mutual joy, we are able to present this proving in a manner that will help us all begin to understand this powerful substance. I also wish to thank them for the abundance of laughter and mutual conviviality our meetings engendered. It was an enormous pleasure and I am sorry it has ended.

For Lotus, I cannot thank enough those "beautiful flowers," Sharon Stanley, D.O. and Tasha Turzo, D.O., who made it their special project and worked with me on many a long evening, stunned at this incredibly intense proving.

I wish to thank my good friend Doctor Jayesh Shah from Bombay, India who obtained the sacred Lotus tincture from Auroville India and gave it to me as a precious gift for this proving. Dr. Shah has also done a proving on this powerful new remedy.

For Anhalonium, I wish to thank Claire Green, N.D. She was one of the early pioneers in helping me to delineate the themes running through the material.

For Ginseng, I wish to thank Naomi Marks, my wonderful daughter. She labored with me on this proving with love, and to learn, as a budding homeopath, how to do provings. I hope that someday she will choose to conduct a proving or two on her own.

For St. Francis Rose, I wish to thank Joan Kandel, D.O., Mark Brody, M.D. and Tanya Baldwin, N.D. for all the hard work of paring down the material to eighteen themes. This proving, as the last one to be done at Hahnemann College, was a momentous project that seemed to require that last push of effort and energy. I deeply appreciate the hard work this group has done on this amazing proving. Most of all, I want to thank Carol Been for supervising all the projects around this proving and keeping it going strong. Left up to me it might have flagged and not made it into this book.

I wish to thank Swami Chetanananda for his generous support of Hahnemann College and Hahnemann College Student Clinic on every level from financial to emotional. Without support like his we could not manage to have a college at all, much less extra projects like student provings.

I also wish to thank Duncan Soule, M.D. for his loving heart and dedicated spirit in arranging and facilitating the provers and proving meetings for the Anhalonium and Lotus provings. It was stunning for me to walk into the room for the Lotus proving and see a beautiful painting full of open lotus blooms on the wall behind the reporting prover's chair. All serendipity, since I alone knew the proving substance was Lotus. Also Duncan helped to manage the horrific response to the Lotus proving that four of the provers had to undergo. To these provers and to Duncan, I am eternally grateful.

I wish to thank Deborah Gordon, M.D. for her excellent skills and willingness to edit and review huge bodies of material, doing it with grace and a smile.

I wish to thank my husband, Roger Morrison, M.D. for his loving willingness to review each of the write up and rubrics sections of this book and make final suggestions and corrections. He is a master at whatever he touches and he helped this book enormously with his eye for detail.

For the earlier provings I had the unstinting help of Micki Elia as editor. She worked cheerfully, editing many long, complex, and often nearly unreadable journals, as well as, long lists of rubrics and themes. She became quite an expert in the art of the repertory and details such as where to put commas and where to put semi-colons. No small task in creating rubrics, a thankless job for which I give her many thanks.

Finally I wish to thank, from the bottom of my heart, Carol Been, M.Div. Carol has thrown herself into this project heart and soul. She researched the Internet and demanded clarity for each natural history, mythological, and historical write up. She has truly made it possible to put out this book at this time through her total devotion and unceasing dedication to the editing and perfection of each fact, each quote, each theme, each proving journal and finally each and every damned rubric. Carol, you are a wonder and I love you for it. I hope homeopaths for 100 years will appreciate you as well.

Keep knocking, and the joy inside

will eventually open a window

and look out to see who's there.

– RUMI

NELUMBO NUCIFERA

Sacred Lotus

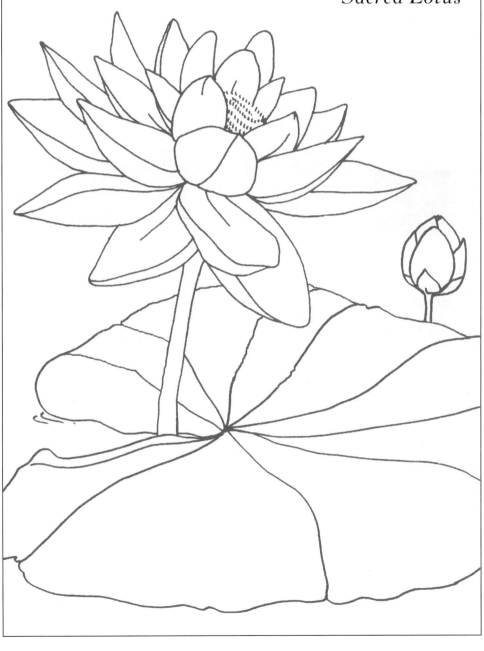

NELUMBO NUCIFERA [NEL NUC.]
Sacred Lotus

Nelumbo nucifera
Family: Nymphaeaceae
Miasm: Syphilitic

The Sacred Lotus, traced as far back as the Cretaceous period (about 135 million years ago), is considered by botanists to be among the first angiosperms on earth. Remarkably, the peoples of its indigenous sources: China, Japan, India, Tibet, ancient Egypt, and Persia, intuitively perceived its place in the origin of flowering plants, portraying the Lotus as the mythic source and symbol of creation. Deeply embedded in the spiritual life of these cultures, the Sacred Lotus, known in some traditions as "the king of all flowers" or "God's place," became a powerful symbol of purity, fertility, and immortality.

Historically, lotus is a generic term that refers to any of two varieties of aquatic plants in the Nymphaeaceae family, Nelumbo (lotus genus) and Nymphaea (water-lily genus). While there are more than forty strains of water lilies, only two true species of lotus exist in the world: *Nelumbo lutea*, the American lotus, or water chinquapin, and the plant of our proving, *Nelumbo Nucifera*, commonly known as Sacred Lotus, prevalent in southern Asia and Australia.

These aquatic plants, with roots firmly fixed in mud, bear an external resemblance. However, there are distnctive features to each. The common water lily's roots and stems are solid like a potato, its leaves and flower float on the surface of the water and after the flower blooms, it withers, and then sinks down and seeds underwater. In contrast, the Sacred Lotus has a hollow stem and rhizome that resembles the spokes of a wagon wheel when sliced. Although filled with air, the stalk is unbending, rising from round, mostly funnel-shaped wavy leaves. The bottom leaves float (**FLOATING**) but most stand from twenty inches to six and half feet above water. Referred to as the "thorny lotus" in Buddhist writings, the neck of the stem is covered with small thorns for protection from insects. (**NEEDLES/SHARP/STABBED**)

Atop the stem blooms a solitary flower, exquisite in pure perfection of color, symmetry, and grace. Blooming two to five days and darkening with age, it opens each morning at dawn and closes late in the day. Chen Chin-yuan, from the

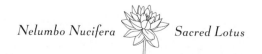

Department of Horticulture at National Taiwan University reports, "The [Lotus] flowers close up to make it easier for the plants to control their inner circulation of water, so as to avoid being affected by the weather, the humidity, or even being touched by people" (*Chin-ju*). Having this remarkable ability to warm itself, the flower can actively maintain a relatively stable core temperature regardless of the external air. "The flower achieves this stability by stepping up its oxygen consumption (and thus heat production) when the air is cold and stepping it down when the air is warm" (*Scientific American, March 1977*). (**INSIDE VS. OUTSIDE**) Few other plants have this ability. In addition, fine hair-like filaments on the leaves repel the muddy waters and keep the petals from discoloration. This provides further protection from contamination by the outside world.

Up to a foot in diameter, each flower usually has between twenty and twenty-five petals. However, there are lotus blossoms with multiple layers, some with a hundred or as many as three hundred petals per flower. A variety called the "many-headed lotus" puts forth multiple flowers having up to five thousand petals per stalk, giving rise to the symbol of the thousand-petaled lotus in Buddhist teaching.

The Sacred Lotus is renowned for being the only plant to fruit and flower simultaneously. Much has been made of this in sacred writings. As extraordinary as this appears, botanists now know that the fruit (a receptacle shaped like a conical pod with seeds inside the holes and resembling a beehive) is not fully mature when it first emerges (*Chin-ju*). The flower still requires insects to gather pollen in order for its fruit to fully ripen. When the fruit is mature, its seeds become loose and the pod tips toward the water releasing the seeds.

These seeds are amazingly hard. In fact, *nucifera* literally means, "having hard seed." This impenetrable outer shell allows them to survive under extremely adverse conditions. Recently, radiocarbon testing has shown that ancient lotus seeds can germinate after more than two thousand years of dormancy. Plant physiologist Jane Shen-Miller who grew a tiny green shoot from a 1,288 year old lotus seed unearthed in China concludes: "This sleeping beauty, which was already there when Marco Polo came to China in the thirteenth century, must have a powerful genetic system to delay its aging" (*Allan*). Steve Clarke, a biochemist who "more than a decade ago discovered that the enzyme L-isoaspartyl methyltransferase (MT) repairs proteins routinely damaged as part of the aging process in plants, mammals, and bacteria," proceeded to find the MT enzyme in ancient lotus seeds (*Allan*). Both researchers believe studying these seeds will provide valuable information about the aging process in plants and humans.

Indigenous to Asia and Australia, the Lotus has been cultivated since the twelfth century B.C. for use as religious offerings, in cooking, and for its therapeutic properties. The rhizomes and leaves, recognized as a cooling agent, astringent, and diuretic, has been used in the treatment of diarrhea, constipation, dysuria, high fever, hemorrhoids, and leprosy. The stamen and seeds, depending on their maturity, treat digestive problems, male sexual disorders and act as an astringent for leukorrhea. In *Australian Wellbeing,* Cheryll Williams reports that lotus seeds have a sedative action, thought to be due to the release of histamines, and prove useful for insomnia, nervous complaints, high blood pressure, and heart palpitations. The flower receptacle, containing an alkaloid nelumbine, helps stop lung, nose and uterine bleeding, and eliminates stagnant blood. Recent investigations have shown the effectiveness of the flowers in lowering blood sugar (*Williams*). The petals are also reputedly used in the treatment for syphilis and liver regeneration. Beyond its medicinal uses, the plant is completely edible.

In spite of the fact that the Lotus no longer exists in the region of the Nile, historians trace its origins to Persia twenty-five hundred years ago. It is believed that trade brought the Sacred Lotus, with its distinctive shape, to Egypt. Eventually this image, pervasive in Egyptian art, architecture, and cosmology, made its way to Greece. Its imprint is still visible on the temple of Olympus and in time influenced Asian art. According to theologian Ikeda:

> Alexander the Great brought Greek civilization to India.... The encounter of Indian and Western civilizations eventually gave birth to the brilliant Buddhist art of Gandhara, which spread throughout Asia by way of China, eventually reaching as far as the Korean peninsula and even Japan.... In a sense, the entire Eurasian continent was united by a grand Lotus Road. The Silk Road was therefore also a Lotus road. (**TRAVEL**)

As the Sacred Lotus touched each Asian culture, its distinguishing qualities became *the* metaphor for spiritual perfection and power. The bloom, closing at dusk and opening at dawn, became the symbol of creation and rebirth. The sun was referred to as a heavenly lotus and the lotus flower as an earthly sun, representing the synchronicity between heaven and earth. The annual appearance of lotus blossoms rising from the mud of the Nile region mirrored another biorhythm, signaling prosperity and continued blessings from the gods. Understandably, the tombs of the pharaohs were, literally and figuratively, littered with lotus blossoms in hope of a similar blessing. Almost every creation myth in the ancient Orient has the Sacred Lotus at its center. Katsuji Saito describes an early Indian legend:

"In the beginning there was only water. From within this water a lotus flower floated to the surface. . . . Within that lotus flower, which is described as a 'golden womb,' Brahma, the creator of the universe, was born. . . . The 'golden womb' . . . contains within it all things in embryonic form, and brings all things into being."

In Buddhism, the heart of a being is likened to a Lotus bud, blossoming when the virtues of the Buddha are fully developed. Thus, the image of the Buddha sitting on a beautiful Lotus in full bloom evokes the awakening of the highest consciousness. Overcoming all causes of suffering and concerns of power, sexuality, and material gain, the Buddha is indifferent to praise or blame, joy or sorrow. (**INDIFFERENCE**) He has perfect equanimity and sees all sentient beings as one. Every attachment that chains one to the endless cycles of birth and death and rebirth is severed.

The Lotus Sutra, thought of as the spirit of the lotus flower, is a Mahayana teaching from India developed in the first century B.C. Given most highly favored status in China around the sixth century and becoming the cornerstone of the constitution of medieval Japan, the Lotus Sutra is considered by many to be the summit of Buddhist teaching (*St. Clair*). Compared to the lotus seed itself, Ikeda believes this sutra, "is like a diamond, unable to be damaged or broken. It can't be destroyed even if someone should fall into the state of hell or any of the evil paths." Its teachings on compassion and enlightenment hold within it the "mysterious law" embedded in all of life and many teachers understand this sutra to be like the Lotus itself, "the origin of origins," "the ultimate principle governing the universe," and a symbol of "the great drama of life" (*Chin-ju; Ikeda*).

With root in the swamp (**HEAVY-STUCK**) and head in the clouds, the sacred Lotus is a symbol of this spiritual purity. It represents the ascendance from darkness into light. Saito explains, "When [the Buddha] is in profound meditation, he emits a great light, each of the rays of this light, becomes a 'thousand-petaled lotus' and on each of these lotus flowers a Buddha is born." In yoga, the thousand-petaled lotus flower signifies the state of *samadhi*, or spiritual ecstasy. (**CLARITY/EXPANSION/AWARENESS**) At the same time:

> Mahayana Buddhism stresses finding a release from worldly affairs while in the world, taking the path of a bodhisattva amid the five filths of the world. The bodhisattvas take the human masses as their "field of blessing" — the muck is luck, evil is good, pollution is purity and no clear dichotomies can be made. Hence, Mahayana Buddhism stresses the idea that "this flower doesn't grow in the highlands but rather it blooms in the vile swamps." The root and flower merge into one, in which there is no

distinction between pollution and purity. Apart from pursuing inner cultivation, meditation, and deep thought, experiencing muck is also a form of cultivation, for it tests one's ability to endure misfortune and to sacrifice. Only by going to hell and being tempered by fire there, can one rise to religious exaltation and radiate the brightest and most beautiful light. (*Chin-ju*)

The connection between these two poles of the spiritual path is also expressed in the mythology of this sacred flower. In some Indian cosmologies, the dawn of the first day rises out of the Lotus center while demonic and serpentine beings reside on the underside of its outer petals. In Chinese Buddhism, the souls of the dead must first rise through the vile swamp before passing through the Sacred Lotus Lake to rebirth.

Similarly, violence features in many of the legends surrounding the Lotus. In a Hindu tale, Padmasambhava, predicted to bring the Buddhist Dharma to Tibet, begins his life as a gift to a king. The king had undergone many trials, including the loss of his young son and the ravaging of his kingdom by famine. Stirred by compassion, the Buddha emanates a ray of light that enters a lake and causes a lotus to grow. Upon the lotus, sits an eight-year-old boy, Padmasambhava, named Lotus Born One. His presence ends the drought and prosperity sweeps the land. As he matures, he becomes known as the Lotus King. Eventually Padmasambhava renounces his family and the life of a king by willfully killing a young boy, so that, according to Indian law, he would lose his throne and be exiled. Through this action, the child, previously destined to a lower rebirth, is reborn in a Buddha's paradise and Padmasambhava is free to pursue his enlightenment. In the land of Zahor, Padmasambhava takes Mandarava, the daughter of a king, to be his consort in accomplishing immortality. When the king learns of this, he is outraged that his daughter had consorted with what he assumed was "a common vagrant pretending to be a holy man." The king has Padmasambhava and Mandarava captured by his army and burned alive. (**KILLING/ANGER/VIOLENCE**) Instead of finding their charred corpses, the king discovers that Padmasambhava has transformed the sea of flames into a lake. On the lake floats a pristine lotus blossom on which sits the Great Guru and his consort, unharmed (*Weidner*).

Despite these more ominous undertones, the Lotus, to this day, represents the height of spiritual power. Yet, the proving of Lotus is one of the darkest provings in the materia medica. Similar to Aurum, the king of metals, and Naja, the king of snakes, this king of flowers bears the mark of power gone awry: murder, suicide and insanity. In the case of Aurum and Naja, it is easy to recognize this darker side, revealed in history and folklore, but not so with the Lotus. These sinister

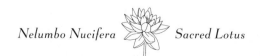

forces on occasion surround the Sacred Lotus but the image of the flower never embodies them.

It is only in Chinese history that the bound feet of upper-class women, imitating the rhizome of the flower and referred to as "lotus feet," directly connect the image of the Lotus to violent forces. Marie Vento, in "One Thousand Years of Chinese Footbinding: Its Origins, Popularity and Demise," writes:

> It is believed that the origin of the term "golden lotus" emerged in the Southern Tang dynasty around 920 A.D., where the emperor Li Yu ordered his favorite concubine, Fragrant Girl, to bind her feet with silk bands and dance on a golden lotus platform encrusted with pearls and gems. Thereafter, women inside and outside the court began taking up strips of cloth and binding their feet, thinking them beautiful and distinguished, dainty and elegant. . . . It gradually became the prevailing style and "golden lotus" became a synonym for bound feet. . . . In its most extreme form, footbinding was the act of wrapping a three- to five-year old girl's feet with binding so as to bend the toes under, break the bones and force the back of the foot together.

This attempt to live up to the highest standard of beauty in the land resulted in life threatening complications, "ulceration, paralysis, and gangrene were not uncommon. It has been estimated that as many as ten percent of the girls did not survive the 'treatment'" (*Vento*). Those who did survive were immobilized by crippling pain and confined to their boudoirs, living entire lives in almost complete isolation. Practically speaking, this procedure eased the imaginations of jealous husbands by guaranteeing the fidelity of these well-monitored women. Culturally, lotus feet became the symbol of eroticism, fertility, and wealth. In fact, having this procedure performed made all the difference in the marriage prospects of a young woman of class. The intense social pressure behind footbinding is reflected in a popular Chinese saying, "A mother can't love her daughter and her daughter's feet at the same time" (*Vento*). After the Cultural Revolution outlawed this practice, lotus feet, once the symbol of beauty and prestige, became a symbol of brutality and shame.

In Hindu, Taoist, and Tibetan scriptures a hierarchy of Lotus blossoms represent a continuum from the most base to the most noble aspects of the human spirit. Each subsequent blossom signifies a chakra, which joins channels of energy that wind around and within the spinal cord, and according to the scriptures, shapes the nature of consciousness and evolution of the human spirit. Through this circuitry of energy, our animal nature and our divine nature are joined.

The first chakra, represented by a red four-petaled Lotus and physically located near the rectum, is the center of the basic human need for survival in the material world. At this level of consciousness, our being has no understanding of itself as an individual or as a spiritual entity. It is analogous to the lotus root, completely submerged under the mud in the water.

> When the energy in this chakra is not activated and purified. . . . We relate to the world out of our particular tribe at the exclusion of everything else. We are almost entirely self-centered and concerned with issues of survival in the material world and the energy manifests in its negative aspects in anger, greed, revenge, collective hatred, lust for power and control, all passions of our lower nature. The need for material security and control is the dominant energy. (*Slotte*)

The divine creative energy or *Kundalini*, once awakened at the first chakra, begins to rise, transforming each chakra from mundane attachments to sex, power, and the self into the great mystical realizations underlying all creation: compassion, truth, creativity, love, wisdom, unity. At the seventh chakra, the pinnacle of consciousness, there is purportedly a release of all negativity, karma, and reincarnations and an infusion of divine light into the individual. (**ALTERED STATES**) Here the being is fully open into the glory of the sun, represented by a thousand-petaled Lotus. This center can be said to correspond to the highest state of the mind or the most disturbed. "It is well known that unsuccessful raising of the *Kundalini* energy instead of bringing enlightenment, throws the whole nervous system into unbalance and can cause madness" (*Slotte*). (**PSYCHOSIS**)

The dramatic and overwhelming degree of deep pathology expressed by many of the lotus provers: suicidal ideations and dreams of murder or being tortured is also prevalent in remedies from the botanically related Nymphaceae and Piperaceae families: Cubeba, Piper methisticum, Nuphar leuteum, Nelumbo nucifera, and Nauchelli. I believe the central theme of this grouping can be expressed as "tension without release." This tension is also revealed metaphorically in the physical symptom of priapism, found in Cubeba, Piper methisticum, Nuphar leuteum, and Nauchelli.

The core issues of the Nymphaceae family are the following:

ACTIVE STATE:

- UNCONTROLLABLE ANGER. EXTREME VIOLENCE. CURSING.
- LEWD and LASCIVIOUS. VOLUPTUOUS THOUGHTS. PRIAPISM.
- EXHILARATION. PLEASURE. CLARITY. EXCITEMENT. ENERGY.

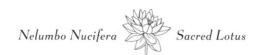

PASSIVE STATE:
- ◆ DULL. STUPEFIED. SLEEPY.
- ◆ INDIFFERENT. DISCONNECTED. BORED.
- ◆ FLOATING. DRUNKEN VERTIGO-like states.
- ◆ GRANDIOSITY. ENLARGEMENT. MATERIALISM. POWER.

The quality of untainted beauty rising above the muddy conditions of the swamp has given the Lotus its metaphoric connotation of mystical trascendence. Representing the noble state of full spiritual enlightenment and revered as a symbol of mystical perfection, the lotus takes its place among the great icons of the world's religions. Like the Cross in Christianity, the Star of David in Judaism, and the Crescent Moon and Star of Islam, the Sacred Lotus bears within it the power, depth, and mystery at the center of the spiritual path. Being able to use this holy icon as a homeopathic remedy is a gift beyond expectations. My hope is that over time we will be able to plumb its depths and find increasingly profound uses for this holy plant in our repertory of sacred plants.

Nelumbo Nucifera **Themes**

Sacred Lotus

- *Psychosis/Inside vs. Outside*
- *Killing/Violence*
- *Irritable/Anger*
- *Sharp/Stuck/Stabbed*
- *Police/Prison*
- *Lost/Travel*
- *Indifference*
- *Clarity/Expansion/Energy*
- *Altered States*
- *Heavy vs. Floating Feeling*
- *Vertigo*

Psychosis/Inside vs. Outside

#2 . . . In my early twenties, I went through a fairly intense time. . . . I'd walk down the street, I couldn't remember where I was, I couldn't talk to people, people would be talking to me but there was so much information that was going through my head I couldn't focus my attention outside of myself long enough to hear people. I felt like it was really an effort for me to stay focused and stay grounded, and if I let myself, I could just float away to that other place again or just really disconnect like that. So it was important for me to stop doing this remedy because it was just too much.

#15 . . . The most notable thing I had was a sense of an awareness of where this patient was at mentally, a sympathy to it and a concern about my own sanity in terms of that I could get into that state, I could sense the state she was in. . . .

#1 There seemed to be all around me a lot of craziness in the air, a lot of people having emotional, little mental problems. . . . One of my friends on the verge of psychosis - very manic, in and out of psychotic state (but not total). She was fine the next day. Another friend gone totally psychotic. Not fine the next day.

#1 . . . I saw a movie the next day called *Event Horizon* that <u>was</u> the worst part of the remedy—it was about all the fears of humanity and violence coming out of people. It was harsh and made me feel almost psychotic. The people in the movie didn't know if the fear, terror, or unknown things were coming from inside them or outside. They were losing the ability to discriminate the difference.

#2 Dream: . . . There were these three large humanoid monsters after us, and they didn't have mouths, they had three teeth and sucker things on their face. And if they caught us they would take our bodies over and basically extinguish our souls, just suck them right out. And so while I was swimming quickly, I didn't want them to catch me but I wasn't afraid, I just didn't want to be caught. And so they were after us for a while. And then the scene shifted again and there was a complete sense of calm, I was outside some sort of civilized camp, it reminded me of a concentration camp. And there was a little girl with long blonde hair there. And there were no signs of the monsters anymore, they were gone, but the little girl was totally vacant and at peace, she had been taken over by one of them. And I had the sense that that little girl was me.

Nelumbo Nucifera   *Sacred Lotus*

#1 . . . Many people seem on the verge of mentally falling apart, emotionally fragile, kind of confused about life. . . . The craziness in the air seems to be at a fever pitch. Everyone seems tired from all the external and internal activities in their lives. I also feel this way. So much going on that it's hard to stay centered or feel very sane.

#1 . . . I felt like everything was closing in here, everyone was acting so bizarre and I felt like I really needed to get out of this environment because I felt like I was absorbing everything around me. It was feeding this inner state in the sense that you could go mentally off balance at any moment. . . .

Killing/Violence

#1 Dream: My mother thought that I was an imposter in my body and wanted to kill me. And there was such an incredible real homicidal rage to it. . . . There was this incredible strength and rage and she was going to kill me. And I reacted to that in the dream, I became very homicidal and I wanted to kill her. I woke up and this dream was reverberating through my psychic system for ten minutes. If she had been in that room, we would have tangled. . . . I'd never felt the chemistry of a dream come so deeply and powerfully into the waking state for such a sustained time.

#14 . . . I started to think of ways of killing myself. I thought of using a gun, but that would be too messy and disgusting. I thought of drowning myself, but I knew that I'd probably struggle and that would be bad. Then I thought that it would be really cool if I could jump into a volcano. But the best idea I had was to jump off a tall building, because as I was thinking about it, I really liked the concept of falling from a really high place, and falling really fast really appealed to me, that that would be like a very wonderful experience to have. . . . I figured I'd go to the airport and board a plane to Hawaii—then go find a building or cliff to jump off. That way I'd just disappear.

#10 Dream: . . . I woke in a hot sweat after dreaming that I had an argument with a girlfriend and was angry at myself in the dream, and threw dishware and glasses through windows, kicked things and shouted for her to go away, leave me in the unsafe place where we were, and that I wanted to be mugged, robbed, and shot. . . .

#14 Dream themes continued to be of competition, warring, threats being made by one group of people towards another; my role as a mediator and/or running and hiding from danger. Guns shot across a yard at an outdoor party. Women being threatened by men, power struggles.

#4 . . . I was agitated, and actually got near violent a couple times.

#12 . . . This is mad like wanting to hit somebody, crying. . . .

#11 Dream: . . . I was demanding to be tattooed across the bridge of my nose with something that said: "LJ did this." And it was to show that I had been tortured and this woman was trying to knock me out so that I could take the tattoo. . . .

Nelumbo Nucifera   Sacred Lotus

#15 . . . at one point, she was describing this fear that she was about to be killed and I felt myself get afraid that she might decide that I needed to be killed. A striking comment was, "I've been liberated but it's a bad deal," and "They're evil, they're all evil." Those were the first words out of her mouth.

#11 Dream: Peeling off a thick layer of skin from lower legs in long, thin strips. Not particularly painful.

#15 . . . She called me in the middle of the afternoon suddenly believing that she was going to be killed by him or that she'd been told by other teachers to kill herself. So she called me thinking that it was her last day alive and wanting me to know that she either had to kill herself or she would be killed. . . .

#15 [Real event]. . . Opened bedroom door—saw mud tracks on floor, sliding door open. Sense of violation, concerned burglar still in house. Searched closets—called police instead of checking for myself like I would have ordinarily done. Heard the robber escape across the roof. Feel a little more paranoid, less strong than usual. Kept everyone on the porch while police searched, worried about gunfire. Sense of vulnerability—fragility of sanity and life.

#9 . . . I feel very agitated, perhaps slightly feverish. I recognize feelings of anger, hostility, aggression, defensiveness. . . .

#7 Dream: . . . Two Indian doctors were desperate and felt they need to attack us to get the remedy. They were not successful in attack and we learned it was a misunderstanding. . . .

#13 Dream: Strange fighting dream—friends and I arming with guns for a conflict. Shots fired through doors. It was nervous excitement. We were gearing up and it was basically a work project but this time with ammo. Yeah, we were going to kick some butt. . . .

#1 Feel very aggressive, irritable today. Feel a little off balance and have feeling that there is danger and I need to be very careful, calm, and openhearted today or I'll get into an ugly situation with someone.

#1 Dream: Another homicidal dream, and I don't remember the content. Somebody was trying to kill me and I wanted to kill them. The same sort of theme. Again, I woke up and this state was strong for about ten minutes after I woke up. Again, if somebody was in the room, I probably would have like tried to kill them. I felt they were trying to kill me. Just amazing, amazing chemistry at work. I think I had a dream on the last proving about wanting to kill somebody. But these were of a whole other order, because those dreams were more the idea or the feeling of doing something. And this dream was that my whole actual physical body chemistry was set in motion to carry out that state. I was just blown away by how strong it was that morning.

#14 Woke from nap after breakfast sobbing. I'm crying, depressed, hopeless, suicidal. . . .

#15 Very antagonistic all day. Thank God the effect of this is decreasing—think I would have gotten into some fights. As it was—patients, attorneys, friends, angry around miscommunication and projection. Had hysterical quality to it.

#15 Dream: Took bomb I had acquired over to friend's house who was a Vietnam vet. Bomb was not loaded—but I was excited that I had it and dismantled it to show everyone the nuclear portion. Feeling of battle excitement—precision of machinery—love of power. I was proud of this bomb that I'd built. And the whole dream had this sense of love of power, of excitement about battle, that I had an understanding of the intricacies involved in building this. I took it over to him, and I unscrewed the top so I could show him how I put this thing together. It was all intrigue and this sense of being on the edge, that this could go off at any time, that I knew how it worked. The feeling was pride and a sense of power over.

#10 The hallmark of my experience during the last couple weeks is extreme anger, depression, wanting to die but not suicidal, it's just that I want somebody to kill me. . . .

Irritable/Anger

#14 . . . I felt, on the one hand, completely belligerent, anticipating conversations with people who'd pissed me off, imagining the entire argument. I was defensive and bitchy as I argued in my mind. . . .

#10 The hallmark of my experience during the last couple weeks is extreme anger . . . I've been very pissed off at people who I've seen, who I've felt, either subjectively or objectively, have done something unjust to me. . . .

#14 This F—ING BAD TRIP will never end!!! Please give me back my NUX!!

#4 There were times of feeling kind of disconnected from the people around me and almost feeling calm and relaxed but knowing that it was just a little more than skin-deep and if someone pushed me I would spit at them very quickly. Like everything's real fine, don't bug me. . . .

#2 I've been extremely irritable. People are aggravating the hell out of me. I'd like to scream.

#4 . . . I was very, very irritable. Everything exasperated me. I work at a college and take care of continuing education programs, and can be quite busy. The phones were ringing off the hook and I finally went out to the office staff and said, "No calls get through unless they're bleeding. You understand me? I will not talk to anyone." And I never do that. I always let my clients get through to me, but I was not going to let them get through to me because I was going to bite their heads off.

#4 . . . [I] was trying to work out a watering system for our yard. We hadn't been maintaining it terribly well and things were drying out. I was wrestling with the hoses around the yard. I was jerking them around and dragging them all over and cussing and screaming. And one of my housemates just loves this garden and thinks it's great, and I said, "I am going to roto-till this m———. I am sick of it." And he was gasping.

#11 Feeling pissy—wanting to hide behind doing routinized things, then feeling benumbed and angry about having to do routine things at work. . . .

#9 . . . Pent-up hostility wants to unleash—I'm trying to stay cooperative though I don't feel like it at all. . . . I feel very agitated, perhaps slightly feverish. I recognize feelings of anger, hostility, aggression, defensiveness. There's a distinct tightness in my solar plexus, pressure on my bladder (even after I pee), and an overall agitation and anxiety. Fear and resentment of petty authority. . . .

#1 Feel aggressive, irritable. Not looking for trouble but not taking any shit. Also feel drugged. . . . A little more sensitive to sounds, vibrations, light, anything in my sensory environment was a little harder to take. And there was a feeling over the next ten days of just trying to process all this stimulus and information, and it was sort of compressing me so that I felt more irritable. . . .

#13 Lost temper at work today. Generally aggravated by circumstances at work. No more Mr. Nice Guy.

#15 . . . Very irritated with noise this evening. Sound of dishes being moved around made me want to yell at the person doing it. Very surprising—realized it <u>had</u> to be proving symptom.

#12 I've been totally agitated when people ask me about my trip because I don't want to talk about it, because I love it here. I just moved home, now I have to leave again. And I exercised late at night because I was agitated, and I thought that would make me feel better. Then when I got into the kitchen, a friend asked me when I was leaving, and I said, "Wednesday," not mean, but just empty, not with a smile or anything. "Are you in a bad mood?" And I was, well, you know, I'm a little bit flipped out because I'm leaving. And she starts telling me all this stuff about why are you upset? You know you're going to a different country, why are you upset? I just looked at her like, okay, I guess there's no reason for me to be upset, and that just made me more agitated. And she goes, "When's your birthday?" And I said, "It's in December." She goes, "Because I've noticed you're so moody and emotional." It was all I could do to not turn around and whack her. I was so mad. I really had to get out of there. This is mad like wanting to hit somebody, crying. Because it felt so condescending. And of course I am happy, but I'm still scared about going too, and I said to her, "You know, I think moving to a different country is always a frightening experience, don't you think?" To have somebody bring to my attention that I had been emotional and moody upset me even more. She's lucky I have self-control, I'm telling you, because my tongue could have lashed out at her so bad.

Sharp/Stuck/Stabbed

#15 As I held the remedy in my hand, the immediate sensation was a sharp, expansive quality, and I had a vision of needles projecting out from my body and a soft greenish-color. . . . Keep thinking of cactus. Something green, spiny. . .

#15 Severe left-sided shooting pain in spleen. . . . Like a single finger poking into subcostal region on left. Broom handle. Had two other people in house, not on remedy, say the same thing.

#14 I drew a picture of how I was feeling. It wasn't conscious, I just sort of started scribbling—there's something really sharp and pointy on the top, and the inside is just like a big scribble.

#11 Sharp pain on inner bone of right wrist—odd.

#15 Like energy shooting out in yellow spikes. . . .

#7 Had abdominal cramps (1) about 8:30 for about 20 minutes. Had suprapubic sharp, cutting pain (3) radiated to left slightly, <<< motion or jarring, >>> sitting with left leg up. . . .

#2 . . . And when I was holding it [remedy] in my hand, it felt sharp.

#7 Dream: . . . When I got back I removed a needle that was inserted in eyebrow of Asian woman. It was infected. I had a similar needle and it wasn't infected.

#14 . . . My tongue has been very sharp and I've even been more violent. . . .

#11 Dream: . . . I was demanding to be tattooed across the bridge of my nose with something that said: "LJ did this." And it was to show that I had been tortured and this woman was trying to knock me out so that I could take the tattoo. But she failed, she was unable to do that. And then somebody came along and said I didn't need to be knocked out. . . .

Police/Prison

#15 [Real event] . . . Came back—opened bedroom door—saw mud tracks on floor, sliding door open. Sense of violation, concerned burglar still in house. Searched closets—called police instead of checking for myself like I would have ordinarily done. Heard the robber escape across the roof. Feel a little more paranoid, less strong than usual. Kept everyone on the porch while police searched, worried about gunfire.

#11 Dream: Family adventure, cars, trying to get out of prison, don't know where daughter/I am. Try to escape via top floor of factory-like building. The whole crew of "police" are an assortment of people who swarm toward us from outside the building. I thought they were the police, but in fact it was just this assortment of different people, different ages and everything like that. Scary. . . .

#7 Dream: . . . I am a cop and they ask me to help arrest a man in neighboring building who left and did not pay bill. I am reluctant to go, as I am not dressed as a cop. As I leave with a black coworker, I am brought two (small and large) wrenches to use if needed against the man. . . .

#9 Dream: . . . Another scene has me walking through what seems to be a prison, though it's outdoors. There's a jungle path, but I'm the lone woman passing by lots of men, and I hope I'm safe. . . .

#9 Dream: . . . G. is driving N.'s car with a few of us in it. N. tries to make him do something illegal. G. doesn't want to do it. A cop catches us as we're entering the property and now we're in trouble, but because we convince the cop that G. is such a careful, good guy, they shouldn't give him the big fine but let him off with a warning. We're all in the dining room (which is outdoors, lined with picnic tables and benches). I'm explaining to the two cops why they should be lenient. . . .

Nelumbo Nucifera   *Sacred Lotus*

# Lost/Travel

#9 Dream: In another scene, I'm following directions to go someplace. I'm in a multilevel city setting. After I park I'm walking by a hotel and some stores looking for a certain elevator that will take me down to the exact spot I'm going. A classy storekeeper—woman—tries to help me and ends up accompanying me to the elevator, because nothing is at right angles or easy to follow with any certainty.

#9 Dream: . . . Afterwards, the vehicle that was going to take us home (a bus?) breaks down in the middle of nowhere. . . .

#16 Dream: I was flying to France but I just couldn't get to the airport on time. I lost my ticket, then I couldn't find the ticket counter when I did get to the airport. There was a gambling casino in front of the airport. It was like a maze to go through to get to the airport. . . . And I don't know if I ever got to the airport. But it was a dream full of anxiety because I had to be somewhere and I couldn't get there. I felt like I was standing out on the edge somewhere watching something I didn't understand. . . .

#10 Dreams: Being in a track meet of a few miles but not knowing the distance around the track; feeling is uncertainty and anxiety. . . .

#7 Dream: . . . Basic feel was of a science fiction epic. I was on another planet with a number of small disgusting insect-like critters. An alien required I catch five of them in order to leave. . . .

#7 Dream: . . . I drop car off during meeting to get oil changed. At one point I am moving a car looking for my car. They had a dining hall at the meeting but I had some trouble finding a seat so went to check on the car. . . .

#9 Dream: . . . I'm back in a car driving to a place I haven't been before, trying to go through (or get out of) a parking lot. The apparent exit from the lot is blocked and I have to go around again. . . .

#4 Dream: Visiting Arizona or Bloomington. Lost my luggage by putting it down and dashing to catch a bus. Can't get a hotel room. It is hot and raining, I am uncomfortable and frustrated. . . .

#3 Dream: Airport dream. Trying to find my way to the gate; running but not getting anywhere; wandering all around; missed the plane. . . .

#12 Dream: I think that I may have had a dream about the morning I went jogging in Glasgow because when I woke up I kept thinking about it. I hadn't thought about it since I did it because I didn't particularly like that city. Plus, I got lost that morning, so it wasn't as enjoyable as jogs I had in other cities on the trip.

Indifference

#4 . . . my wife became ill. She had a severe stomach problem, and the only significant part to that is that my wife never vomits, she's totally afraid to vomit. And she vomited for two days straight, several times. And it was weird. But also she was very anxious about that, and it was kind of like, you go in the bathroom, and you vomit, and if you need to, you drink some warm tea and have some toast. Any other time I would ask, "Do you need anything else?" I was not going to support her in this. It was like, I'm sick, I'm vomiting! Yeah, so what? Go in the bathroom, do it. Usually I would very much be right there with her through any type of physical trauma that she had.

#2 My friend was thinking about killing herself and going through this intense time. Usually I'm fairly compassionate with people. So, although I would be nice with her and stuff, inside I was thinking, "Oh, can you just get over it, I've had it with this stuff. I don't want to deal with this, you're whining." I'm not usually like that. I'm usually fairly empathetic and very caring, and I just wanted people to stay away from me. . . .

#4 My choir director, who took me to Romania when I was a kid and had been my personal voice teacher for ten years, died in a car accident a couple of days ago. It's the type of situation where I knew I couldn't get there, but usually I would have made an effort to find out where's the funeral home, what donations need to be made, should I be sending flowers, etc., etc. And I called an old choir friend and said, "Let me know what you need done and I'll do it," and I removed myself from the situation. And that's not typical of me.

#4 Dream: A common thread was a dream that morning when I woke up preparing to have sex, but it was like a totally non-sensual/emotional thing. It was like, okay, get the bed made up, lay out the condom, is the lighting right. There was nothing romantic about it at all. And I noticed that that was the theme there.

#15 . . . So when I walked into the house there was this lack of connection and, in my own self, a sense of an incredible drain on my energy just being around this situation. And I could feel myself getting into the space she was at. She was essentially completely disconnected from this reality and she was hearing voices, believing she was getting these high-frequency sounds. I'd try to talk with her, and she'd have me be quiet while she tried to listen to these voices. My feeling with it was being unable to connect with her. There was a huge void between us.

#1 . . . I'm usually so compassionate . . . but this time, they were talking about killing themselves maybe, and they were kind of having a psychotic state, and I just felt overextended, I didn't want to be sucked into it, I didn't really feel much compassion. It was just like, you know, enough, I've heard it before.

#2 . . . I didn't feel really connected with people. Like I felt like I couldn't make a strong connection with them, and didn't.

Clarity/Expansion/Energy

#15 . . . Went to very deep place treating [another person] (osteopathically). Entire anatomy became tubes and line of light. . . .

#1 Elevated energy, light high-octane energy . . .

#7 . . . relaxed feeling . . . Slight warm and tingly feeling in area of chest, some expansion.

#6 I had some very positive experiences early on, of things looking very sharp and clear and colors being very bright and pleasant. I also had the experience of just looking at people around the house and having the strong experience that these people were all angels. Just looking at them and every person looked completely beautiful or handsome or just, you know, magnificent. It was a wonderful experience, actually. It was quite strong.

#16 . . . Felt very good . . . and not concerned about very much, just breathing good and feeling like I had no problems. And then from then on, I continued to have good energy, the congestion seemed to go away and I feel peaceful, pleasant, relaxed and feeling good. . . .

#7 Dream: Something about psychic abilities—reading minds.

#2 I'm waking up with a clearer head. Usually, in the morning, I have mind-fuzz for about an hour. I am much clearer.

Altered States

#14 . . . I definitely was feeling elated. As I was eating my breakfast, I felt stoned, I was laughing with people, I was giggling. And later on that morning I was studying and I had a really, really hard time concentrating. It reminded me of smoking pot, which I did for many years. I would be with drool hanging out the side of my mouth, not focusing on anything. And I had to prepare for my second-year board exams. I thought, I really can't just let myself space out like this, I have to really work to concentrate. I had to keep reeling myself back in. My attention would go off and I'd stare out the window and I'd look at the trees and I'd start seeing the branches moving and I'd be kind of like moving with the branches, and then I'd go, okay, wait a minute, come back to what you're studying. So it was like an extreme dissipation of my attention.

#1 Elevated energy, light high-octane energy. Rather like very good cocaine. Feel very good in general.

#4 Upon taking it, the next day I felt fine, in fact, pretty light and cheerful and almost a little buzz, like I'd had a joint or something . . .

#15 . . . I felt a tremulous vibration all over, like a high buzz you get with a lot of coffee, like a double espresso kind of buzz, everywhere. And immediately after that, my mind seemed to slip into almost a strange kind of stupor. I described it as being between asleep and awake, not really able to engage but not asleep. . . .

#4 . . . I felt drunk, I felt like my head was spinning, I was very distracted, I had trouble physically moving around, staying focused. . . . When I felt really dizzy and drunk, I had the flashback of the first times when I drank. I drank quite heavily when I was young and started when I was fourteen. I would often feel very numb in the face and warm. And I noticed that my face was numb and warm, it was like, god, I'm fourteen and I'm drunk again.

#6 Dream: I had a dream of marked confusion of time and identity where I thought it was 8:00 in the morning and it was actually 3:00 in the afternoon, and I just could not get the time straight. And someone said, "No, it's 3:00," and then I would go, "Oh, it's 7:00," or something, and it was just this real confusion of time and there was no way I could orient myself by the sun or anything, it was just very confusing. And a friend of mine who's very sweet and demure turns out to have a secret life as a punk rocker. It was so surprising to me because it's someone I know fairly well. So it was this strange identity that came up in this dream.

#7 Dream: . . . Then I woke my wife up with that [crying out or moaning], and I reassured her. I said, "Don't worry, it's just the proving," and I was okay. Thought I got up to write dream down. Was going to use light of computer screen and couldn't turn screen saver off. Asked wife to help. Then woke up. I asked wife if I had talked with her and she said no. Very strong experience—like drug, and wanted to have again.

#7 Dream: Working on house. (In real life, construction of roof continues.) There is small square tower with shingle on top that another individual is trying to complete and may abuse the power of it. By entering, can pass between times—into other times and/or dimensions. (Again, the theme of something appearing ordinary having unusual power.)

#13 Just one time I had a jittery dizziness. I did acid twice in college, I was kind of a nerd, but it was a bit of a flashback of that. . . .

Heavy vs. Floating Feeling

#9 . . . I couldn't keep my energy low (it was all above the chest), and my head and upper body felt thick, dense, heavy, slow, it was a very bad combination. . . .

#14 . . . And every time I tried to wake myself up, I just felt like someone was throwing me back down into my bed. I just didn't have the energy to even sit up. And this would go on, every ten minutes or so. I'd try to get up, but I just couldn't get up.

#8 Dream: A lot of little dreamlets, mostly horn-related (just returned from a week-long music festival in Coos Bay on Sunday), that were heavy and "thick" in nature. I'd wake up tired, feeling the need to roll over and re-collapse heavily into bed. . . .

#7 Somewhat heavy feeling in body.

#7 Dream: Woke up about 11:25 p.m. Laid in bed and did not want to get up to write things. Heavy, immobilized feeling but not unpleasant. Could feel dream drifting out. Had a thought about getting a message. I only recalled theme of turning back and forth, from side to side, which I did, but heavy sensation.

#14 . . . I went into meditation. And as I sat there, I felt like I was floating, like I was a balloon. . . .

#15 . . . It was like I was floating up, but not in a nice sense, not like some of the other provings. They were a lot more fun. This was just sort of diffuse anxiety and not sure where I was in myself.

#4 . . . I had this image of those compasses you have on dashboards sometimes where they're kind of floating in water. Like my mind was here but it was floating in water and I could turn here but my mind was still over there and I might turn over here and it was over there. It was like it was never in synch, everything was always floating in this little thing I call my head.

Vertigo

#6 I sat up first thing in the morning and the whole world spun vigorously. I had intense, intense vertigo, like I've never had before in my life. I had to basically grab the ground and lie down immediately. Incredibly intense. I would try to sit up again and it would happen again; I would sit down and it would be okay. That symptom has actually persisted since that time; it has become slightly less intense during the preceding twelve or fourteen days, but the modalities of it are: vertigo, always spinning to the right in a clockwise fashion, worse bending my head forward, very much worse with any pressure on the occiput in the back; initially worse turning the head from side to side, although that's no longer a symptom. This was accompanied by nausea and malaise.

#4 Dizzy, feel drunk and woozy. I am relatively calm, but irritable or exasperated. I had this image of those compasses you have on dashboards sometimes where they're kind of floating in water. And so it was like my mind was here but it was floating in water and I could turn here but my mind was still over there and I might turn over here and it was over there. It was like it was never in synch, everything was always floating in this little thing I call my head.

#6 Teaching hatha was really a nightmare on two occasions. Doing floor poses and having my head against the floor, doing some lying twists, and the whole room was just violently spinning. And the vertigo was associated with some kind of disorientation, and also nausea, and that nausea has persisted also slightly over time.

#9 At Saturday Market (mid-afternoon) I had a very strong experience. The crowds and heat and sun were *awful*. Since I couldn't keep my energy low (it was all above the chest), and my head and upper body felt thick, dense, heavy, slow, it was a very bad combination. I almost felt like fainting, not from light-headedness, but because I was so max-ed out, needing *to get out of there*. It was all too much for me. I was extremely agitated and uncomfortable. I had to get out of the sun and every time I saw a patch of shade I darted for it.

#13 Only thing today was a jittery dizziness as I was squatting to finish some concrete—perhaps it was the fluorescent lights. . . .

#11 Lots of dizziness over the past few days when I move from sitting to standing position.

NELUMBO NUCIFERA RUBRICS .... *Sacred Lotus*

MIND AFFECTIONATE; wife, with
AILMENTS from;
  business; failure
  crowd, in a
  reproaches
ALTERED STATES
  cocaine, like she is on
  coffee, like had been drinking
  drunk, as if
  LSD, flashback, as if
  stoned, felt as if on marijuana
AMBITION; much, ambitious
ANGER; irascibility; easily
  reproaches, from
ANTAGONISM; herself, with
  others; with
ANXIETY
  anticipating
  conscience, of
  exercise amel.
  family, about his;
  work
CAPRICIOUSNESS
COMPANY; alone, while agg.
    desire for
  working, while
CONFIDENCE; want of self
CONFUSION of mind
  cannot tell what is real and what is not
  dissociation from,
  identity, as to his
    depersonalization
  loss of self-knowledge and self-control
DEFIANT
DELUSIONS, imaginations
  angels, seeing
  cactus
  danger; of
  hand;
  hands, holding something sharp
  needles coming from own body
  neglected duty, his
  suffocated, she will be
  time; passes too quickly
  work; accomplish the, cannot; over-committed

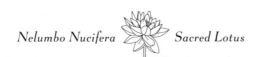

DESPAIR
DISCOMFORT
DREAM, as if in a
DREAMS
  accidents
  acrobats, swinging from trapezes
  airport, rushing to gate
  aliens, distant planets
  amorous
    looking for sex encounter
    phallus, of
  animals, of;
    bees,
    birds
    bugs
    dogs
    snakes, spiders
    spider webs
  anxious
  arrested, of being
    cop
  ashram
  batteries
  beating, someone is beating his friend
  boat, upside down
  body, body parts
    face
      distasteful expression
  bomb, nuclear, building a
  boyfriend, of
  business, of
    projects
    tedious
  calling out
  cars, automobiles, of
    accidents
    defective
  churches
  clairvoyant, prophetic
  cleaning
  companies
  confused; awake, half
  crazy, going
  crimes;
    other's of
  criticized
  dancing
  danger
  dog catchers
  earthquake
  eating distasteful or bland food
  emotions
    exciting
    fearless

exertion; mental
falling
  high places, from
  white abyss, into
family, own
  reconciliation
food; uneaten
friends
  pursuing, unable to connect
  seeing, of
fruit; gathering poisonous cherries
guns; shots
hiding, of
horses
hospitals
house, houses
  built
  lost
hurried; impatient
impendingdisease
  own disease, his
  sick people
insects
insults
intoxicated
intrigue; that his character is one of
irritable
jealousy
journey; bus, by
  car, by
  difficulties, with
  dimensions of time, through
  distant regions, in
  railroad, by, while starving
  spaceship, pleasant
killing
looking for people
lotus, of a
meeting, business, of
menopause
money; gold and silver, of
monsters
  sucking out essence of soul; with sense of calm
murdered; of being
  by his mother
  desires to be
murdering; father, her
  mother, his
music
nakedness, about
nature, of
office
old friends
parties, of

people, of
  assembled, conference
  black
  pleasure, of
police
political prisoner
power; love of
prison
procrastination
proving remedy
psychotics killing themselves
quarrels; with loved ones
relatives
  getting married
religious
running;
  in rain
  repeated, on track
schoolmate, meeting of old
scientific
servant, he is, to influential persons
sex; preparing to have
ship, of
shooting
shot, of being
singing
skin, peeling
spinning
stealing; food
steaming heat
stool; efforts at
striving
tattooed, of being
teaching
theatre, but could not see
threats
time lost, sense of
travel
trees; of, cutting
  leaves falling off
turning around
starvation
vehicles
violence
violent rage
violent, tendency
visits; to old friends
vivid
voodoo
waking, of
walking, of
water; swimming in
wedding
work

   wounded war veteran, cooking for
   worlds, changing
EXCITEMENT, excitable
   morning
   tendency; intoxicated, as if
EXERTION; mental agg.
EXTRAVAGENCE; emotions, of
FEAR; diverting the mind on, keeping herself busy, amel.
   injured, of being
   insanity, of losing his reason
   murdered, of being
   people; of, anthropophobia
FORGETFULNESS
HYSTERIA; anger, from
IMPATIENCE; with others
INDIFFERENCE, apathy
   death, to
   duties, to
   welfare of others, to
   wife, to
INSANITY; others, of; difficult
INTENSITY; emotions, of
IRRITABILITY; morning
   aggression, with
   anxiety, with
   business, about
   company, in
   conversation, from
   easily
   intense
   noise, from
   touch, by
   trifles, from
   work, about
JEALOUSY
   irrational
KILLED, desires to be
LOATHING; work
MANIA; everyone else is, as if
MEMORIES, of childhood events
MERGING OF, self with one's enviornment
MOOD; changeable, variable
POWER; love of
RELAXED feeling, letting go
REPULSIVE mood
RESTLESSNESS, nervousness; tendency;
   rest, when at
   worries, from
SADNESS
   anxious
   despondency, dejection, mental depression, gloom, melancholy
   suicidal disposition, with
SCHIZOPHRENIA; paranoid
SLOWNESS; purpose, of

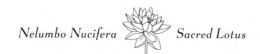

Nelumbo Nucifera   *Sacred Lotus*

                    STUPEFACTION, as if intoxicated
                      between awake and asleep
                    SUICIDAL disposition
                      throwing himself from; height, a
                    THOUGHTS; *clearness of*
                      collect, cannot
                      rapid, quick
                      stagnation of
                    TIME; passes too quickly, appears shorter
                    UNSYMPATHETIC, unscrupulous
                    VULNERABLE, emotionally
                    WEEPING; easily
                      remonstrated, when
                      tearful mood
                    WORK; *aversion to mental*
                      difficulty in
                      fatigues
                      impossible
                      indifference, with
                      pressured difficulty in
                      too demanding

VERTIGO   BENDING head; forward; agg.
                    DIZZINESS
                      Morning; agg
                    FLOATING, as if
                    HEAT; from
                    HOLD to something, must
                    INTOXICATED, as if
                    MOTION; from
                    MOVING the head
                      side to side; agg.
                      suddenly; agg.
                    NAUSEA; with
                    PRESSURE ON OCCUPUT; agg.
                    REST; amel.
                    RISING, from
                    SIT UP; cannot
                    SITTING, while; agg.
                    SPINNING SENSATION
                      violent
                    SUN; heat of, from
                    TURNING, on; agg.
                    VIOLENT

HEAD   HAIR; affections of
                    sensation, oily
                    HEAVINESS, sensation of
                    LARGE, sensation of

HEAD PAIN GENERAL; night
                    CONSTANT; continued
                      forehead, center of
                    CONTRACTING

	catarrhal
	closure of frontal sinuses, due to
	dull
	migraine
	ENLARGED; sensation as if
	LOCALIZATION
	forehead
	left side
	occiput, extending to
	vertex; morning
	sides; right
	PRESSING; forehead

EYE   DRYNESS; morning
       waking, on
    HEAVINESS
    LACHRYMATION
    PHOTOPHOBIA; sunlight
    REDNESS
    SWELLING; lids
    TIRED SENSATION

VISION   ACCOMMODATION; defective, headaches, with

EAR   DISCHARGES
      crusts
      sensation of
      watery
    ITCHING in; right
    PAIN; aching
      right
    STOPPED sensation; right
      noises, cracking

NOSE   CORYZA; nose;
    DISCHARGE; morning
      right
      watery
      yellow
        morning
    FULLNESS, sense of
    OBSTRUCTION
      night; wakes him
      right
    SINUSES, complaints of; catarrh
    SNEEZING

FACE   *DISCOLORATION; red*
      flushes
    NUMBNESS
    PULSATION

Nelumbo Nucifera   *Sacred Lotus*

MOUTH	DRYNESS; night *NUMBNESS;* tongue
TEETH	CLENCHING teeth together; constant inclination to in evening
THROAT	MUCOUS; morning PAIN; stinging uvula SCRATCHING; morning TENSION; talking, while
EXTERNAL THROAT	TENSION

STOMACH	APPETITE; diminished
	  increased, hunger in general
	    night
	ERUCTATIONS; foul
	NAUSEA; morning
	  afternoon
	  sleep
	  after
	THIRST
	  extreme
	  unquenchable; constant
	THIRSTLESSNESS

ABDOMEN	DISTENSION; morning
	  drinking water, after
	  gas, by
	PAIN; general
	  hypochondria; left
	  iliac region; left
	  pubic region; cutting; stitching, sticking
	  spleen; boring
	TENSION; hypochondria
	TIGHTNESS of liver region

RECTUM	CONSTIPATION; morning DIARRHEA; morning; seven a.m. FLATUS HEMORRHOIDS; painful, very
STOOL	DRY HARD ODOR; sweetish PIECES; hard ROCKS; like SOFT
BLADDER	URGING to urinate; morbid desire; night URINATION; frequent; night

URETHRA PAIN; burning
    urination; during

MALE ERUPTIONS; rash
PAIN; burning
    urination; during
SEXUAL; desire; diminished

FEMALE COITION; painful
    dryness, from
MENSES; copious
    clotted, coagulated
    dark
    flow; absence of, only in
    late, too
    painful; beginning, at

SPEECH & VOICE
VOICE; hoarseness

RESPIRATION DIFFICULT
    breath; taking a deep; agg.
    exertion; after
    expiration
    inhalation
    water, as if under

CHEST CONSTRICTION; morning
HEAT
PAIN; sore, bruised; mammae
PALPITATION of heart
RELAXATION, sensation of
TIGHTNESS, around chest
    Morning; agg
TINGLING
WARMTH, sensation of
WEIGHT; on, as if there were a

BACK ITCHING; dorsal region; eight p.m.
STIFFNESS; morning; lumbar, lumbosacral region

EXTREMITIES AWKWARDNESS
COBWEB, on ulnar surface of arm; sensation of
DRYNESS; foot
HEAT; foot
ITCHING; fingers
RESTLESSNESS; lower limbs
STIFFNESS; morning; rising, on and after
    ankle; morning, on rising
    foot
    lower limbs
    wrist; morning

Nelumbo Nucifera   *Sacred Lotus*

EXTREMITY PAIN
    ACHING; knee; right
    SHARP; wrist; right
    SORE, bruised
      exertion, after
    UPPER LIMBS; shoulder

SLEEP
    INTERRUPTED
    POSITION; side, on
      side, on; right
    SLEEPINESS; afternoon
      five p.m. agg.
    SLEEPLESSNESS
      one a.m.; until
      fright, from
        of monsters, fear
    UNREFRESHING; morning
      dreams, from
    WAKING; difficult
      afternoon
      early, too
      siesta,
      midnight, after
        four a.m.

FEVER
    HEAT; cold showers; amel.

PERSPIRATION
    ODOR; pungent
    PROFUSE

SKIN
    ERUPTIONS; red
    ITCHING; mosquito bite, after
    SWELLING; sunburn from

GENERALITIES
    COLLAPSE
    EFFICIENCY increased
    ENERGY; strength increased
    EXERTION; physical, agg.
    FAINTNESS, fainting;
      crowded, in a; street
    FLOWING sensation; water, of
    FOOD and drinks;
      bland food; desires
      chocolate; aversion
      fats and rich food; desires
      ice; desires
      meat; desires
      plain food; desires
      sugar; desires; evening
      sweets and fruit; desires
      water; cold, desires
    HEAT; sensation of
    HEATED, becoming

HEAVINESS; external; rising from a seat, on
  internal
HYPERACTIVE; on rising
ILL; sick feeling
INTOXICATED; sensation, of
LASSITUDE; tendency
LIE down; inclination to; afternoon
PAIN; muscles;
  motion; agg.
RESTLESS
SENSITIVENESS; sounds, light, and vibrations
SLEEP; short sleep; amel.
SLUGGISHNESS of the body
SUN; exposure to
  sunburn
  sunstroke
WEAKNESS, enervation; afternoon
  anxiety; with
  irritability, with
WEARINESS; all day
  morning
  evening
  night
  tendency
WEATHER; hot agg.

Nelumbo Nucifera   *Sacred Lotus*

JOURNALS .... *Nelumbo Nucifera*

EDITOR'S NOTE: *Punctuation, abbreviations, and individual stylistic nuances of the original journal entries have been preserved wherever possible.*

Prover #1 • Male • 37 years old

Day 0
- Dose one, around 10:00 p.m.
- Elevated energy, light high-octane energy. Rather like very good cocaine. Feel very good in general.
- Some pressure in upper-center of forehead.
- Some slight pain in lower left side. It was very light and happened maybe six times over a couple hours; like somebody taking a pen and poking me. It didn't really hurt, it was more a sensation. It was so immediate and localized after the remedy that I associated it with that.
- Dream: Of being in fearless situations. Somehow I ran into a bunch of spiders somewhere. And instead of being scared, I really don't care for spiders too much, I was kind of okay about it. I was thinking rationally and I just got out of their way. I don't really remember much of the dream, but I remembered feeling like I wasn't too afraid. And also I kept kind of running into spider webs over the last three weeks and seeing spiders a lot. And for some reason, that just kept coming to me during this proving.

Day 3
- Dose two.
- A little boost in energy, but that's all.

Day 4
- I actually had the same word-for-word experience as M. with somebody completely different than the people that they've mentioned, and I felt the exact same way as M.

Day 6
- Dream: My mother thought that I was an imposter in my body and wanted to kill me. And there was such an incredible real homicidal rage to it. She had a knife in one hand and something in another, and there was this incredible strength and rage and she was going to kill me. And I reacted to that in the dream, I became very homicidal and I wanted to kill her. I woke up and this dream was reverberating through my psychic system. For ten minutes, if she had been in that room, we would have tangled. It was unbelievable. I'd never felt the chemistry of a dream come so deeply and powerfully into the waking state for such a sustained time. It was incredible. And it didn't worry me at the time, it was just,

wow, this is happening and this is not usual. The part that was the juice of the dream was an incredible violent rage and this homicidal quality, but very clear and powerful. With a knife or maybe a hammer. I can't remember. She had something in the other hand, I can't remember what it was, but she definitely wanted to finish me off.

Day 8
- Feel aggressive, irritable. Not looking for trouble but not taking any shit. Also feel drugged.
- A little more sensitive to sounds, vibrations, light, anything in my sensory environment was a little harder to take. And there was a feeling over the next ten days of just trying to process all this stimulus and information, and it was sort of compressing me so that I felt more irritable. It was definitely kind of tough, a sense of uncertainty about what was around the next corner all the time, a real sense of everything in my life being up in the air, both literally and figuratively. Things changed so much in my life, so rapidly over the last few weeks, and I don't really know where anything is. And that's a good thing, but there was definitely a sense of danger and a sense of being careful about the whole thing. Like a time for potential growth but also to be very careful not to get entangled with any aggressive things that came out or any emotional things or any thoughts that would take me away from my center. I had to really work at that over the next couple weeks and it was imperative for me to stay out of big trouble. I would have gotten in things with people or in situations with myself in my own mind that would have been hard to get out of if I had fed those sorts of thoughts. Like getting angry at somebody for something that probably wasn't true in reality, or deciding to feel a certain way about a situation I really wasn't clear about. I felt like I really couldn't afford to label things or pin down causes to experiences or I'd be in big trouble. I just had to stay very quiet, clear, and sweet in my heart to stay out of big trouble.

Day 7
- Feel very aggressive, irritable today. Feel a little off balance and have feeling that there is danger and I need to be very careful, calm, and open-hearted today or I'll get into an ugly situation with someone.
- Dream: Another homicidal dream, and I don't remember the content. Somebody was trying to kill me and I wanted to kill them. The same sort of theme. Again, I woke up and this state was strong for about ten minutes after I woke up. Again, if somebody was in the room, I probably would have tried to kill them. I felt they were trying to kill me. Just amazing, amazing chemistry at work. I think I had a dream on the last proving about wanting to kill somebody. But these were of a whole other order, because those dreams were more the idea or the feeling of doing something. And this dream was that my whole actual physical body chemistry was set in motion to carry out that state. I was just blown away by how strong it was that morning.

Day 9
- Feeling irritable, aggressive, a little wild.
- Energy level very pumped up—revved.
- Stool much drier.

Day 10
- There seemed to be all around me a lot of craziness in the air, a lot of people having emotional, little mental problems, people really going through the grinder with a lot of issues, and people really feeling off balance. A lot of people having problems. And some of them would talk to me about it and other people I would just see and notice. Or I'd run into a lot of people around here during the day and it was a very hard time for most people.

Day 11
- Same state—irritable, a little pissed off.
- One of my friends on the verge of psychosis—very manic, in and out of psychotic state (but not total). She was fine the next day. Another friend gone totally psychotic. Not fine the next day.
- I've noticed a depressed sexual urge over the last couple weeks. Fairly extreme for me.

Day 12
- Dry stools.

Day 13
- Continuation of state. Many people seem on the verge of mentally falling apart, emotionally fragile, kind of confused about life. Major events and themes in everyone's lives seem to be in transition.

Day 14
- The craziness in the air seems to be at a fever pitch. Everyone seems tired from all the external and internal activities in their lives. I also feel this way. So much going on that it's hard to stay centered or feel very sane.

Day 15
- Went for an eleven-mile hike—it helped ground me a lot. I was so glad to go. And that really shifted the whole thing. I felt like everything was closing in here, everyone was acting so bizarre and I felt like I really needed to get out of this environment because I felt like I was absorbing everything around me. It was feeding this inner state in the sense that you could go mentally off balance at any moment. But that day I did a lot of physical hiking and work, and it really helped ground a lot of the energy. And then there seemed to be a shift after that.

Day 16
- A shift seems to have happened. I feel more grounded and less crazy inside. I've been doing a lot of physical work, which is helping a lot.

Day 17
- Feel more stable, less irritable, less angry.

Day 18
Additional notes:
◆ Loss of appetite for sweets; very unusual for me.
◆ Over-sensitivity to sound, light, etc.
◆ Remedy shifted after meeting, but still fairly strong. I saw a movie the next day called *Event Horizon* that <u>was</u> the worst part of the remedy—it was about all the fears of humanity and violence coming out of people. It was harsh and made me feel almost psychotic. The people in the movie didn't know if the fear, terror, or unknown things were coming from inside them or outside. They were losing the ability to discriminate the difference.
◆ For the next few days again, irritable, aggressive, feeling a little wild. A lot of energy with no specific reason attached to it or motive, very pumped up but not knowing really what to do with it. I had written down the word revved. Like revved up and nowhere to go. I also noticed that my stools were much drier and harder during the last ten days of the proving.
◆ I also noticed a depressed sexual urge in the first couple of weeks, and when S. said that having a feeling mainly from the upper body, that really describes an accompanying physical state to that. It's just being more aware of the energetics from the chest level up and less about the sexual things.
◆ During this whole time period I've been working very hard physically, outside. I was grateful for that, because it really helped me have much more of a groundedness during this period, and kept me a lot more stable. Even though I felt like my mind was just wild, it didn't bother me too much sometimes because I was physically tired and that took a lot of the energy edge off. The irritability continued up until now.

| **Prover #2 • Female • 32 years old** |

Day 0
◆ Right before I took the remedy my energy level was just a little lower than usual and I wasn't feeling very well, I was just starting to get sick. Like the beginning of a virus. I took the remedy fairly late on Saturday night, maybe around 11 p.m. And when I was holding it in my hand, it felt sharp. I put it in my mouth and it left my mouth and tongue numb, like some kind of really strong mint or something that was really strong. It numbed my mouth out. About four minutes later my face and body became completely flushed, a lot of heat went to my face directly after taking it. Prior to taking the remedy, when held in my hand I was unable to hold the bottle firmly. I had a soft grip. There is a pulsating, circular feeling while holding the remedy that runs up my left arm.

Day 1
◆ Was feeling a little lonely/sad this afternoon, missing the comforting arm of a lover/boyfriend. Haven't felt that way for awhile.

◆ Dream: I had a fairly intense dream the first night after I took the remedy. It started in my aunt's house and everything was shrouded. There were people moving around and there was a strong sense of foreboding. Everything was covered in sheets and mirrors had sheets draped over them. And there were a lot of people milling around kind of talking in really low tones, you couldn't make out what they were saying. And then the scene shifted all of a sudden; I was outside with two other people next to a really wide river and the climate was very warm. Immediately we went into this river and started swimming, and I could feel the water going right over my skin. There were these three large humanoid monsters after us, and they didn't have mouths, they had three teeth and sucker things on their face. And if they caught us they would take our bodies over and basically extinguish our souls, just suck it right out. And so while I was swimming quickly, I didn't want them to catch me but I wasn't afraid, I just didn't want to be caught. They were after us for a while. Then the scene shifted again and there was a complete sense of calm, I was outside some sort of civilized camp, it reminded me of a concentration camp. There was a little girl with long blonde hair there. And there were no signs of the monsters anymore, they were gone, but the little girl was totally vacant and at peace, she had been taken over by one of them. And I had the sense that that little girl was me. Completely at peace. But I was watching it from a distance. And so that day, I guess I was feeling a little lonely or sad, just missing contact with another person. And I haven't felt that way, that kind of loneliness, for a while.

Day 2
◆ For the first time—maybe ever—I am not craving sugar and chocolate. I haven't had either for the last couple of days, and I'm not tearing my hair out like I usually am. Usually after staying away from chocolate or sugar for a couple of days, I want it a lot, but the craving was gone.
◆ I got my period that day, and usually I have cramps that start to creep down my legs and it's usually a horrible experience for me. But I had hardly any cramping, and that was a significant change.
◆ My mood—I was lonely, I felt like I had less patience for the people around me, like I really had to work to relax and be accepting. People were starting to bug the shit out of me. That was also one of the prevalent things for me with this proving.
◆ I'm waking up with a clearer head. Usually, in the morning, I have mind-fuzz for about an hour. I am much clearer.
◆ Dream: I am in a political environment. Friends (sort of) with one of the Kennedy brothers. I stop by their house to get some of my clothes. I have the distinct impression that I am not of their social class. Then the scene shifted again, and I was rollerblading outside of Central Park in New York. A couple of friends from college were ahead of me and I kept trying to catch up to them and I couldn't connect to them either. It was just like I was reaching out to touch them and I couldn't make contact. And then, separate and apart from that, I felt like I was not myself with people, like my personality wasn't flowing out, I wasn't connecting with people.

Day 3
- A little sluggish. I think in general, I need to rest—the last couple of weeks have been hectic.
- People are getting on my nerves, I have less patience for them. I'm usually fairly patient when I'm at work, I like the people around me, but it was really hard not to snap at people or just to tell them to shove off because they were really aggravating the hell out of me. My earache was gone that day.

Day 4
- I've been extremely irritable. People are aggravating the hell out of me. I'd like to scream.
- Everything feels like it's pushing in on me. Like I have too much to do, too many people making demands on me, too many commitments. I would like to take a vacation. I am tired out.
- I am helping to organize the neighborhood picnic and do not have as much free time as I normally do. However, I usually have more patience, and don't feel so boxed in. I feel pressure from all sides. What's the pressure from? It doesn't seem like external events are really warranting feelings like that.

Day 5
- Was extremely exhausted for most of the day. Not irritable, though. Still am not having sugar/chocolate cravings like I usually do.
- I'm feeling like the virus is gone.
- Still feel like I'm over-committed. My reaction to this is to do nothing—not make my bed, not make phone calls, not listen to my messages, not open my mail, not do my laundry. My room has become a pit. I can barely stand being in it. I haven't done my chores this week either, and didn't water the plants. At about this time, I gave D. a call, wanting to antidote the remedy or figure out how to antidote the remedy, because it was getting fairly intense, the feeling of being over-committed.
- My sweat smells weird. It's sharper—more pungent, as if it belongs to somebody else. Like I didn't recognize my own smell.
- Dream: I could remember only fragments. I was the person in charge and I had responsibility. I think that my sisters were there. But we were in this room and we had to go someplace and there was this vagrant wandering through, this woman with lots of cloths and scarves, and she was in and out of our apartment, looking through the things when we weren't around, just lifting things. And I was the one who had to tell her she had to leave and to get out. Scenes kept shifting—sometimes we were on a train in a sleeping booth. And I saw this dream through a fuzz, as if I were standing/watching from a distance. A lot of times in my dreams I'm right there. But I felt like this paralleled a lot of things that were going on in the day, in that while I was very irritable, I didn't feel really connected with people. I felt like I couldn't make a strong connection with them, and didn't.

Day 6
- Feeling of not being able to get enough oxygen out of the air.
- Intense irritability.

Day 8

♦ I went to the beach and I got a really bad burn on my left ankle, you can still see it. And S. told me it was pretty bad second degree burns. And my ankle swelled up to be quite big. This was on Sunday, and the picnic was on Tuesday.

Day 10

♦ I had to be nice to people at this picnic. In the meantime, I'm in agony with my ankle and I was coordinating the raffle. And so, calling out prizes and then having 400 people jump on me like bugs, sucked. And my ankle was hurting and at the same time, to get above that and to try to be nice to them and not to yell at anyone and to trick myself into the fact, oh, you're in a good mood, you're going to have fun, don't get sucked into that, because I knew that if I let myself sink into it, it would be all over. About 8:30 or 9:00 p.m., when people were packing up, I just told the person getting a ride, I need the ride home, can you walk? All I wanted to do was come home—be driven home. My ankle was just becoming huge. It was probably the worst burn I've ever had.

♦ I stopped writing things down because it was a way for me, in my mind, to antidote this remedy and to not do it anymore and to not participate. Just because it felt like I was getting crushed down, and by not writing on it and not focusing on it, it was a good way to divert myself.

♦ I snapped at someone that I worked with. And it felt like it would be better for me to just not focus on the yucky stuff but just to try to breathe and feel good and focus on nice things, because if I kept focusing on the symptoms, I was just going to go ballistic and start yelling, because I didn't want anyone to ask me any questions, I wanted to be left alone. And I have a job where I have to be talking to people all day long and be nice to people, and it was easier for me to take myself out of the picture.

♦ Another thing that has happened throughout the remedy was that I felt like I couldn't breathe, like I couldn't get enough oxygen out of the air. Like even though I'd take a deep breath, I felt like I was under water or something, and I still feel like that today. It's gone throughout the whole thing. Intense irritability.

♦ One other thing I have noticed in the last week or two. I really have to focus on staying grounded because I could easily picture myself, that feeling of being disconnected from people could get magnified and, you know, I think you mentioned psychotic break earlier. In my early twenties, I went through a fairly intense time where I couldn't remember where I was. I'd walk down the street, I couldn't remember where I was, I couldn't talk to people, people would be talking to me but there was so much information that was going through my head I couldn't focus my attention outside of myself long enough to hear people. I felt like it was really an effort for me to stay focused and stay grounded, and if I let myself, I could just float away to that other place again or just really disconnect like that. So it was important for me to stop doing this remedy because it was just too much.

♦ My friend was thinking about killing herself and going through this intense time. Usually I'm fairly compassionate with people. So, although I would be nice with her and stuff, inside I was thinking, "Oh, can you just get over it, I've had it with this stuff. I don't want to deal with this, you're whining." I'm not usually like that. I'm usually fairly empathetic and very caring, and I just wanted people to stay away from me. I felt like I was over-committed. It's not that I have that many more things going on than usual, it's just that I've been unusually grouchy and prickly.

◆ My friend was out of control, or approaching the outer limits, and I did not want to open to that because I didn't want to get sucked into it. I mean, if she's sobbing hysterically, I knew that I could get pulled into that state myself.

Prover #3 • Female • 41 years old

Day 1
◆ Dream: About a friend's young daughter, no details.

Day 2
◆ Dream: Doing dinner clean up, putting away food. All the plates were uneaten.

Day 3
◆ Dose two (of the remedy).
◆ Dream: Drinking a beer while riding in a bus. A friend comes in and says "Having some suds?!" Get off the bus, boyfriend is standing on a street corner. We go down into a subway together and talk to someone about subway fares. Later, back on the bus, talking into a dictaphone about the earlier dream, when I get to the part about "having some suds?" everyone on the bus starts laughing.

Day 4
◆ No symptoms.
◆ Dream: I was teaching dance lessons (the jitterbug) in a gymnasium.

Day 5
◆ Dream: At a soccer game, women's ashram team, friend stops play and announces that she has to leave early. We leave together. On the way out we run into another friend, someone has made a giant cake shaped like a soccer ball. She is tasting and analyzing the cake.
◆ Dream: Running in the rain.

Day 6
◆ Dream: Music lessons.
◆ Dream: Tours of the ashram.

Day 8
◆ Dream: Cooking and dehydrators.

Day 10
◆ Dream: Airport dream. Trying to find my way to the gate; running but not getting anywhere; wandering all around; missed the plane. (One of my recurring dreams.)

Day 11
- Dream: Osteopathic treatment with S. She said I had been getting better but now my pelvis is out of whack again.

Day 17
- Dream: Dream about driving the bobcat.
- Dream: I was struck by how mundane they were.

Day 19
- Dream: Packing for backpacking. Trying to figure out how to carry a bowling ball.

> **Prover #4 • Male • 39 years old**

Day 1
- A bit foggy between 4:00 and 8:00 a.m., clear the rest of the day.
- Some stiffness in low back, but did a lot of gardening and hatha yoga.
- Dream: 4:00 a.m. I was traveling at night by car, there was a small accident. Tea party. Child and mother on a bike carrying a ladder too.
- Dream: 5:00 a.m. Horse farm. Someone is preparing for sex.
- Upon taking it, the next day I felt fine, in fact, pretty light and cheerful and almost a little buzz, like I'd had a joint or something, but nothing really major.
- Dream: A common thread was a dream that morning when I woke up preparing to have sex, but it was like a totally non-sensual/emotional thing. It was like, okay, get the bed made up, lay out the condom, is the lighting right. There was nothing romantic about it at all. And I noticed that that was the theme there.

Day 3
- Spinning, distracted, agitated, angry (this is <u>NOT</u> common!). Near violent.
- Slow.
- Migraine in the a.m. with stuffy sinus (common form of headache).
- NOT hungry.
- Stool loose (uncommon with migraine, usually constipated).
- The big reaction for me was day three. I had a difficult night, I woke up at 4:00 in the morning and the dreams weren't terribly significant. I remember, I was dreaming about a retreat and all the decorations and what colors they were. They were all colors of gold and silver and images of nature, leaves, shells, waves and things. Need to change clothes in a train station stairway—like a vagrant; Jim B. offers a ride home. I felt drunk, I felt like my head was spinning, I was very distracted, I had trouble physically moving around, staying focused. I was agitated, and actually got near violent a couple times.

Day 4
- Dose 2. Felt fine, in fact a little bit light and giddy for a day or two after that.
- Dream: Visiting Arizona or Bloomington. Lost my luggage by putting it down and

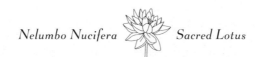

dashing to catch a bus. Can't get a hotel room. It is hot and raining, I am uncomfortable and frustrated. Could not get back to sleep so went to the gym.

Day 5
◆ Dream: I was living in a small dorm-type room with a roommate. The roommate's family comes to visit and I am working at the desk and it is a mess. The family seems to be hungry and waiting to have a discussion in private. I offer to leave so they can finish.

Day 6
◆ Dream: 4:30 a.m. Images of dogs and dog-catchers.

Day 7
◆ Gardened today and hit left big toe with hoe, it bled. Low back is stiff.
◆ Dream: 4:00 a.m. It is spiritual teacher's birthday and there is a special cake outside for a party.
◆ Dream: I am taking a shit and have an ecstatic experience and a poem regarding spiritual teacher comes to me. I run outside in my robe and spray paint it on the wall and fence.

Day 8
◆ Dose three.
◆ Mind quite clear, despite being up early, not sleeping and being very busy all day.
◆ A bit stiff from gardening, my feet hurt, low back is stiff (back is not new, sore feet is rare), this may be the gardening. The toe hit with hoe yesterday is still sore.
◆ Dream: 5:00 a.m. Visiting a clerical/administrative office where they take registrations (conferences and workshops). The people all are new to me, but seem ready to go.
◆ I slept poorly.
◆ Slightly burnt from being out in the sun while gardening and not using sunblock, and itchy due to sweating and heat.
◆ On what would have been the third day following taking the remedy again, I just had energy to burn. In fact, I did brunch and dinner that day here, so I was up at 5:00 a.m. in the kitchen, and then back in the kitchen again at 6:00 p.m. And for me, usually standing on the hard floor really wears me out. I was very relaxed and didn't mind it, and did both duties fine. Had slept very poorly, gotten up early. So that's common. I usually get annoyed and sore.

Day 9
◆ Dizzy, feel drunk and woozy. Relatively calm, but irritable or exasperated. I had this image of those compasses you have on dashboards sometimes where they're kind of floating in water. Like my mind was here but it was floating in water and I could turn here but my mind was still over there, and I might turn over here and it was over there. Like it was never in synch, everything was always floating in this little thing I call my head.
◆ General energy very low.

- Headache in the a.m., dull thud the rest of the day. My face feels numb, like when I first got drunk back in high school.
- Stomach is fine (my migraines and headaches usually have a stomach component, so this is rare).
- Very stiff low back and thighs (hamstrings), feet ache in the joints and heels. I am stiff and ache everywhere. My feet are dry and hot (unusual, usually the opposite).
- The fourth day after taking the second dose, I woke up again dizzy and drunk and woozy. I was very, very irritable. Everything exasperated me. I work at a college and take care of continuing education programs, and can be quite busy. The phones were ringing off the hook and I finally went out to the office staff and said, "No calls get through unless they're bleeding. You understand me? I will not talk to anyone." And I never do that. I always let my clients get through to me, but I was not going to let them get through to me because I was going to bite their heads off.
- I had a migraine, very stiff. It was not a good day. On that day, I left work early and lay down on the bed at five o'clock. I'm not a nap-taker at all, like once every six months I take a nap. I lay down for a second, I was really, really tired, and I was out like a light and slept till 9:30 at night, totally dead to the world. Woke up very groggy. It was my dinner clean-up night and I didn't give a damn that I didn't participate. I'm usually very conscientious about getting there or having a substitute, but slept through it, gone. And got up and then was able to get back to sleep at around 11:00 o'clock. Slept very poorly, if at all, going back and forth from being hot and cold all night. New sprinkler running outside may have kept me up and caused me to need to pee frequently. Felt anxious all night.

Day 10
- Slight headache on right side behind the ear, but fine. I am slow today.
- Sneezed a lot.
- Hamstrings still tight. Hips ache in the a.m. Took a walk and felt better.

Day 11
- I'm noticing on day eleven that I'm beginning to have difficulty making decisions. I commonly decide how many brochures I'm going to print or who's going to get this training, or I review people's credentials and tell them they're going to need more certification or less certification. And I kept reviewing these people's portfolios and then I'd ask another faculty member to review the materials. I'm usually not one who feels I need lots of people's opinions to validate my decisions. And it was like I just didn't have a clue. That's not like me.

Day 12
- Dream: I go to a sale at a store and want to buy a lamp with University of M. insignia on it, and it is on the top shelf. I am waiting in a cashier line behind a boastful black man who is buying a sports car for his daughter and is trying to get it gift-wrapped.

Day 13
- Dream: I visited a friend in a big old house and she had been beaten up by a housemate

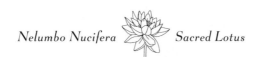

who practiced voodoo. I was upset and insisted that she move out immediately. I gathered an ashram moving crew and they were perplexed as to why we were doing this so suddenly. I explained that this was for her personal safety.

Day 14
◆ Some burning when urinating, may be passing gravel, this is common with kidney stone condition.
◆ Dream: I am starting to study in a college. There are lots of details to manage (applications, schedules, registration, etc.). I am hanging out with friends and really not getting it. I am late for everything, class and assignments. I am slow and unmotivated, etc.

Day 15
◆ Some burning when urinating, may be passing gravel.
◆ Dream: There is an election and there are questions for the kitchen on the ballot. I visit the kitchen staff with a copy of the ballot.
◆ I am sitting up at night and my mouth is dry.

Day 16
◆ Mind slow, quiet, foggy—and a little irritable—difficulty making decisions.
◆ Woke up with a headache. Took Excedrin and gave myself a combination self-osteopathy treatment and liver pack with ice pack on back of head, and felt better within 45 minutes.
◆ Mouth is very dry.
◆ Sacrum tight in a.m., it hurts and is stiff. Legs are stiff, especially hamstrings.
◆ Dream: I was looking for a parking place and couldn't find one. It is difficult and frustrating.
◆ Woke up again foggy, irritable, migraine. Definitely not having a good day. I had realized that this was a Monday, and that over the weekend for three days in a row I had had a caffeinated iced tea drink. I had given up caffeine six months ago and thought well, that was stupid, you don't take caffeine. But again, I'd been kind of feeling like I was okay, so why not have some caffeine. Again, having difficulty making decisions. And migraines are linked to caffeine for me.

Day 17
◆ Difficulty making decisions.
◆ Woke up very horny.

Day 18
◆ Fine, a little testy, but fine. Difficulty making decisions.
◆ Woke up very horny.
◆ Dream: 2:30 a.m. I am producing a comedy show and need a Friday Night act. I am looking at a list and trying to decide between Cosby and Gleason.
◆ Dream: 4:30 a.m. The organization I work for tried to hurt me and I argued with our past president and newly appointed co-executive director (my replacement).

Day 19
- Dream: I am watching a parade with a family while someone trades with me. We all hide sometimes in a furniture store.

Day 20
- Difficulty making decisions.

Day 21
- Dream: Had to go out of town and am concerned regarding our garden—who will care for it and when?
- Dream: Tim S. goes on trip to NYC and comes home and tells us about it. Describes large brick mansion, like Hampton Palace outside of London.
- There were times of feeling kind of disconnected from the people around me and almost feeling calm and relaxed but knowing that it was just a little more than skin-deep and if someone pushed me I would spit at them very quickly. Like everything's real fine, don't bug me. I was aware of this and so I was constantly working in ways to minimize that. And I didn't have real strong emotional reactions.
- I felt drunk, like my head was spinning. I was very distracted, I had trouble physically moving around, staying focused. I was agitated, and actually got near violent a couple of times.
- At one point, I had come home a little bit early and was trying to work out a watering system for our yard. We hadn't been maintaining it terribly well and things were drying out. I was wrestling with the hoses around the yard. I was jerking them around and dragging them all over and cussing and screaming. And one of my housemates just loves this garden and thinks it's great, and I said, "I am going to roto-till this mother—. I am sick of it." And he was gasping.
- I did remove 14 bags worth of waste that day. I was into pulling things.
- The other significant thing is that on this day and other days when I had reactions, I got migraines. I'm prone to migraines. I've been through a period with a naturopath that had pretty much cleared up that condition, I wasn't getting them very frequently at all. But they came back, they were strong, and the difference for me was my body—my migraines are always linked with a bloated stomach and constipation, and those two symptoms weren't present. I just had a migraine.
- I have a kidney stone condition, and a couple times I started having burning sensations when urinating, which is common when I'm passing gravel. But again, that hasn't bothered me for a long time, so that's the old symptom returning.
- Not feeling romantic or sexually inclined at all during this period; couple times waking up in the morning feeling like I would like to have sex, but just nothing there.
- When I felt really dizzy and drunk, I had the flashback of the first times when I drank. I drank quite heavily when I was young and started when I was 14. I would often feel very numb in the face and warm. And I noticed that my face was numb and warm, it was like, god, I'm 14 and I'm drunk again.
- At some point during this couple-week period, my wife became ill. She had a severe

stomach problem, and the only significant part to that is that my wife never vomits, she's totally afraid to vomit. And she vomited for two days straight, several times. And it was weird. But also she was very anxious about that, and it was kind of like, you go in the bathroom, and you vomit, and if you need to you drink some warm tea and have some toast. Any other time I would ask, "Do you need anything else?" I was not going to support her in this. It was like, I'm sick, I'm vomiting! Yeah, so what? Go in the bathroom, do it. Usually I would very much be right there with her through any type of physical trauma that she had.

◆ Other instances that were unique, was watching other people go through severe conditions, and each time asking them key questions to see that they were okay but not at all feeling that I would invest myself in supporting them. My mother has metastasized cancer, diabetes, high blood pressure, and severe arthritis, and called up and said, "The doctors feel I have congestive heart failure," which is what killed my father a year ago, and, "What should I do." And I said, "What did the doctor tell you to do?" And she says, "Ah, you know, less salt, drink more, exercise and take my medicine." I said, "Uh-huh, good. Call my sister, if you need me to do something and be there for you." And both my brother and sister called me and said, "Oh, Mom's much better now." But they were very anxious and had to spend a lot of time and energy with her calming her down, and usually I would have called her twice a day to check in. And this time, not once, it's like, you're fine. You know what this disease is, you know how to deal with it.

◆ My choir director, who took me to Romania when I was a kid and had been my personal voice teacher for ten years, died in a car accident a couple of days ago. It's the type of situation where I knew I couldn't get there, but usually I would have made an effort to find out where's the funeral home, what donations need to be made, should I be sending flowers, etc., etc. And I called an old choir friend and said, "Let me know what you need done and I'll do it," and I removed myself from the situation. And that's not typical of me.

◆ At my office, we were in a situation where my boss is a bit of a workaholic and has very high standards. I've only been there a year and a half, but I've seen her basically fire or insist on people leaving very quickly if they didn't meet her standards. And there was a person who she'd decided she didn't like, and over this period it fell to me to either let this woman know that she will be fired or to interest her in expanding her career elsewhere. And I was able to do that, I was able to convince this woman that she wanted to take a job elsewhere and let's see what we can do, and help her draw up her resume, the whole bit. And it was interesting that I didn't feel terribly committed to either of them. They both had different goals and it was kind of like, okay, you're very tense and you're going to get all upset about when she's leaving and how she's leaving and how quickly, and I don't care. And the other one was, you know, I'm being outed, what's going to happen to me; it was kind of like, well, you're going to find another job. And the two of them have continued to have this hailstorm. The other one got a job and is leaving this next week, which is before anyone asked her to leave, and the boss is furious because it's too soon. Usually I take these things very seriously, and I was just not involved at all.

Prover #5 • Female • 47 years old

Some general observations about how I was during the first four days of the proving:
- Headache.
- Nausea.
- All energy in upper chest and head.
- Pounding heart.
- Frequent urination at night.
- Physical agitation.
- Extreme discomfort.
- Hot, achy eyes.
- Thirst that couldn't be quenched.
- Self-deprecating attitude.
- Restless sleep, with lots of tossing and turning.
- Extreme aversion to disorganized, crowded, noisy places.
- Aversion to sun (normal, but exaggerated).
- Lack of hunger.
- Desire for simple foods, and trouble digesting easily.
- Need for more sleep than usual; naps at odd times.

Later:
- Alertness, energy, vitality.
- Compression, intensity.
- Over my head.

Day 18
- Spiritual teacher's talk/signing. Class was very profoundly deep and relaxed, no concern or upset from his talk.
- Saw Chinese massage therapist. He seemed more harsh than usual, talked about relationships and his marriage.

Day 20
- Slammed arm into car door.

Prover #6 • Male • 45 years old

Day 1
- Went sailing in afternoon with friends—had a wonderful time—felt very peaceful and contented, "at home" in myself. Everything looked sharp, clear, colorful, like a movie.
- Energy good—mood fine. Had a good run in early evening—felt strong.
- Copious flatulence in the afternoon otherwise unexplained by dietary indiscretion. This was nearly odorless and without discomfort.

Day 2
- Agitated in the morning. Feeling restless/hyper—quite uncomfortable—in the morning. This dissipated by afternoon. This was partly related to realistic financial concerns, but the response seemed excessive.
- My afternoon run was much more tiring than usual—I stopped for a few minutes in the middle to catch my breath—sweating profusely.
- Very much enjoyed the company of my friends, who seemed extraordinarily handsome and beautiful in appearing like angels.

Day 3
- Dream: Of a large underwater camera with robotic legs that was amazing, but it needed a battery pack that I had trouble finding. S. and S. also had a camera they loaned to me, and it needed batteries as well. I spent most of dream looking for batteries. Some feeling of impatience—wanting to get on with the activity.

Day 5
- Mood good.
- Some increased flatulence, but may be explained by rich diet of nuts and dried fruit while hiking.
- Some discomfort in right knee—along medial joint line, possibly in response to stresses of walking on uneven terrain.

Day 6
- Dose two at night.
- An uneasy day of rest after a hiking day—felt restless and dissatisfied with camping spot. Worried it wasn't the best possible spot to camp.
- Got many mosquito bites which are terribly bothersome, itching, causing lumps all over my body—reaction seems stronger than usual for me.

Day 7
- Felt peaceful and happy most of day. Several episodes of losing things and finding them again during day.
- Dream: I had a dream of marked confusion of time and identity where I thought it was 8:00 in the morning and it was actually 3:00 in the afternoon, and I just could not get the time straight. And someone said, "No, it's 3:00," and then I would go, "Oh, it's 7:00," or something, and it was just this real confusion of time and there was no way I could orient myself by the sun or anything, it was very confusing. And a friend of mine who's very sweet and demure turns out to have a secret life as a punk rocker. It was so surprising to me because it's someone I know fairly well. So it was this strange identity that came up in this dream.

Day 8
- Travel day while on vacation from Three Sisters Wilderness to Mt. Hood. Feeling tired and hot midday, but then hiked three and one-half miles with 60-pound backpack in

the afternoon and spent three hours in evening photographing wildflowers. High energy despite being tired.

Day 9
- Dose three at night.
- Dream: About Paul McCartney coming to the ashram. We had a nice chat, he gave me a bunch of clothes as a gift, and I was supposed to run around to do some errands, but I kept putting them off (procrastinating).

Day 10
- I sat up first thing in the morning and the whole world spun vigorously. I had intense, intense vertigo, like I've never had it before in my life. I had to basically grab the ground and lie down immediately. Incredibly intense. I would try to sit up again and it would happen again; I would sit down and it would be okay. That symptom has actually persisted since that time; it has become slightly less intense during the preceding twelve or fourteen days, but the modalities of it are: vertigo, always spinning to the right in a clockwise fashion, worse bending my head forward, very much worse with any pressure on the occiput in the back; initially worse turning the head from side to side, although that's no longer a symptom. This was accompanied by nausea and malaise.

Day 11
- Continued vertigo when sitting up from supine or bending head down while standing or pressure on occiput. Overall intensity less, so I ventured to teach my hatha yoga class in late afternoon—only to find the vertigo was incapacitating—I had waves of spinning and nausea and could barely get through the class. I briefly admitted to class what was happening—to explain why I was losing my balance on simple standing postures.

Day 12
- Continued vertigo symptoms, although intensity slightly less. Modalities the same. Vertigo symptoms tend to be worse on waking in the morning and in the evening when tired.

Day 13
- More vertigo, less bothersome but still bad when bending forward or sitting up from supine.

Day 14
- Continued vertigo symptoms on sitting up in bed and when bending forward. Not so much when turning head anymore.

Day 15
- Quite hot today (90+ degrees)—which is intolerable to me.
- I feel energized by the seminar and new understanding it brings. Quite tired in evening—heat is oppressive—hard to concentrate on a case I'm working on.
- Continued vertigo on bending over to pull book out of my bag while at seminar.
- Thirst increased—ice water tasted very good.

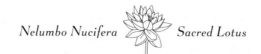

Day 16
- Still dizzy on sitting up in morning—although it resolves quicker than in past. On lying down on floor to try yoga exercises, immediately on pressing occiput to floor, I had a sudden wave of vertigo at approximately 2/3 of original intensity. Not having nausea at present.

Day 18
- Continued vertigo.

Day 21
- Still having vertigo, approximately 1/2 the original intensity, same modalities (pressure on occiput and to lesser extent bending head forward).
- I had some very positive experiences early on, of things looking very sharp and clear and colors being very bright and pleasant. I also had the experience of just looking at people around the house and having the strong experience that these people were all angels. Just looking at them and every person looked completely beautiful or handsome or just, you know, magnificent. It was a wonderful experience, actually. It was quite strong.
- I also was on vacation during this, and I won't do that again. Had very strong reactions to mosquito bites. There were a lot of mosquitoes, and I usually get some reactions, but I had huge welts from them and they were terribly itchy.
- I didn't have very many dreams during this proving at all, which was unusual.
- Teaching hatha was really a nightmare on two occasions. Doing floor poses and having my head against the floor, doing some lying twists, and the whole room was just violently spinning. And the vertigo was associated with some kind of disorientation, and also nausea, and that nausea has persisted also slightly over time.
- The symptoms tend to be worse on waking in the morning and in the evening when I'm tired. Also seems to be a little bit worse from heat and dehydration. I've been consciously trying to tank back up and get enough fluids because I was thinking maybe it started when I was on vacation, got dehydrated. I wasn't quite sure what maybe caused it. It is a little bit worse when I'm dehydrated.
- I was at a conference at the beginning of this week, and the bending forward modality had gotten better. And then I reached under the table to grab my book and the whole room was really spinning and I had to kind of again brace myself to not fall off the chair. It's a pretty intense symptom, actually.
- I had difficulty concentrating on work activities.
- My thirst was quite a bit increased and I very much enjoyed ice water, which I don't normally do. And it's been hot, but that was different for me. So the main thing is this vertigo, which persists.

Prover #7 • Male • 52 years old

Day 0
Dose one.
- Before taking remedy, I held it to see if I could get any vibration. I felt like it relaxed me a little bit.
- Took remedy at 10:00 p.m.—relaxed feeling.
- Slight warm and tingly feeling in area of chest, some expansion.
- Dream: 1. Woke at 1:00 a.m.—levels of reality blended—I had trouble getting up and could feel dream elements fading away as I was analyzing dream. Felt a message was being given and wondered if plant remedy. 2. As getting back to sleep noted very warm and threw off covers. In dream had pleasant warm feeling in chest, felt immobilized and then felt like body spontaneously making large jerky movement of right side 90 degrees from "astral body" lying on left side, like kriya. I was sleeping on my left side, and I felt like my physical body was moving and my astral body was staying there. And I also felt that I was crying out or moaning in my sleep. Then I woke my wife up with that, and I reassured her. I said, "Don't worry, it's just the proving, and I was okay." Thought I got up to write dream down. Was going to use light of computer screen and couldn't turn screen saver off. Asked wife to help. Then woke up. I asked wife if I had talked with her, she said no. Very strong experience—like drug, and wanted to have again. 3. Dream—interviewing people at work. They start to tell me about proving dream. I tell them to stop or it will ruin proving. At work—very crowded, sorting very tiny silverware. At bank I am telling teller how hot it is, can literally see steam.
- Awoke 5:00 a.m.—pulsation in face and neck for a couple of minutes. Recalled dream of taking course with institute people. About to take test. Talking with friend—noncompetitive and laid back. Scene shifted to conference. People very friendly. Looked like caring for or use of pets. Very pretty—fantails. Some of the people were going to chant in a.m.—(which I didn't want to do) and they had slices of bread with peanut butter on edge.

Day 1
- Less time urgency.
- Increased thirst in afternoon and evening.
- Dream: Woke up with alarm clock and had to sit to recall dream. Basic feel was of a science fiction epic. I was on another planet with a number of small disgusting insect-like critters. An alien required I catch five of them in order to leave. I succeeded but had deceptive feel to it. Scene shift—got back to general office at government. Like a hospital overcrowded with people, and I had trouble finding a place to sit to go over mail. Another job I did not like was I was supposed to oversee a dentist's work to see that he was ethical. Later I learned I was going to have to go to Far East. I had mixed feelings but looked forward to food. After I awoke I felt like I slept just two hours.

Day 2
- Time passed quickly during meditation (also with sleep the previous night).
- Dream: Mixture of two themes. One had to do with studying differential of materia

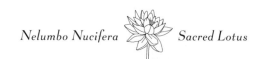

medica. Looked at sulphur vs. natrum sulphurica. Also looked at calcarea muriaticum, and thuja. Somehow Paul Herscu was involved—giving complex cases. This discussion and work on presentation materials alternated with the work setting, which had a Germanic militaristic setting. Lots of silly regulations. For example, about toilet paper. I broke the regulations. Another fragment of dream, I parked at a bowling alley—the police had bowling league. On way out I couldn't find car—not where I put it. Woke with frustrated feeling.

Day 3
- Dose two.
- Saw very little effect except mind—more mellow, laid back.
- Tired. Took nap—only slightly refreshed.
- Warmth in chest—pleasant.
- Somewhat heavy feeling in body.
- Dream: Woke up about 11:25 p.m. Laid in bed and did not want to get up to write things. Heavy, immobilized feeling but not unpleasant. Could feel dream drifting out. Had a thought about getting a message. I only recalled theme of turning back and forth, from side to side, which I did, but heavy sensation.
- Dream: Recalled after woke up at 12:53 a.m. Hot relaxed feeling in chest. Slight dull frontal headache. Eyes tired. Part of dream: Had to get back to room at night with no clothes. Embarrassing. But I succeeded. People ignored me if I got out of way. Idea of back and forth again. When I got back I removed a needle that was inserted in eyebrow of Asian woman. It was infected. I had a similar needle and it wasn't infected.
- Woke at 3:30 a.m.—was working with a professor. He offered to take us to lunch but he was trying to avoid expense and so took us to cafeteria. Drove car. On the way, critical of drivers. (He was from NYC.) We had to take off shoes and put in footholds of earth to get to cafeteria. I didn't want to but did and showed him the way.
- Another fragment: We're at ceremony on long table. I had to sit on table at one end—embarrassing to be exposed. Ceremony involved successive people moving towards me but stopped halfway—I felt relieved. At one point we are surprised a hand calculator worked better than a personal computer. Again feeling of immobilization but turning side to side.

Day 4
- Dream: Working with a lot of people to build gambling casinos in New York City. There was one game setup with several people behind different concessions. Trying to sort out how to do and how much money it would make emphasized.
- Dream: A big meeting with foreign experts—very dynamic speakers. Some concern about info—whether should be government agency vs. a different group. Presentation interesting—something about building and saving resources. I drop car off during meeting to get oil changed. At one point I am moving a car looking for my car. They had a dining hall at meeting but I had some trouble finding seat so went to check on car. When got back looked like different group in dining hall. I took a lemon pastry but it had taste like cardboard. Feeling was our lack of enjoyment.

- I decided on day four to take another dose of the remedy because I really liked the feeling it gave me the first time. So I took it again. I didn't see much affect at that time, but I did feel mellow and laid back, and that's basically how I was feeling during the day as I looked back on it. And again, I got the warmth in the chest, pleasant, but a somewhat heavy feeling in the body at that point.
- Woke up about 11:25 p.m. and was lying in bed, and I did not want to get up to write the things down that I was dreaming about. I had a heavy immobilized feeling, but it wasn't unpleasant, and I could feel the dream drifting in and out of a dream state. And then I had a thought about getting message. I only recalled the theme of turning back and forth from side to side, which is what I had in the first dream.

Day 5
- Dream: Something about psychic abilities—reading minds.
- Dream: Son and I visiting. Go to massive movie theater with an enormous brick stairway. I hear some guy say they are ripping us off in the parking lot place. Something about predictions from pieces of chocolate. Movie not that good and we leave. Wanted to make sure and so go a second time and park in expensive lot again. Scene shifted to class, students would hold hands in a line or circle to better get impressions of music. I don't join in until end of music class. Another scene shift—I am working at a restaurant washing dishes. I am a cop and they ask me to help arrest a man in neighboring building who left and did not pay bill. I am reluctant to go, as I am not dressed as a cop. As I leave with a black coworker I am brought two (small and large) wrenches to use if needed against the man. We go through weird vertical tube escalator/elevator and find the man—an attorney. A theme in this dream: I was also trying to go to movies and restaurant but somehow our timing was off and we kept missing each other. Scene shifted to restaurant—again friend was at a different table. On menu was an unappetizing desert of fruit, rice pasta, and cheese.

Day 6
- Scratchy throat. Slight hoarseness to voice.
- Dream: Working on house. Second dream: At train or bus depot. Had a change of clothes and had to go back and get them. I was using certain materials (at one time like bread rolls, another a canister of gas.) I try to conserve and not use. We were eating. A black man offered me his beer—there was a shortage of food. Again hot dog rolls came up in this part of dream. Later on go through closet at front of institute to get to clothes left at station (kind of a back door to station.)

Scene changes—in older part of house I am using sink and unsure if it has garbage disposal. Theme of cannisters—some kind of synthesis of discarded materials—material part and nonmaterial part! At one point in dream was with soldiers and I had large gun (like the movie, *Men in Black*). I'm playing with it, but doesn't fire (awesome destructiveness not unleashed).

Scene shift—sent a card to GP for professional meeting—speaker shows it off. It included toenail clippings and was colorful. A member of audience looks at it and unfolds it so he can't put back together (I'm disgusted). I get to go to space station. Very relaxing—games, music, swimming pool!! I feel like real vacation. Something goes wrong with space station—come down and land in Iowa near base with missiles and nice high school. I get separated from wife and go to concert. Person in audience didn't believe I was in space station. Talking with woman and cracks develop in earth (? disaster). We travel quickly down alley in car and meet undercover cop. Feeling—these and other dreams, usually enjoyable and pleasurable.

Day 7
- Throat still scratchy, less hoarse.
- Dreams: Something about visiting with east coast friends. Converse over dinner and trying to find out headlines for next day.
- Dream: Eating and talking. We ate light at one meal because were going to eat a second meal at institute. Computers were on desk at meal. Scene shift—I am educating a man. He says he thinks he was a Ph.D. I ask him where he was born. He won't tell. I ask why he won't tell and he refuses to answer. Scene shift—going to proving meeting. I forgot journal and some people had three journals!

Day 8
- Still laid back.
- Dream: I helped friend with German homework. He got good grade. Teacher then verbally critiques notes I used to help him, as if it was assignment I turned in (which it was not intended). I felt this was unfair.
- Dream: A number of scene shifts. One part involved a physician we may be having join our group. He had fancy pager with code numbers for many situations. There was a certain dissonance with him. He wears a suit, not holistic, and loved fishing (asked if I did fishing—which I haven't for years). Shift to robbery involving thirty people. I wander off (as I did not want to participate). They reject me later. Scene shift of a trial of a young girl who was an outcast but was not really guilty of crime accused of. Details I cannot integrate into dream. At one point I was up in a tree.

Day 9
- Dream: (In real life remodeling is being done on our house). An object, shaped like this /\, in black, somehow was a certain remedy (explosives). We were arguing over what it means. Meanwhile, *Saturday Night Fever* background music is going on.
- Dream: Went to India with another person to heal them with the above remedy. Some secret ritual involved. (In real life I had gone to talk on ritual the night of dream.) Two Indian doctors were desperate and felt they need to attack us to get remedy. They were not successful in attack and we learned it was a misunderstanding. We then worked together. Scene shift—We were supposed to deliver flowers. I couldn't find ones for friend—there seemed to be a mistake. Later standing in cafeteria line waiting for food—talking about mistake.

Day 10
- Dream: I was working on my house with Native Americans.
- Dream: Taking course. Two friends get big position at California company. We are

getting ready to go to dinner and I am asked to help move a fish tank. I agree but say I want to stop off at Chinese restaurant on way to get catfish that they serve. One of my friends has a child who will be going to Harvard, Stanford, or Sorbonne in France.

Day 11
◆ Continue to be laid back. Less time pressure.
◆ Dream: Working on house. (In real life, construction of roof continues.) There is small square tower with shingle on top that another individual is trying to complete and may abuse the power of it. By entering, can pass between times—into other times and/or dimensions. (Again, the theme of something appearing ordinary having unusual power.)
◆ Dream: I am fixing breakfast as man with no legs (lost in war) is taking insulin. I think to myself, I am going to be healthy when I am his age. I arrange to meet patient at my other office because more convenient for them. I am taking bus to work. I comment to wife about the ecology of a bus (who sits in the back, front, etc). She tries to make me shut up. I note certain rule that allows to sit in back. Scene shift—Two relatives who are going to get married. Talking with two sons who are worried about cost of fixing up house.

Day 12
◆ Less judgmental and more affectionate with wife.
◆ Dreams: Myself and others set out for big meeting. One fellow had packed a set of weights in styrofoam. There was an enormous meeting hall. Members of audience picked at random for certain contests or game. Middle-aged woman and I were picked to select items as a team. I feel we have very different tastes, but I picked baby lima beans and two other food items. In returning from meeting, some chose regular transport, but I got back by entering small room and propagated instantly in mysterious way. (This room is similar to room in upper part of my house being remodeled.)
◆ Dream: Saw woman in office on Saturday. She was upset and wanted me to hold her hands. I notice a swarm of bumblebees in office. I tell her we'll talk outside building but I never get there, as first I try to get maintenance to do something about bees. I run into Mike (old colleague). We leave to get his car but it needs to be towed. I say I need to get back to see patient. In process go to dining hall—has large wood doors (like castle). A number of empty chairs at table. I was late but still some people there. I try to get out four eggs that are in a "synctrium??"—I just want two. Scene shift—I am teaching two young men. One is very silly, teasing and ridiculing me. I ask if he was taking his lithium. Scene shift—Getting ready to leave early in morning to bring son to airport. We were making breakfast. I was having two halves of pepperoni pizzas with pockets like pita bread, and they could be worn like slippers. I put two pieces of cheese in skillet and think I should have used two pieces already in skillet.
◆ I note on day twelve I continue to be laid back, feel less time pressure, and seem to be more physically affectionate but not necessarily more sexual. And I'm not a particularly touch-feely type of guy, but I was more in that mode, and seemed to be more conscious of other people's needs during this time, less irritable.

Day 13

◆ Had abdominal cramps (1) about 8:30 for about 20 minutes. Had suprapubic sharp, cutting pain (3) radiated to left slightly, <<< motion or jarring, >>> sitting with left leg up. Might have been better with meds but I decided to sit at computer and reassess pain—pain left. I thought during the pain, "Here I'm building this nice house and ill health could interfere with it."

◆ Dream: The tone and feeling of this dream seems different from what I have been having. A psychologist colleague, who I am friends with, is in a different group that is coordinating with my group. I have become head of a psychiatric unit. He is shouting across a field, things I have disclosed to him and he's distorted. I feel he's trying to bait me and I don't respond, but some people in my group do. We get together to eat and I comment how my school beat his in football in a joking way. He becomes apologetic and we arrange to have lunch at his house. A man outside house is injured and ambulance takes him to hospital. At one point I am on psych unit. A nurse is trying to get on the unit as a patient. I try to avoid making decision due to "conflict of interest." I felt she was feigning to avoid problems. I have cynical view of project or unit and felt it is political gambit. Scene shift—I know general way and see woman who appears like Dionysus and lady is agreeing with what I am saying about my observation. Attending woman doctor irritated by me and says I should go to medical school if I am so interested in medicine. I say I already have (I felt like remarks were disingenuous).

Day 14

◆ Dream: I was consulting on patient who was depressed. (Colleague had asked me about a depressed patient before my dream.) The name of a patient I saw in consultation in real life came up. Scene shift—I was going to office but had to stop at store. Was buying laptop computer. Woman who was supposed to wait for me goes buying books at same time. Scene shift—With physician and he is making exaggerated remark about sexual experience and I say maybe you're just more experienced than me. I was climbing up a small stack of circular stones and then rotated while sitting on them to get up raised embankment to office. There are a lot of people sitting around rocks, a crowd.

◆ Dream: Saw a girl about eight years old—very adult-like she had a narrow nose and dark hair. She hallucinated in past but has been on massive medications in past. (In real life I saw a patient who had also been overly medicated by another psychiatrist.) I had trouble typing. So somehow the number 250 came up. In another fragment I had come back from vacation, four straight patients did not show and I was trying to find out why. Again I was doing some consulting. Scene shift to going for dinner, but I have to get some of the food out in the fields of the host. I see friends gathering tomatoes for the dinner as I am driving by in car.

Day 15

◆ Stuffy nose when I went to bed at 9:30 or 10:00 p.m., my nose was very dry and I found it hard to breathe. It was even interfering with my sleep. It was worse with the heat. But it seemed like it went beyond what I would usually experience if it's hotter than usual. It's almost like feeling like I couldn't get enough air.

◆ Dream: (Awoken by pager 2:30 a.m. Very tired and try to get back to sleep.) In dream pager goes off and problem with timer on it and clock radio, so can't go to sleep because alarm will be inaccurate. Try to fix it and need to get battery. My son was awoken and is just a three-year-old child in dream. I finally go to store. Clerk won't take a $20 bill I had in pocket but will take Visa. I had forgotten wallet and I say, "F____." He says, "Now I won't take Visa." I feel I understand his position and tell him. He then tells me story of religious conversion related to Air Force experience. His sleeves have two wings or corporal insignia.

Scene shift—Two girls who may have leprosy. One thin blonde girl is being pursued. Tries to blend into crowd by running but it is obvious she is not well. I am also a fugitive (for unclear reasons). I have her sit down and I try to get her help. As I disappear into crowd she goes to microphone and asks for help. At first I am upset she did this but then I realize she was trying to provide a distraction so I wouldn't get caught. At some point I had a fragment of dream where I was on statue talking to black man about statue for Martin Luther King. They take part of statue I'm standing on (for view) and use it for Martin Luther King statue where there are other heroes, but confederate heroes of Civil War.

Day 16
◆ Dry and hard stool, bent in shape of colon (curved, not straight) for last three to four days.
◆ Dream: Had dream of two lawyers insulted by term "whore-yers." Join two gangsters. Later killed. Story then got re-run from beginning.

Day 17
◆ Right lower quadrant supra pubic pain due to distension by gas. Was present when awoke 4:00 a.m. Disappeared gradually by 7:00 a.m. Also had some antacids—neutral effect on pain.
◆ Cobweb—single strand sensation on inner ulnar edge of left elbow that goes away if brush or rub lightly, but then returns. Occurred in early evening and lasted just a few minutes.
◆ Dream: Traveled to old 1890's style shop. Somehow kids were involved and we, in a contest, try to guess the weight of short chunky woman cooing like a bird. Also tried to put outline of hats over three birds—then throwing some objects in a game but I don't want to participate. In another fragment of dream, I get Catholic-type mail. I attribute to consulting with Catholic Social Services. In another part of dream, priest is having a meal of bread. Someone comments, "This is not realistic food for this group," i.e., they would not be eating this. Priests turned in uniforms to go incognito.

Day 18
◆ Notice a tendency to be more physically affectionate. I'm not a touchy-feely person usually. Also more considerate and giving, in regard to son, mother-in-law, and non-relatives.
◆ Dream: Something about using the herb hypericum. Was in form of bare twigs. Somehow was using to help in building house. Something to do with wiring.

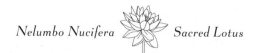

Nelumbo Nucifera   Sacred Lotus

Day 19
◆ Cobweb sensation in same part of left arm. Occurred midmorning and around 9 p.m.
◆ Dream: I'm sitting in library reading technical books on a variety of topics. Some I am familiar with and others are unusual names. A group of med students come in and want orientation to library. I apologize that I can't help because I am not on staff. I joke with their leader with put-down joke about New Jersey. (We are on the west coast.) Scene shift—In hospital, and two workers speak to patient in foreign language but use the word "die" and he reacts hysterically. Investigators think nothing is wrong—patient just hysterical—but actually a medical scandal is going on and patient is seriously affected. Scene shift and I am working in the emergency room—it is outside and starts to snow. I like it but coworkers don't. I feel confident in handling the situation.

Scene—Irritable patient (I treated in real life with sulphur and he did well). He notes has sleep atony. He and friend watched television show and figured out this is what MK had. He is disgusted I didn't pick it up. So am I. Scene shift—helping to prepare tacos. I suddenly realize I am naked and manage to find a pair of cut-off jeans to wear. I leave to do workout, but can't find Nordic Trac—disappointed. Something about lycopodium being used for a structural problem—not in a sentient being.

Day 20
◆ Dream: Worked on house, helping some people shop for food. Scene shift—I am seeing patient and her husband. While they are talking I am polishing shoes and I get polish on suit. (I don't wear a suit to office.) They go to get something to help and I try to get out stains. When they come back we finish session, but ran over usual time. I charge them for just a regular session. Next patient doesn't show. Fragment—someone drew cartoons with caricatures of stars—one is Jimmy Stewart. Scene shifts—Taking exam. Feel I did well and was going to turn in but noticed I had not signed name on test. Have trouble finding pen, then can't get one that works or right color. Then my test paper got misplaced among other papers. I finally find it but it seems messy from the same.

Day 21
◆ This morning from 6:45 until about 7:30 a.m. I felt the cobweb sensation on left arm again.

Prover #8 • Male • 43 years old

Day 1
- A little down and irritable, which I'm sure is sleep and energy related. Feeling a little atrophic at work and that I'm not doing much that's creative or engaging.
- Despite sleeping in this morning, I've been very low on energy today. Especially noticeable without an afternoon coffee pick-me-up. Black tea jut doesn't do it.
- Woke up with the beginnings of rash around genitalia (moisture collected there last night). Treated with baby powder this morning. Don't think it's remedy-related. (Rash did not return.)
- Dream: A lot of little dreamlets, mostly horn-related (just returned from a week-long music festival in Coos Bay on Sunday), that were heavy and "thick" in nature. I'd wake up tired, feeling the need to roll over and re-collapse heavily into bed. In one dream, I remember showing my mouthpiece and another practicing device to friends of G.'s at some gathering. The last dream involved going down to University to fetch an old horn and bicycle of mine. It involved using some strange neighbor's phone to facilitate getting those things.

Day 2
- Still very sleepy today, despite the fact that this is the first time in about six months I've had two consecutive eight-hour nights of sleep. Still nodding off during class tonight, so I'm gonna try for a third straight early-to-bed evening.

Day 3
- Dose two.
- I skipped dinner after having just a little salad last night, and went to bed instead around 8:30 p.m. I tossed and turned for about two hours before finally nodding off, even after practically sleeping through evening meditation. The plus side is that I felt better and less bloated (better posture) during morning meditation. And it's my third consecutive eight-hour night of sleep—a new record.
- Dream: The dream I remember is the beginning of a meditation retreat. This one was being held in a theatre/arena-like church. And J was up at the pulpit leading everyone in the singing of a popular tune that everyone knew, except me.

Day 9
- Emotional upper.

Day 11
- Minor emotional downer.

Day 13
- 28-mile bicycle ride. Emotional upper.

Day 17
- Opera horn audition. Major emotional downer.

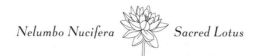

Prover #9 • Female • 47 years old

Day 1
- I definitely started having a reaction within about three hours.
- Mood not light, but rather heavy and full of anxiety. I'm having such an intense reaction to the remedy this soon, will it go away or will I be stuck with it for a long time? I did not impose this mood on anyone; it was strictly internal. Days after the fact, I recall that I expressed some self-deprecating remarks (more so than normal) during the voice workshop. It took me a really long time to relax, but I was very glad that we had that workshop because we did about an hour and a half of relaxation exercises, which was really helpful. I perspired very heavily during that workshop.
- The first thing that happened with me was getting a headache, which is typically what happens with me, that's my weak point. The headache was dull and thick, constant pain in the center of my forehead, with dull pain in the back of the head and a similar quality pain circling but not behind my eyes. This is very different from my normal headaches. And as the day progressed, pain settled in the upper right head and also slightly above both temples. It was a constant dull pain that made my head feel constricted and heavy and very large. Also had pain in neck (right side), as per usual when vertebrae are out and shoulder/neck muscles tight.
- The other thing that happened physically, right away I noticed that all of my energy went to the upper part of my body, from my chest and above (heart, throat, and head). My heart was pounding. Hard to relax. I had the headache. My throat got very dry, I had a lot of thirst for several days that I couldn't really quench. So that was very significant.
- General energy level low, at times agitated. This feeling only lifted when I did voice class workshop in the afternoon and spent a couple of hours doing relaxation exercises, after which I felt much lighter, happier, even liberated. But that feeling did not last long, and I sunk back into the agitated, unpleasant, uncomfortable state that predominated today.
- I had excess mucous in the mornings when I woke up, but then I would be dry later.
- Nose stuffy upon waking: left nostril more blocked than right, easily expelled mucous (as per normal). Eyes heavier than usual during day, part of the headache picture.
- By early evening throat was tight; it was a real effort to relax there and bring energy to areas below.
- Drank several glasses of water during the night, but not very much during the day. Appetite not very high.
- My appetite was different. I felt this for several days, I had very low appetite and contrary to usual, I wanted very bland foods. I didn't want sugar, salt, spice. I wanted very plain, bland foods. And I did have trouble digesting, and I had a lot of gas and bloating and loud belches and like that. So between the lack of hunger and being really thirsty and not being able to quench my thirst, it was an extremely disturbed digestive system.
- Solar plexus tight on waking.
- In the evening, partner discovered that my upper back (between and above the shoulder blades) was rough textured and red—some kind of rash.

◆ Dream: Slept a bit restlessly, getting up twice to pee. Slept mostly on right side, back, and front. (Night before, after taking remedy.) Woke from disturbing dream at about 4:45, went to bathroom, came back to write it down, and didn't go back to sleep again.
◆ Dream journal by bed: Dreams of proving. Sense of pressure and intensity. Activities surrounding spiritual teacher's birthday, but also specific to the proving. What do I feel? Agitation, some start of headache. Former boss and former job are mixed in here. I'm being asked to do something that takes a great deal of effort and I'm resistant but know I'll do my best anyway. It involves some notes and sketches scattered all over a page that I'm not ready to work from but am required to, even though I'm not ready. I'm trying to be very observant about what's going on in me, but I can't tell what's the proving, what's the birthday, what's something else. Pent-up hostility wants to unleash—I'm trying to stay cooperative though I don't feel like it at all. There are lots of people around, the environment is very disorganized.
◆ When I wake up I have a headache in the center of my forehead, pain around, but not behind, my eyes, my heart is beating strongly (pounding), I feel very agitated, perhaps slightly feverish. I recognize feelings of anger, hostility, aggression, defensiveness. There's a distinct tightness in my solar plexus, pressure on my bladder (even after I pee), and an overall agitation and anxiety. Fear and resentment of petty authority. All very pronounced. Did about 40 minutes of tension release, then got up to do hatha yoga before morning meditation.
◆ Took a half-hour nap at 6:15 p.m., which is very unusual.
◆ Skin tone looked somewhat flushed, pinker than normal across cheeks and chin, but in mid-day I checked and had no fever; in fact, temperature was 97.6. I was rather cold in the afternoon.
◆ Perspired heavily during voice class workshop (1:30–5:00), but that has happened in earlier classes too.
◆ The other thing that happened, starting from the first night and through the several days where my reactions were the most intense, was that I had to pee several times during the night—three or four times. Which is pretty unusual.

Day 2
◆ Agitated, very uncomfortable both mentally and physically. Everything felt like work. I asked proving physician at breakfast if I could purposely antidote the remedy if it gets too bad, and he said yes. But I want to stick it out a little longer if I possibly can.
◆ At Saturday Market (mid-afternoon) I had a very strong experience. The crowds and heat and sun were *awful*. Since I couldn't keep my energy low (it was all above the chest), and my head and upper body felt thick, dense, heavy, slow, it was a very bad combination. I almost felt like fainting, not from light-headedness, but because I was so max-ed out, needing *to get out of there*. It was all too much for me. I was extremely agitated and uncomfortable. I had to get out of the sun and every time I saw a patch of shade I darted for it.
◆ Energy levels generally low.
◆ During the night my headache got much worse—sharper pain on right side with a very slow throb, like a wave. I couldn't release in or around it. Finally took two Tylenol

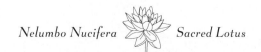

at about 3:30 a.m., which helped some but not entirely. (Usually I can't take Tylenol for a migraine.) I ended up taking Tylenol four times during the day. By evening the headache was concentrated in the front of the forehead and high in the temples. Sinuses were draining, and I was blowing my nose quite a bit. I put a cold washcloth on my forehead, which didn't exactly help, but the sense of quiet and containment was good.

◆ Eyes were hot when I woke up. Right nostril partially clogged when I woke up. I blew my nose—felt like the sinuses were swollen. Clear mucous (as usual).

◆ Throat felt dry and tight most of the day.

◆ The dominant sensation upon waking in the morning was *nausea*, which lasted quite a while. Very unusual for me, except during some migraines.

◆ I wanted to avoid anything complex, spicy, or difficult to digest. I wasn't all that hungry. Felt thirsty but couldn't quench my thirst. I wanted something very simple, so I got a raspberry seltzer, which I was not able to drink very quickly. The liquid did not feel as though it quenched my thirst at all. Dinner was a BBQ at a friend's house. I ate quite a bit, but wasn't exactly hungry and didn't feel like it went down all that well.

◆ Digestion not very good at all. Lots of gas and heavy, smelly burping at night.

◆ Did not have a bowel movement until mid-afternoon. Stool slightly hard.

◆ Went to bathroom about three times last night (more than normal).

◆ Again upon waking there was a sense of a pounding heart (though it was not racing) and tightness in the upper body (above the mid-chest), thickness and discomfort from there on up.

◆ Sleep/Dream: Couldn't read more than a page before turning out the light the night before—eyes hurt. Headache and needing to pee woke me up several times during the night. In one dream fragment I remember from the middle of the night, I'm on call in a store at the register. It's a very tiny, cramped space. There are workmen coming and going who buy coffee or snacks. I'm also trying to snatch a snack now and again. I can hardly remember any details of this dream, but there's a scene where I leave to walk or drive someplace and it's all World War II vehicles, but they're new. There's also a summer camp scene where I'm to work in the kitchen with a crew that includes two ashram women, and there are lesbian overtones but no overt sexual content to the dream. The headache persists throughout, making it difficult to remember what's going on, what's just happened, or to direct the dream at all. I'm cognizant, however, that I want to remember so as to record—but even when I wake up to pee it hurts so much I can barely look at the numbers on the clock. It's an extremely uncomfortable sleep. Some parts of the night I'm outside the covers. I try sleeping on my back, sides, stomach, but no relief from the pain.

◆ My mood was very heavy, full of anxiety, but it was strictly internal. I had excess mucous in the morning when I woke up, but then I was dry later. My throat was tight.

◆ The other thing was that, besides the physical and mental agitation, I noticed that I had a very self-deprecating attitude. I would have to say that's a previous symptom that came back pretty strongly during the days that all the physical symptoms were the most intense. And by day two, I had serious nausea, although I didn't throw up.

◆ My headache got worse during the night. By that evening, the headache was concentrated in the front of my forehead, high in the temples. My sinuses were draining. My eyes were very hot and achy. I had a pounding heart again. My eyes were very agitated. I couldn't read; my eyes wouldn't stay focused on the page.

Day 3
- Knocked out today by the headache; stayed home and did the bare minimum necessary.
- Partner wondered whether we might both actually have some sort of flu, because he also is not feeling up to par (burning and red eyes, low energy). But we are quite certain my symptoms are remedy related. I am wondering if some of my severe reactions today are due to dehydration. T. says, "Never again!" I do too.
- Low energy. Got up in the morning to give my car key to my sister-in-law (I ducked out of our plans to spend the day together); this took a lot of effort. Then spent most of the day lying on the couch, either watching TV or sleeping (had to sleep at two different points during the day, for about an hour each time). This is pretty much my nauseous headache routine. But I felt very restless and uncomfortable.
- During the night my headache shifted to the left side (exactly the opposite of the normal progression for my headaches). I took Tylenol twice during the day (ran out). As the day went on the headache settled in the center, high up in the forehead. Partner felt my head in the evening and said it was hotter than usual.
- When I got up during the night to go to the bathroom, my mouth was dry but I couldn't drink much water. During the day I made some bean soup and crackers (the only food that was in our cupboard), but I could hardly get any of it down. I was not able to drink more than a glass or so of water during the day. But T. gave me some watered down fruit juice and that was fine. After my yoga class I was able to eat.
- Went to the bathroom at least three times during the night.
- I felt rather weak.
- Shoulders and neck extremely tight (common with my headaches) for the whole day. Low back was okay, however (contrary to usual). After dinner, when watching TV with partner, I noticed a great degree of physical agitation in my legs.
- Dream: Woke at about 3:00 a.m. and had a visual memory of a dream fragment that was simply partner making a face of distaste (sticking out his tongue) and seeing it through the eyes of my niece as hideous. I also had an experience at about this time of some release in my chest that enabled me to bring my energy lower.
- Completely knocked out by the headache. Very low energy. My headache shifted to the left side. Usually, my headaches start on the left side. And I was still nauseous.
- In the evening, partner noticed that I had a rash on my upper back; the skin was all bumpy and red. I looked at it in the mirror. It wasn't itchy or anything. But that was just for a short while.
- Every night I had to get up a zillion times to pee. I had lots of dreams. All the dreams had similar sorts of themes to them. They were all ashram-related, they were always two or three people that I know featured in the dream as bit players. Physician is in this one. Dream: I'm very sleepy, all I can do is close my eyes and lean against something or lie down. I'm not exactly sick, but suddenly I'm in a hospital. There's me and one other new patient getting settled in my room. All the other patients are there for routine operations or birth; they're very chatty and bright. All I want is silence and

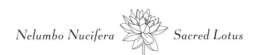

Nelumbo Nucifera   *Sacred Lotus*

rest, and I'm totally non-responsive and limp. I want to be moved to a quiet place, but even the doctor doesn't understand me. Finally, I'm walking down the corridor which turns into a road, and I'm walking back to the ashram, but now it's a compound with several buildings and I can't find where I'm supposed to stay. I do see a friend of mine, she's going someplace I can't get to. My physician is rushing off with someone else to a new building that's just opening, he's going to pick a nice room. I'm basically left on my own with no place to be and no energy to make a place for myself.

Day 4
- It felt as though the remedy basically worked itself out and my normal balance was restored by later in the day.
- General and gradual elevation of mood during the day, until I was really quite chipper by late afternoon.
- In the morning, even before leaving the house to collect keys, etc., from my brother, I had a strong desire to take a brisk walk in the cool shade (circumstances prevented this), as if to channel all that agitated energy into healthful movement.
- Through the day energy level gradually grew, until by the end of the afternoon I was quite perky and upbeat and ready for anything. Had a lot more energy functioning throughout my body, and felt like I was operating at about 95 percent capacity.
- Left-sided headache during the night; eyes were still a little sensitive and achy. During the day the headache gradually disappeared (by mid- to late-afternoon it was almost entirely gone).
- Jaw clamped during the night.
- During the night whenever I went to the bathroom I noted that I was thirsty, but I didn't really want to drink much. Ate nothing for breakfast and some sushi for lunch. By dinner I had a good appetite and ate with relish.
- During the morning I was offered a Triscuit, which I would normally love, but I found it totally unappealing and ate only one bite. By evening everything back to normal in terms of what I wanted and didn't want to eat.
- Got up several times (maybe four) during the night to urinate.
- During the night I couldn't relax my neck, shoulders, or jaw at all.
- Dream in early morning: There's a kind of reunion happening somewhere in Massachusetts that I've never been before—it's for friend's family, and also a bunch of former ashram people from long ago, and a bunch of Boulder guys who all have such a similar look and feel to them that it makes you wonder if people are attracted to different places based on qualities of personality, attitude, or behavior they share. (They're kind of "soft.") It was very obvious. I can't find partner when friend comes by, so I tell her to sit on the bed, and by the time I do find him, she's gone. She tells me that the next day is another reunion for current students that spiritual teacher is going to be at, but it's in a different place, and she quickly (too quickly) describes where it is and how to get there. So I become very worried about how to get there—who can I get a ride from. Meanwhile, preparations for the second party are underway and all the women it seems are busy with tasks related to it—decorations, plates, etc.—except for me. I offer to help but it's kind of too late, because it slows them down to have to spell it out to me. Eventually I'm

sitting outside with partner at a picnic table. In the distance, over woods, fields, and hills (with a slice of cityscape off to one side), is Mt. Hood and another mountain, both snow-capped. I see an airplane flying and as it gets closer I see it's not a small plane but a toy plane. I look for a boy but don't see anyone operating a remote. Women friends are going through a door and I call out in a panic to ask who's going that I can catch a ride with. Friend says she doesn't know but I can check with so-and-so, and then she's gone. I woke up from this dream sometime around 7:00 a.m. but didn't get out of bed for 20–30 minutes.

Day 5
- Feeling back to normal. Finally! Felt really good.
- Cheerful.
- Energy high.
- I didn't have to go to the bathroom last night.
- Dream: Guests to the ashram have some work to do, which I set up for them. There are several bizarre scenes—in all, I'm with others, doing the tasks but kind of as a warm-up. Once it's in the bay at a waterside restaurant where you can "swim" with leaping fish (porpoises?) to whom you're connected by a rope. You go way up in the air, and then splash into the water. Only one or two people in our party get to do this. Another scene has me walking through what seems to be a prison, though it's outdoors. There's a jungle path, but I'm the lone woman passing by lots of men, and I hope I'm safe. A third scene has me climbing balconies off a building, and somehow my spiritual teacher is connected, so maybe it's the ashram and this is a guest suite. In each scene I'm with a few others discussing the project (like at the restaurant we're not actually eating a meal), and there are other groups of people there too that have nothing to do with our mission. At the restaurant, for instance, we encounter two women who are wearing outlandish, seemingly tasteless clothes, but they are very critical of my too-plain and conservative look, and after some discussion I buy into the notion that their dress is probably better than mine for this experience. The prison scene has me wearing a very short dress that's some flowing, light, white fabric, and, while it's very comfortable, I'm concerned that it's too provocative.
- Basically, since day five, I've had a lot of energy, I've been very well-organized, very clear-headed. I still had a few symptoms that persisted, like the agitation in my eyes. And in the few days after I had my hair done, a lot of people complimented me on how good I looked, and I thought it was just from my hair, but I really was feeling good, and my skin tone always reflects my energy level, and my skin tone was really good. And by day six, partner and I were joking about maybe it was really the remedy that was making me look and feel so good. I was feeling like my body worked through all this stuff in a matter of days and I could really feel every stage of it happen. And then, afterwards, there actually was a qualitative shift in my energy level.

Day 6
- I was almost euphoric at moments during the day. My mind was moving rapidly.
- A woman came to where I was working at the end of the day to see S., and I recognized

her middle name as being the last name of a family that used to live in my neighborhood when I was an extremely young child. They moved away when I was five or six years old. And, indeed, this was a girl who was one of my friends up until the age of six. And I remembered her—she didn't remember me at all. But that makes sense because she's a year older than me, I was a little kid. I remembered her whole family except for her oldest brother; I remembered what her house looked like, I remembered the house they moved to two towns over, I remembered going to her birthday party the year after she moved and the music they played and the furniture, everything. I remembered what her father did for a living. I have pretty good long-term memory and not very good short-term memory. But this was unusually acute. I was more impressed by it than anyone else.

◆ Dream: Remembered in fragments only, here in random sequence: Spiritual teacher—weaving. Friend discovers a lovely embroidered and jeweled cloth hanging on the line. He realizes he's been using the loom incorrectly. He gives away so many things off a long shelf. Asks me to give people the record albums—I hesitate (So many! So generous! How to decide who gets what?) and in that moment people come and it's all gone, I won't even get one. We're in a boat reminiscing about the very earliest days. Friend, it's said, was born in Puerto Rico ... friend loaned spiritual teacher money for his first trip. Other friend has helped in some essential way.

We're in a very big dining room, like a cafeteria, in a corner from which I see only a tiny portion of the room. Friend is explaining a process for us to calculate how much garbage we've generated over the last year; as I'm finding a scale to weigh my sample bag, she's explaining something to a person who is friend's new girlfriend, something about his nature that indicates to me she still keeps an eagle eye on him—not that she still wants him, but it's just her way; she wants to be helpful but to me it reveals an unsuspected attachment.

Running through a huge lobby area, a dog comes to me happily (a small German Shepherd), then a slew of Rotweilers run to another door and administrator says, "Better get them out of there," (a huge audience is gathering and we don't want anyone to get hurt or freaked out). That's why I'm late when teacher is giving things away.

I feel closer to spiritual teacher, more of an "old-timer," but learning and not as quick to respond as those used to serving him. I'd like to demonstrate that I can be useful and helpful.

Day 7

◆ After dinner I was agitated and a little anxious about my workload.
◆ Had good energy today, but feel I'm over my head a little bit.
◆ Dream: I had a good sleep and woke up cheerful. Three dream fragments: 1. G. is driving N.'s car with a few of us in it. N. tries to make him do something illegal. G. doesn't want to do it. A cop catches us as we're entering the property and now we're in trouble, but because we convince the cop that G. is such a careful, good guy, they shouldn't give him the big fine but let him off with a warning. We're all in the dining room (which is outdoors, lined with picnic tables and benches). I'm explaining to the two cops why they should be lenient. We're overheard and the other ashram people spontaneously

start singing or applauding G. to show love and support. N is really pissy about it but we tease him lovingly. G.'s arrest is so remarkable that a local Massachusetts newspaper covers it; I see the article. 2. I'm back in a car, driving to a place I haven't been before, trying to go through (or get out of) a parking lot. The apparent exit from the lot is blocked and I have to go around again. I go through a narrow lane and finally get to the street, but it's very busy and I'm glad I'm only turning right and not crossing it or going left. 3. In another scene, I'm following directions to go someplace. I'm in a multilevel city setting. After I park I'm walking by a hotel and some stores looking for a certain elevator that will take me down to the exact spot I'm going. A classy storekeeper—woman—tries to help me and ends up accompanying me to the elevator, because nothing is at right angles or easy to follow with any certainty.

◆ I felt like I was starting to overextend myself or something, but I had so much vitality, and so much that I hadn't been able to do in the intense part of the reaction to the remedy, that now I was ready to do things. More dreams, lot of work; decided that I wasn't going to record my dreams anymore because they were getting to be variations on a theme.

Day 8

◆ I continue to get compliments about how good I look. People say it's the hairstyle, but I think I'm very healthy right now and brimming with energy, so that's really what it's about. Partner suggests in the evening that maybe it's really the remedy, and we both laugh at that one. What an irony that would be!

◆ Energy excellent.

◆ Dream: Retreat and its problems. 1. Double booked space for S. and my prenatal yoga class (finally resolved at the last minute). 2. Family friends, father and daughter visit and I didn't know it (I see them from above through a glass wall). 3. Partner wants to go to a movie the last night of the retreat. I wear a life jacket (thick foam vest) with nothing underneath; I'm self-conscious about exposing myself. We are on a very high shelf or loft. A security videocam finds us and I notice our faces are projected on the wall right next to us (but it's at a sharp angle so I don't see it until well along in the evening), plus it captures our voices, so everyone can tune in even though we thought we were pretty much isolated from everyone. I don't much like the movie, just did it for partner. Afterwards, the vehicle that was going to take us home (a bus?) breaks down in the middle of nowhere. Partner has his plane ticket to leave the next morning on his business trip and is able to somehow use it to get out. Couple are there and say they're renting a car to drive to Jupiter, Florida, the next day, and maybe they can rent it in this little town, but all the Avis agency has is a more expensive car, not the model they wanted. So logistics get sticky and we may have to stay overnight at a tacky hotel (which costs about the same as this car). I wake up before it's resolved, but am starting to be anxious about getting back by morning to resume my retreat duties.

Day 9

◆ Dream: Decided not to record my dream, though it was vivid, but they all seem to be following a pattern of characters and types of situations and moods and self-image.

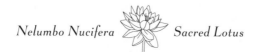

Day 10
- Good mood continues.
- I'm able to work hard and sustain my energy all day. I've noticed that I'm not taking naps any more—no mid-afternoon drop in energy.

Day 11
- A long day of work, but fun.

Day 12
- Had sex this evening, but I was very dry and the contact hurt. Decided to buy some KY for the future.

Day 14
- Energy strong, but taxed. For instance, when I came home (briefly, I expected) in the mid-morning to take care of some things, I ended up spending well over an hour taking care of lots of personal business—dog duty, arranging housing for the evening, making and getting a few phone calls, etc.—before rejoining them for a late breakfast.
- Menses: Heavy flow.

Prover #10 • Male • 40 years old

Day 1
- Dreams: 1. Being in a track meet of a few miles but not knowing the distance around the track; feeling is uncertainty and anxiety. 2. Being in a moving vehicle which is somehow defective, e.g., parts falling off, paint and siding peeling; same feeling of anxiety.

Day 2
- Hot and agitated all day at office.
- Tired and slept longer in morning than usual.

Day 4
- Awoke at 3:15 fearful and had to turn on lights and check closet; fearful about being attacked by monsters.
- At work felt very hot and agitated all day.
- Rearranged room completely—moved furniture and unsatisfied with present configuration.
- Energy low. I want out of this—don't want this to continue for three weeks.
- Direct sun during jog felt burning at 5:45 p.m.
- Dream: Woke at 3:15—very unusual—also that I woke in a hot sweat after dreaming that I had an argument with a girlfriend and was angry at myself in the dream, and threw dishware and glasses through windows, kicked things and shouted for her to go away, leave me in the unsafe place where we were, and that I wanted to be mugged,

robbed, and shot. Woke up and felt depressed and fearful. Felt like I did in childhood. Stayed up for one and one-half hours, ate potato chips and watched TV.

Day 5
- I feel like getting room configuration settled, buy new furniture and get rid of other.
- Last night slept badly—tossed and turned all night—woke up unrefreshed and don't really feel like going for a hike.
- Woke up with tight chest and difficulty taking deep breath.

Day 6
- Hot all day. Direct sun seems oppressive. Tired all day—didn't go hiking as I had planned because of bad night sleep.
- Slept three hours Sunday afternoon—unusual. Did not awaken but still feel tired. Woke with mild, center of head, headache.

Day 7
- Told by another that I felt hot—unsolicited stranger.
- Dream: About timber cutting and some distress.

Day 8
- Depressed because of slow business.
- Still hot all day; of course, the day was hot also.
- Still fitful (sleep) but did not wake up; still a little tired despite enough hours of sleep.
- Dream: Of working with others on a large structure like the bowels of a large steel ship; hot; fire; then notice that a submarine must burn off the paper stuck on its hull as it starts to submerge.

Day 12
- Dream: Living in large, complex, convoluted house with big alienating feeling. People traveling through the building to find people not found.

Day 13
- Energy level: Tired all day—low stamina and ran out of energy where my legs and breathing became very weak and shallow.

Day 15
- Heat dissipated.
- Trouble breathing—asthma felt during jogging.
- Dreams: Wandering around St. Andrews church (mythical). Walking on cliffs high above church and gardens; falling off cliffs while yelling to friends on church grounds.

Day 16
- Fear.
- Aggravation of asthma.

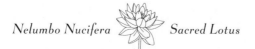

Nelumbo Nucifera   *Sacred Lotus*

- Mental confusion.
- Extreme anger.
- Depression.
- Wanting to die, but not exactly.
- Suicidal—wanting to be killed.
- Pissed off at people who do injustice to me.
- Hot and sweaty.
- Tired because sleep is very disturbed.
- Bad dreams.
- Really, really agitated.
- Anxiety.
- Reversion to feelings when I was committed.
- Took naps during the day on day two and three, which was unusual.
- Client lying to me—so angry and obsessed with company and withholding dollars incident that I haven't been able to do anything else at work for last two weeks.
- Contraction.
- Coinciding events—two mothers going insane in the world, loss of money, loss of control
- Dream of fighting and cutting foot.
- Resistance to writing in this journal.
- Reversion to feelings of involuntary commitment.
- Anxiety.
- Business—deception and technical bad debtor incident.
- Feeling better during this meeting—able to let go of the feelings.

Day 18
- Jogging was labored and felt extreme weakness and hard breathing during exercise—even with medicine.
- The hallmark of my experience during the last couple of weeks is extreme anger, depression, wanting to die but not suicidal, it's just that I want somebody to kill me. I've been very pissed off at people who I've seen, who I've felt, and either subjectively or objectively have done something unjust to me. I've been very hot and very, very sweaty, perspiring a lot. I've been extremely tired, had a lot of difficulty sleeping. I've only taken one dose of the remedy, and I think it pretty much dissipated after about two weeks, about fourteen days. Well, with the possible exception of earlier.
- I've had very disturbing dreams, ones that have made me wake in the middle of the night unable to sleep again, extremely agitated, and fearful enough that I've had difficulty going to sleep for the rest of the evening. All this is really unusual for me because I'm usually not like that. And I've recognized at the time that these are all unusual, and sooner or later the realization has been that it's probably the proving and nothing else other than that, but it's been disturbing. I've had a lot of aggravation of my asthma. I've had difficulty exercising and running, which is what I like to do.

Prover #11 • Female • 40 years old

Day 1
- Feeling down—pre-period? Longing to get back into my room.
- Eyes and lips felt very dry this morning.
- Very slight soreness in throat from dryness in morning, 10:00 a.m. Uvula stingy as if postnasal drip in afternoon. Called a candidate for a job at my office and throat got all tight as I talked to him.
- Rich mayonnaise sauce on crab sandwich was unappealing at lunch. Skipped dinner—felt fat, no appetite.
- Bump on outer knuckle of index finger of right hand.
- I had a lot of vivid dreams the first night. This was weird, I don't think I've ever had a dream like this. I dreamt that I was cleaning a kitchen and I had this big, huge sheet pan in front of me that had a flat cake on it, and at one end there were these trees with leaves falling off. I pulled a very regular diagonal strip of the cake off and then these black women came and danced along the strip. It was very festive and celebratory.

Day 2
- Ear pain, right ear at 9:30 a.m. Sore on inside right cheek.
- Sharp pain on inner bone of right wrist—odd.
- Woke at 4:00 a.m. to pee.
- Dream: I had three dreams that were more like the dreams that I had during the whole rest of it. I was demanding to be tattooed across the bridge of my nose with something that said: "LJ did this." And it was to show that I had been tortured and this woman was trying to knock me out so that I could take the tattoo. But she failed, she was unable to do that. And then somebody came along and said I didn't need to be knocked out. 2. Another dream was that they built an addition to the ashram right outside my window and blocked all the light out. 3. All the ashramians were sitting around in this big stadium and J. and M.'s baby burped (J. and M. do not have a baby). Somebody said, "Guess who," and then everybody laughed.

Day 3
- Dose two.
- Feeling depressed.
- Eyes felt dry upon rising.
- Lots of tightness in throat when I interviewed a job candidate today.
- Feeling restless about food. Nothing is satisfying.
- Menses: Late.
- Felt stiff upon rising.

Day 4
- Feeling out of sorts this morning, cranky. Felt much better in afternoon.
- Break in gum in right lower jaw.
- Back of mouth still stingy/scratchy in morning—throughout day.

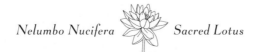

Nelumbo Nucifera   Sacred Lotus

◆ Dream: Reconciliation of a family where the father had been a drunk. The dream started with a fight, but then the brother in the dream called the mother back at some point and that led to the reconciliation, kind of broke everything. It was a good feeling in that dream.

Day 5
◆ Dried out feeling in eyes (morning on rising). Very short pain in left ear. It went away.
◆ Uvula still stingy—as if I'm about to get sick (morning on rising).
◆ I seem to be eating a lot whether I'm hungry or not. Want sweets.
◆ Menses: Still no period.
◆ Dream: Teaching singing to a tall man. Same scene as in a previous dream.

Day 6
◆ Dose three.
◆ A little anxious—around work issues.
◆ Stingy feeling in uvula gone.
◆ Wanted to eat a lot. Minor stomach upset late afternoon, 5:00 p.m. It passed quickly.
◆ Dream: Picked off a scab created by a cold sore. It was huge. I waved it around.
◆ Dream: A long hose (I watered yesterday).

Day 7
◆ Feeling low all day—craving personal attention, not doing anything about it.
◆ Nap in early afternoon.
◆ Ear ticking. Headache today—dehydration?—built slowly from base of neck to entire head, behind eyes.
◆ No period yet.
◆ Dream: Picking cherries and then sorting them on a big sheet pan—we were looking for poisonous ones—the stuff on the sheet pan looked more like tomato sauce than cherries. A long party. Another scene with a beautiful gray cat.

Day 8
◆ Steady.
◆ Nose, especially on right side, is congested.
◆ Lots of dizziness over the past few days when I move from sitting to standing position.
◆ Dream: I can't make any sense of them, so it couldn't have been a very vivid dream: complex; take apart site; Japanese meal at a conference; beautiful hike; play piano.

Day 9
◆ Felt slightly guilty for not working hard at work.
◆ Dream: About menopause.

Day 10
◆ Throat scratchy in the morning.
◆ Woke once in night to pee.
◆ Dream: Lots of bugs crawling all over me. Tiny, tiny ones on my hand. I was told they

would disappear in an hour. They did. The dream was repeated. Fascination; minor revulsion.

Day 11
◆ Breasts are tender last several days.
◆ I've been wanting cooler showers recently. Maybe it's just the heat.

Day 12
◆ Tired in late afternoon because I haven't been getting enough sleep.
◆ Breasts very tender the last several days.
◆ Dream: Peeling of a thick layer of skin from lower legs in long, thin strips. Not particularly painful.
◆ Dream: Attended wedding of a friend whom I haven't seen in well over ten years.

Day 13
◆ Lips are dry—I'm picking at them again.
◆ Scratchy, stingy throat again.
◆ Breasts are very tender.
◆ Woke many times during night: 12:10, 12:30, 1:00, 4:17.

Day 14
◆ A lot of congestion in the morning.
◆ All my joints felt achy this morning.
◆ Woke up in the middle of the night thinking about work.
◆ There were four of us that went out to Larch Mountain to see the Perseid meteor shower. I had this little flashlight, and it reminded me of the story of the last time I got high, which was a long time ago, and I told the story. It's happened in the past that I've told the story and it's almost as if everybody gets high, and that's exactly what happened. All four of us got totally giddy. I don't tell that story very often, but it had the same effect that it always does.

Day 15
◆ Head felt very congested in p.m.
◆ Slept for four hours in afternoon—but this was after staying out 'til midnight to watch the Perseids and then getting up at 6:00 a.m. to go do a 30-mile bike ride, and then going to a brunch and drinking a mimosa.

Day 16
◆ Feeling pissy—wanting to hide behind doing routinized things, then feeling benumbed and angry about having to do routine things at work. Want to crawl in bed and hide/sleep. Feeling depressed, lonely, out of it.
◆ On Saturday I bought a sports bra for the first time ever because of the bike ride I did on Sunday and the tenderness in my breasts. I wore it to work on Monday—Thursday of this week, with a T-shirt over it. But on the way home I just wore the sports bra.

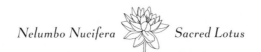

Loved the sun on my back. This felt daring and a bit out of character for me.
- Throat very scratchy/stingy upon arising.
- I crave crunchy.
- Dream: Family adventure, cars, trying to get out of prison, don't know where daughter/I am. Try to escape via top floor of factory-like building. The whole crew of "police" are an assortment of people who swarm toward us from outside the building. I thought they were the police, but in fact it was just this assortment of different people, different ages and everything like that. Scary. This woke me at 2:08.
- Dream: A boat ends up upside-down in the water—we have to right it.
- Dream: I'm driving really fast along a curvy road. My car goes out of control, but I manage to keep it upright and not to crash. No one can believe the car ended up where it did. It seems impossible. Then a tow truck gets the car out easily. A lot of danger inherent in those dreams, and fear.

Day 17
- Feeling quite judgmental about myself and others. The first thought that enters my head when I see someone is some picky thing I don't like about them.
- Breasts are a lot less tender; still no period.
- Dream: I went to a personal shopper. She dressed me in a wizard outfit with a train that you could hitch up and tie around your waist. In real life I am going to a personal shopper tomorrow for the first time ever.

Day 18
- Bit of crampy feeling in the morning, breast tenderness gone. My period came today. I've had regular periods all my life, and in the past six months I've missed two. And so I'm wondering if maybe I'm starting menopause even though it's early, but my mother's menopause was also very early.

Day 19
- Woke up at 4:40 a.m. Couldn't get back to sleep. Energy quite good all day.

Day 20
- Scratchy/stingy throat in the morning.
- Dream: I was traveling with my mother. We had to wait inordinately long to check out of a hotel. She waited in line while I packed her things, which included a number of small figurines and ceramic pots in addition to usual clothes, etc. Made me sad that she had to bring so many "reminders" of her life with her.
- Itchy skin on my fingers last couple of days.
- The major physical symptom I had, and it was very consistent, was that my uvula was very stingy and scratchy. And I had a few throat things, and also had dry eyes.

Prover #12 • Female • 22 years old

Day 1
- Jealous to the point of tears for no good reason.
- The major things I noticed after I took the remedy are that I got really jealous for no reason. I'm not normally a jealous person. I can get a little bit jealous, but mostly I just get a little bit sad about it. But this was like I totally got upset, I would get into tears—and then I'd get even more upset because I realized I was being stupid about it.
- I was totally moody and emotional. I can be moody, but not in as great fluctuations as I have been. I'll be totally happy and bouncing off the walls and then five minutes later I'll be in tears that the smallest thing would just trigger.
- I don't know if that's just stress about leaving or if it was the remedy, but for the whole time I was taking it I was a wreck. Then I'd get even more upset because I thought it was the remedy.
- I was totally crazed because I knew that when I left I needed to be really centered and focused, and so then I was upset that I was totally off balance emotionally. I felt like I had all the same emotions that I had when I was 16, just completely felt terrible about myself, totally. I totally felt like a Natrum muriaticum again. I didn't like being in my own skin, that kind of thing. I've been trying to exercise more and more to get rid of that feeling.

Day 2
- Dream: One of the first dreams I had was that L and I were arguing about who takes better care of my grandparents. She told me that they said they'd rather have her take them to the airport than me. And I was really upset about it. She was getting ready to go and I was pleading with her and crying, "No, please, don't do this." You know. Totally weird. I was totally upset. I was crying, pleading with her—I wasn't mad, I was more like really sad and hysterical that she was taking that position. But I don't normally feel like that for her, you know.
- Dream: I think that I may have had a dream about the morning I went jogging in Glasgow because when I woke up I kept thinking about it. I hadn't thought about it since I did it because I didn't particularly like that city. Plus, I got lost that morning, so it wasn't as enjoyable as jogs I had in other cities on the trip.
- Moody and emotional today. One minute sad and the next minute bouncing off the walls. I have so much anxiety and excitement about moving to Mexico that my emotions are a roller coaster.
- My whole body was sore today from new exercises I did two nights before.
- Sweaty armpits in the air-conditioned office, but didn't feel hot. Started late afternoon and stopped around 7 p.m.
- Difficulty with morning movement (stool).
- Bloated in the late morning. Decreased appetite. Eyes bigger than desire to eat.

Day 3
- Still moody and easily brought to tears.

♦ Dream: There was an earthquake late at night while I was out somewhere with my friends, and then when I came in the house—the house was a little bit different, but when I came in, everybody was downstairs congregating about it, and my spiritual teacher was down there and he flipped out. He said he was so worried about me because he couldn't find me and he was really upset with me that I was out and didn't tell anybody.

Day 6
♦ Still easily tearful. Tolerance level is very low. Things are really getting to me.
♦ I was a total slug today. I had enough sleep, but still was very tired all day.
♦ Didn't have a movement in the morning (stool).
♦ Had a treatment today and it made me feel even more sluggish. It also aggravated the tension in my neck. So I had a headache the rest of the day. I felt really anti-social today. I really didn't want to talk to anybody. It was a major effort to even smile.

Day 7
♦ Going on at least eight days straight of crying at least once per day. I know it's not menstrual because my cycle ended two weeks ago. Even if it were, I've never been so emotional for no good reason.
♦ Only an afternoon movement again (stool).
♦ I felt rested today. Overall, I felt much better than I did yesterday.
♦ Dream: I was recently in a wedding for one of my friends. And afterward I was really sad about it because I knew that I wouldn't see my friends for a while after that. I had a dream that I was in the wedding again, but it was really like a gothic wedding and somewhere during the ceremony, this hole opened up in the ground, and I just fell into empty space. And that was kind of weird. I felt totally helpless, it was just like this vacuum, it was totally white, there were tracers of speed. That was the only light that was in there. And there was nothing to grab onto. I don't know, it just felt totally out of control, but I know that there was some kind of monster thing happening, like chasing and stuff like that. That was a really freaky dream.
♦ Usually when I do cry, it's for a reason, something motivates me. And for the past two weeks, when I cry, it's triggered by something totally without merit. Like one morning, I was five minutes late to work, and my dad got this really intense look and said, please try to be on time, if you worked for anybody else you would be reprimanded. And I just turned around and started bawling and went to the bathroom. And it wasn't even bad, that was mellow for him. And usually I just shrug it off. Something little would happen and it would just set me off. But then like yesterday when something major would happen, I'd be fine through it, but then maybe later something little would set me off.
♦ Yesterday I got lost for an hour and a half. And usually that would flip me out, I'd get really tense and totally upset that I was lost. And I was totally cool through the whole thing. And then when I got home, an hour later, I can't even remember what happened, I think I talked to somebody on the phone, a totally normal conversation, and then I sat there for 20 minutes just staring at the wall and I started bawling. So I don't know if maybe I've had like a lag time on my stress or what.
♦ Vaguely I can think of having a conversation with somebody, but I didn't like the

conversation, and I was fine through it. I usually have a hard time not showing that I'm upset. My dad was giving me a lecture about going to Mexico and what I should do and, I'm 22 years old, why is he telling me this. And then I think like two hours later I just started bawling about it. Why doesn't he trust me or why doesn't he have faith in me. And then the whole conversation just made me more nervous about the trip, because then I realized that all of my fears about holding his business relationships basically in my hands, it was more crucial, and before I had only realized it myself. I can be moody but not that drastically, you know, like it will be day to day, not five different moods within one day.

◆ I've been totally agitated when people ask me about my trip because I don't want to talk about it, because I love it here. I just moved home, now I have to leave again. And I exercised late at night because I was agitated, and I thought that would make me feel better. Then when I got into the kitchen, a friend asked me when I was leaving, and I said, "Wednesday," not mean, but just empty, not with a smile or anything. "Are you in a bad mood?" And I was, well, you know, I'm a little bit flipped out because I'm leaving. And she starts telling me all this stuff about why are you upset? You know, you're going to a different country, why are you upset? I just looked at her like, okay, I guess there's no reason for me to be upset, and that just made me more agitated. And she goes, "When's your birthday?" And I said, "It's in December." She goes, "Because I've noticed you're so moody and emotional." It was all I could do to not turn around and whack her. I was so mad. I really had to get out of there. This is mad like wanting to hit somebody, crying. Because it felt so condescending. And of course I am happy, but I'm still scared about going too, and I said to her, "You know, I think moving to a different country is always a frightening experience, don't you think?" To have somebody bring to my attention that I had been emotional and moody upset me even more. She's lucky I have self-control, I'm telling you, because my tongue could have lashed out at her so bad.

Prover #13 • Male • 41 years old

Day 1
◆ Dose two.
◆ When I took the remedy, I did have some topical itchiness on my upper back, that evening and the next morning. It's summer and I'm working outside, so I'm drinking a lot, but the next day I felt quite bloated as a result of that. That was more so than usual.
◆ Strange fighting dream—friends and I arming with guns for a conflict. Shots fired through doors. It was nervous excitement. We were gearing up and it was basically a work project but this time with ammo. Yeah, we were going to kick some butt. Vivid dream of architecture—houses. Carpentry, too. Awoke with brief headache, gone after I got up.
◆ As soon as I took the remedy last night my back started itching—all over my back. Tonight at about 8:00 p.m., same again.

Day 2
- Dose three.
- Back to work, still aggravating, but mood surprisingly good. Notice an occasional giggle, not characteristic.
- Bloated feeling after drinking water, more so than usual.

Day 3
- Sore right foot—muscle sore. Also left forearm same. Evening, forearm worse. Occasional soreness in knees but brief. Fleeting aches in inner thighs—deepish—muscular. Not on skin.
- Not much sleep last night—I stayed up 'til 1:00, so afternoon nap then uncharacteristic cup of tea. Don't recall dreams.

Day 4
- Left forearm still sore, pang in inner thigh. A very normal day except for the forearm.

Day 5
- Dose four.
- Enervated all day.

Day 6
- Dream: Wedding.

Day 7
- Elbow better with aspirin during the day.
- Renovation dream, combo of work and home situation, the usual.

Day 8
- Dose five.

Day 9
- Tired today. Nothing unusual however.
- Dream: Dreams about hiking.

Day 10
- No symptoms except sore elbows/forearms—better with aspirin or ibuprofen.

Day 11
- Only thing today was a jittery dizziness as I was squatting to finish some concrete—perhaps it was the fluorescent lights. It didn't last long, nor was it pronounced.

Day 12
- Dose six.
- Relatively fitful sleep last night. Woke a few times, up at 4:00 a.m.

Day 14
- Sore forearms as usual.

Day 15
- Snot in right side of head. Congestion.

Day 16
- Still congested—yellow mucous like after a cold in a.m.
- My forearms getting a bit less sore. Better with ibuprofen or aspirin.

Day 18
- Morning mucous—right nasal again.
- Dream: Dreamt about a snake last night.

Day 19
- Lost temper at work today. Generally aggravated by circumstances at work. No more Mr. Nice Guy.

Review:
- Itchy back.
- Soreness.
- Mucous.
- I also experienced some in my right foot and some fleeting aches in my inner thighs. Those were deepish and muscular, not on the skin. But that went away very quickly. I've got this forearm thing that feels almost like tendonitis, which I've had once, and that's the only thing I can compare it to. And that persisted, however it was better with aspirin and/or ibuprofen.
- Just one time I had a jittery dizziness. I did acid twice in college, I was kind of a nerd, but it was a bit of a flashback of that. It could have been hypoglycemia, but I was squatting, finishing some concrete and there were also fluorescent lights, so who knows. But I did have a jittery, trippy feeling at one point. But that was very brief and during the day, and not anytime near a dose, really.

Prover #14 • Female • 35 years old

Day 1
- Dose one.
- I took the remedy on Saturday morning at 6:12 a.m., right before I went into meditation. And as I sat there, I felt like I was floating, like I was a balloon. I definitely was feeling elated. As I was eating my breakfast, I felt stoned, I was laughing with people, I was giggling. And later on that morning I was studying and I had a really, really hard time concentrating. It reminded me of smoking pot, which I did for many years. I would be with drool hanging out the side of my mouth, not focusing on anything. And I had to prepare for my second-year board exams. I thought, I really can't just let myself space out like this, I have to really work to concentrate. I had to keep reeling myself back in. My attention would go off and I'd stare out the window and I'd look at the trees and I'd start seeing the branches moving and I'd be kind of like moving with the branches, and then I'd go, okay, wait a minute, come back to what you're studying. So it was like an extreme dissipation of my attention.
- Drank three cups herbal tea and now water, and it's only 10:15 a.m. Usually not thirsty in the morning. Throughout the proving period, I was extremely thirsty and dry.
- After eating tuna salad, green salad, and coleslaw for lunch, I had minor abdominal cramping and throbbing lumbar spasms. Fifteen minutes later only back spasm remain, about a five intensity on one to ten scale. Lasted one-half hour. Breakfast digested well.
- I noticed that my feet were freezing cold, like ice cubes, even though the room was warm and the rest of me was warm. And while my feet do tend to get cold in the cold weather, they don't when it's warm out.

Day 2
- Eyes (margins) very dry while sitting outside.
- Digestion seems okay except constipation. Lots of small stools that hurt when they come out. This is not new but is worse than usual.
- Woke on my right side with left nostril completely blocked up.
- Dream: Dreaming about an outdoor party and I'm asking T. if she'd like me to help with the cooking. Woke to my dream and I feel pretty refreshed—unusual because I normally wake very slowly and feel depleted when waking. Took nap from 5:30–6:15, < after nap, groggy, tired, etc. Also left nostril stopped up again; slept on stomach with right knee bent, head turned to the right.

Day 3
- I seemed hyper-reactive to comments today. I was more outwardly expressive, whereas usually I feel it but don't express anger and frustration. Also in one case took it very personally when the comments <u>may</u> not have been intended that way. Overall, I felt a little depressed today. Wouldn't you, if many old symptoms reappeared, ones recent and long ago?!
- I had the sensation that all the work that I'd been doing with remedies and Chinese medicine most recently was all coming undone, i.e., face breaking out, bloating and

poor digestion, vaginitis, etc. I really despaired about this, because I thought, well, I didn't really think this would happen with the remedy and there had been a lot of different things I was working to resolve that I really felt like were just coming right back to me. They came back to the nth degree. Worse than they had been previously. Or at least it seemed that way.

♦ Hair is much oilier than usual. Someone told me today that I didn't look like myself. I looked in the mirror and indeed I looked strange but couldn't really describe how.

♦ Thirst is unquenchable. Abdomen is more bloated, rigid, and constipated than I've seen in a long time. After eating lunch, both stomach and abdomen bloated. Difficult exhalation. Basically, many old symptoms that existed in the past have come back strongly. After eating, sighing, spaced out, difficulty with exhalation, tension in solar plexus.

♦ All mucous membranes are very dry, extremely dry, like I'd been in the desert. My eyes are dry and I'm thirsty. Again, I don't normally have a lot of thirst. Especially noticed vaginal dryness. Face is breaking out with pimples again.

♦ The third day is when things started to go downhill. This morning and on several other mornings, I would get up, I'd go to meditation, I'd go back to my room, and I was completely knocked out. I had to lie down and sleep for between a half hour to an hour and a half. I couldn't get up and do anything else. And every time I tried to wake myself up, I felt like someone was throwing me back down into my bed. I just didn't have the energy to even sit up. And this would go on, every ten minutes or so I'd try to get up, but I just couldn't get up.

♦ Also on the third day I started to get really reactive to everything, like hyper-reactive. I was outwardly expressive, whereas normally I'll feel it but I don't express it always. I just couldn't help myself, I couldn't hold back. And I remember there was some interaction with a group of people and some conversation going on, and I took it personally. Later on I thought, well, maybe that wasn't really something I should take personally, but I sort of held onto it for a few days, like it was eating away at me, even though I wasn't sure if it was something I should have taken personally. Like I thought it was some criticism of me even though it may not have had anything to do with me.

♦ The anxiety that I was feeling was always worse after I ate, and I had this kind of full, bloated feeling and a compressed feeling in my chest. Difficulty exhaling. Feeling a lot of tension in my solar plexus.

Day 4

♦ Woke from nap after breakfast sobbing. I'm crying, depressed, hopeless, suicidal. I can't concentrate while studying. I'm trying to study for my board exams and I'm going through this. Struggled all morning to focus enough so I could study. Was re-reading every sentence eight to ten times. I felt like I couldn't absorb what it was I was trying to take in. Afternoon—slightly depressed (after exercise) until meditation class. Shifted to being much lighter and higher, again, S. suggested I "carry on" with the proving.

♦ Exercised for one and one-half hours, aerobic including weights. Feel more stable emotionally after that. I studied while exercising. Sometimes it's easier to study in motion. I usually don't have the energy to work out this long!

♦ After breakfast I have maxillary, nasal, and frontal achiness, particularly on the left side.

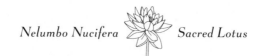

◆ Food craving: Ice cream sundae with hot fudge and lots of whipped cream (didn't have). Hungry for frequent, small meals. Hungry for fruit, like berries, peaches, bananas, etc.

Day 5
◆ Depressed; after exercise for 45 minutes, better. I began to feel anxious about exams also, at the same time as the depression—both got better after exercise.
◆ Mind much clearer, quieter later in the day. Meditation was balloon-like this evening.
◆ Craving at 11:30 a.m. for thick, rare steak with baked potato, butter and sour cream. Appetite all day is vigorous—I FEEL HUNGER!
◆ Dream: I'm in Chinese medical clinic, reading T.'s tongue and taking her pulse. She had her mouth open and her tongue stuck out, and I was taking her pulse and I was discussing the signs, the things I was observing with someone else that was there.
◆ During meditation I had the sensation of being elated and floating.

Day 6
◆ Today I had the distinct experience like I was fourteen all over again; my first memory of being a teenager whose hormones were beginning to f—k up my body and emotions. It was almost like this moment of realization when you're a teenager of holy shit, I can't believe this, no one told me it was going to be like this! Your hormones are changing. You can just feel all that chemistry going on in your body. I felt, on the one hand, completely belligerent, anticipating conversations with people who'd pissed me off, imagining the entire argument. I was defensive and bitchy as I argued in my mind. On the other hand, I had this overwhelming sense of the harshness, the brutality of life, the utter hopelessness of living, of becoming an adult, and it depressed me entirely. It was the feeling of what pain was to come for the next ten years.
◆ Also this morning I ate something small that made my stomach bloat, and instead of stopping eating, I continued to eat a whole bowl of rice, vegetables, etc. until my abdomen was completely distended and uncomfortable. I was thinking, "I'll just throw it up." When I was fifteen I became bulimic, and continued to do the binge/purge thing until I left for college, age 18. So this morning after eating this food that made me *very* uncomfortable, I went to the bathroom and started to get ready to vomit. I cleaned the toilet, washed my hands, and pulled my hair back. Then I looked in the mirror and said, "This is going a bit too far, I don't think I really want to do this." So I didn't. I went back to my room and began studying again. That was the closest I've come to vomiting because I had eaten too much in many years. I think when I was on the Tuberculinum I did it once.
◆ I had a real aversion, a dread of working today when I went to my job in the kitchen. Sometimes I feel resistance to working or studying or whatever it is I need to do, but I kind of work through it and I generally feel better from exerting myself in some way. And this day, it was just unbearable. I felt lazy and I didn't want to have to put the effort into it. And I was finding ways to avoid doing the work in a sneaky kind of way.
◆ 9:00–10:00 a.m. is the worst time of day—when I'm having the most acute "whatever."
◆ I feel very averse to consolation—and usually I like to be comforted.

- Went out for a hot fudge sundae with P. and C. tonight. I had mint ice cream, hot fudge, whipped cream—YUM! It has been a long, <u>long</u> time. After eating the ice cream my stomach was fine, in fact better than when I ate fruit etc. this morning.
- Burning during urination. Return of old symptom.
- Dream: About studying for board exams (muscle types: slow glycolytic vs. fast oxidative).

Day 7

- This work is f—-ing difficult. No wonder not many people can maintain it. Boy is it worth it though. To think of where I'd be without this practice (meditation).
- Much more stable today than any other in last week.
- Sleepy <u>all</u> morning, napped from 1:00-2:30. Every time I tried to wake, I felt drugged.
- Completely bloated abdomen, about three inches wider than usual, even before eating breakfast. I'm doing a castor oil pack to see if it can get things moving.
- Very dry vagina, difficulty having intercourse—I've never had this problem before.
- While I was sitting in meditation, I had a sort of collective flashback of art school. I never had a lot of confidence in my work and I always took things that people said very strongly. And a lot of times people just could see that I was vulnerable and they would say something nasty because they got a kick out of it. And I remember times when teachers would make really cutting comments in front of other students, or friends of mine had made comments that really hurt, it was like they all came back to me in that moment, all those comments at the same time, of the most stabbing criticisms and the harshest, cruelest comments, mostly from men. Everyone had something completely nasty to say, even friends of mine who were artists. And I wrote down, I feel all of those comments like a big, heavy, stinking layer of shit flaking off of me. I felt the accumulation of hurt and rejection and pain of those many experiences. And after I had the sensation of this caked layer flaking off of me, I had the sensation that I was being scrubbed with this bristly brush until I was shining, like I had this metallic skeleton that was completely cleaned. It was a positive feeling, like this gunk had fallen away.

Day 8

- This will be the last remedy proving for me for many years. Interesting, but not worth f—-ing myself up for. I'm planning to have coffee today. D. says it usually doesn't help reduce symptoms but I don't care any more. I feel most of this experience has been as a result of the retreat, stirring many layers up. The remedy may have pulled certain flavors to the forefront. I really feel stupid for having done this proving while being under so much academic stress. I talk myself into thinking I'm superwoman, that I can do anything and everything. That's why I need <u>NUX</u>!!
- C. and I had a good talk about how we communicate. I was able to tell him some things about his behavior that I haven't wanted to deal with so far. His need for attention, what it's like to study with him, etc. It had the result of us being less reactive and emotional and even simplifying our interactions. Finally. He recently took his first constitutional remedy.
- I feel like there's an hourglass spilling sand and it's running low now. Not much time. Racing to cover material I haven't yet.

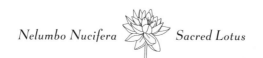

Nelumbo Nucifera   *Sacred Lotus*

◆ I had the experience of quieting my mind in a way that I haven't before. In meditation class I was pissed off at someone who has "creative kriyas" endlessly through entire class. I couldn't stop reacting to her ridiculousness. Finally I began to feel the teacher's quiet penetrate through my agitation. It was remarkable, as I realized what being one-pointed means. Being one-pointedly quiet and completely calm.
◆ Depressed and fed up with how much I have to try to remember for five 50-question exams. Anxiety and fear of forgetting all. This is a return of old symptoms but not really as bad as in the past. <u>Intensely</u> painful meditation.
◆ "Exercised" for an hour. Very fatigued physically tonight, but in a good way. Not exhausted but just tired.
◆ I'm eating like a freakin' pig. I think I've gained weight. I have no will power at all.
◆ Still dry and thirsty; also my eyes were so dry in meditation class I could hardly keep them open. Constantly blinking.
◆ I seem to be constipated every other day, then okay every other day.
◆ Felt a weight on my chest as I watched television after dinner cleanup tonight. I couldn't take full breaths—like my ribs wouldn't expand.
◆ Spasms in back, neck; ribs are out; pain. My neck is out of alignment again, probably from violent kriyas during meditation. My hamstrings are so tight they hurt. It hurt to get out of bed this morning (again, same but <). Ribs are out also.
◆ Dream: More studying dreams. After lunch I passed out for one-half hour and dreamt of the beach, and of a wave coming over me, like I was going to drown under it. I was slightly afraid.
◆ Skin has been itchy; bottoms of feet, legs, arms, face, back, etc.
◆ The next day I had two decaf coffees hoping that I would antidote the remedy, and it didn't make a bit of difference. The eighth day was a work project day, so everyone's out in the sun, gardening and doing other stuff, and I was sitting inside studying, and it was driving me nuts. And I just had to get away from the house and all of the energy that was here, I had to go away somewhere and escape from what I had to do. I don't often have that feeling.

Day 9
◆ Exercised for an hour; in general my exercise stamina is better on this remedy—I don't get exhausted during exercise.
◆ Constantly eating, still, no will power at all.
◆ Back very painful and stiff this morning. Fifty minutes of hatha helped—best hatha practice in months. Very slow and quiet and gentle.
◆ I've bitten all my nails down to the quick, return of symptoms, pre-Nux, while studying.

Day 10
◆ Feels like the remedy is really wearing off now. Can't come up with interesting symptoms.
◆ Aversions, food: Cakey, doughy, yeasty, carbohydrates, especially refined; greasy, heavy.
◆ Desires, food: Sweet and crunchy, i.e., chocolate, well-baked cookies.
◆ Dream: More study dreams.
◆ Skin: Mucous membranes and skin very dry.

Day 11
- Last night I was crying and feeling completely agonized about just having a body. All the things that you have to do to take care of your body, you have to clean it, you have to exercise, you have to put clothes on, etc. Feeling so earthbound in this dense thing that gets so much attention. Resentful that I had to give so much attention to something that was so mundane. I started to think of ways of killing myself. I thought of using a gun, but that would be too messy and disgusting. I thought of drowning myself, but I knew that I'd probably struggle and that would be bad. Then I thought that it would be really cool if I could jump into a volcano. But the best idea I had was to jump off a tall building, because as I was thinking about it, I really liked the concept of falling from a really high place, and falling really fast appealed to me, that that would be a very wonderful experience to have. But not the ashram roof, because spiritual teacher would be pissed, plus I'd probably just become paralyzed from the neck down. I had an image of him punching me in the face as I "came to" in my hospital bed. I may sound joking here but I was seriously considering it. I figured I'd go to the airport and board a plane to Hawaii—then go find a building or cliff to jump off. That way I'd just disappear.
- This morning I was still feeling disgusted with my physical life, but I came back to my room and found someone had left me a "good luck" pencil for board exams, and I was SO TOUCHED by it.
- At the exams I wasn't really too nervous—as the day went on and I fatigued I got more tense, especially the 2:30-3:30 exam—I was starting to space out and my eyes cross, etc. There was a lot of tension in the room but I felt really grounded and really focused, like I was there to do a job and to get it done. So even though all the preparation was a real struggle, once I actually got there I just did it. Afterwards we went for ice cream (coffee ice cream with hot fudge, whipped cream).
- Tonight I'm devastated again. Completely depressed about leaving spiritual teacher for ten days. Was so beautiful tonight sitting out on his deck, flowers on the table, wisteria branches trailing down from the ceiling, drinking wine and feeling a cooling breeze against my skin. Now I'm packing in my room and I'm hot and agitated and my back is completely locked, one big piece of metal from neck to knees on the back side.
- This F—ING BAD TRIP will never end!!! Please give me back my NUX!!
- Nasal passage so dry I have to pry boogers out with my nails. I hate the feeling of something hard and dry in my nostrils. I also had a lot of sinus pain.
- I'm disgusted with myself for eating so much these past ten days. My stomach is huge. Now I feel grossed out by food unless it's meat, wine, salad, fish, or seafood. I'm going to scream if I have to eat another rice, beans, and cooked squash meal.
- Pain in gluteus max and med, radiates down rear thighs. Lumbar pain. I feel swollen—my feet, hands, whole body. Dry, hot and swollen like a cactus.

Day 12
- Dream: I dreamt I was working at a (school?) clinic that was in a large house with huge bedrooms that were turned into clinic rooms. I was looking at myself in a mirror and noticed I'd gotten fat. Not just as in I'd gained ten pounds. I mean, FAT. Like, blubbery, slabs of fat hanging over my belt—in the <u>back</u>. I waited until nobody was around and

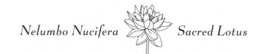

pulled up my skirt in disbelief. Flab was hanging over my belt. I thought how COULD I NOT HAVE NOTICED I WAS GETTING SO BIG?! I stood next to a very tall person and asked him, "How come you let me get this big? I'm short (I was less than five feet tall) and I can't handle as much food as you can." I didn't have time for depression; I was still in shock. I was walking along, I felt like I was in my normal body, but when I looked in the mirror, the image was completely different.

Day 14
♦ Headache tonight. Occipital, especially right side, throbbing, radiating up to temporal area. Return of symptoms. Had three vertebrae adjusted. Two of them, C2/3, keep becoming misaligned, every other day. Sometimes I casually turn my head and they just slip into misalignment. Other times my muscles start to spasm and eventually the neck bones move. Same but much worse symptoms.
♦ C. told me tonight that I've been making noises after falling asleep, shortly after. I sounded like "a cat in distress," a moan that is whiny.

Day 15
♦ Dream: Sitting in a park with friends from school; on a swinging chair; looking out onto a foggy scene, an orchard. We wandered to an old house that turned out to be a hospital or something where my grandfather died. I went to see the room he was in. The building was in the process of being demolished but I could still go to the room. There was a basin that gave information about how big his stool was, his body measurements, etc. It almost felt like his body was there but I didn't see it. All the walls were pulled down, scaffolding and studs were all you could see. The color sky blue was in there—I don't know what it was connected to but I was looking at it and admiring it for a long time, 'til I woke up. It was a dark, dirty building and the floors were partially pulled out, all the walls pulled down.

Day 16
♦ I feel this remedy brought out all the most negative feelings I have about myself and human beings. I hated myself and everyone else on this remedy. My tongue has been very sharp and I've even been more violent, i.e., punching C. He asks me to punch him but usually I don't.
♦ My vaginitis is back, full blown, after I tried to resolve it for six months and it was finally gone. Mostly causes itchiness on the outer labia, some inflammation to the vagina and urethra.
♦ Everything is very dry. I feel drier than I ever have. My skin on my left foot (bottom) is cracked and rough. Right foot is okay.
♦ Dream: Spiritual teacher was teaching me from a thangka [Ed. Tibetan painting], and as I woke up I was thinking that I have to love myself.
♦ I also noticed in general that while my energy seemed to be in general heightened, that I also had to take naps. Like I would have these crash periods where I would have to take a nap and I would be completely exhausted, and if I was driving I had to pull over and have someone else drive. There was an occasion where I went on vacation and I had to

help move some things into this new place we were staying. Everyone was carrying things into the house for an hour and a half or so. And after lunch there was more work to do, but I couldn't even sit up, I had to lie down and I slept for an hour and a half, then I slept on the ride home.

Day 17
- Energy very low when I woke, or, got woken around 10:00 a.m.! Took an energizing bath with bath salts and essential oils and now I feel much better, awake etc.
- I've been coughing a dry cough for several days.
- Went to bed last night with my left eye inflamed. Woke up with what looks like conjunctivitis. I have a small opaque spherical blob of mucous on the inner edge of my left pupil, and ciliary injection medially. It doesn't hurt, and I have sticky opaque mucous. I've never had this, that I can remember. And it ended up lasting for a few days.
- We walked in the sun this afternoon; about 2:00 p.m. menstrual cramps began. I took two Advils and cramping continued to grow in intensity. What followed was a return of old symptoms to the nth degree. The cramps were at eight, on a scale of one to ten, until they went up and off the scale for several hours. I threw up twice. I got really scared before I threw up because my whole body felt like it was going to explode and like I was going to self-destruct. And I had to call C into the room because I was afraid, I didn't know what was going to happen. I couldn't be alone. Undigested food came up. I was shaking and crying when I could cry, and I had this feeling of remorse, like I was really sorry for something that I'd done or some way that I'd been bad. And then the next day the flow was heavier than I've ever had in my life.

This has happened before many times before I got remedies, between age 28 and 30 mostly. The last time I threw up was years ago. What was remarkable is that as soon as I remembered acupuncture points for LIVER 3 on the foot and pressed them, my whole body calmed down and the cramps subsided within ten minutes. I slept for a couple of hours.
- Dream: Dreamt much last night but nothing noteworthy or significant.

Day 18
- I stopped to check my tampon and was practically hemorrhaging. As I began to change my tampon, two very large clots dropped to the ground. Everything else went into a plastic bag, but my hands were covered with blood. We decided to go home. Basically I continued to gush blood and clots for several hours. Later that afternoon we went to a lake to go swimming and sunning, and the bleeding slowed. There was no pain with the heavy flow, but I've rarely experienced this heaviness of flow before.
- Was up most of the night restless, exhausted, muscle tension, etc. Got about four hours sleep.

Day 20
- Overall I had more sharpness and arguments with C. than ever before, which ended up resolving ultimately. We talked about what it felt was going on between us. In the end I feel now that I'm closer to C. than before.
- Spaced out during conversation; vulnerable; sarcastic.

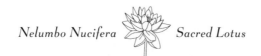

◆ Desires: Carbonated drinks—soda and soda water, beer, etc. I <u>NEVER</u> drink carbonated stuff.

◆ Weight gain of about three to four pounds in six weeks, which continues after having taken Nux 200C; my clothes feel uncomfortable and my belly is noticeable to me, it pokes out. I am eating about two to three times more food than it seems I need to eat, sometimes eating as much as four times before 1 p.m. Snacking before bed on dessert, etc. This is beginning to worry me, disturb me that I have a complete lack of control. I tried to fast on vegetables for three days and then hoped to change my appetite. But since I broke the fast, I've been eating out of control worse than ever.

◆ Dream themes continued to be of competition, warring, threats being made by one group of people towards another; my role as a mediator and/or running and hiding from danger. Guns shot across a yard at an outdoor party. Women being threatened by men, power struggles.

◆ Excessive resistance to doing the work of meditation, most noticeable around 6 or 6:30 p.m. Wrenching emotional states that drag me around. Despair, dense and powerful self-hatred as I have EVER felt. Crying about my utter worthlessness as a human being. Depression worsening in the evening, hysteria at night. Emotional state best in the morning. Asking my partner why he likes me, what is there that could possibly interest him in me? Do I have any qualities that he finds at all interesting? Am I at all attractive? Unhappy—in fact, miserable! Lack of interest in doing a good job, working hard, like it's not important, nothing is important. Avoidance of people.

◆ Total lack of sexual desire. I'm not even deserving of sexual activity. Less sexual excitement physically while in the act but more verbal, using language that is more daring than usual. It's more of a mental experience. Feeling stuck, sluggish. Happy to say, as soon as I took Nux, this shifted and moved to a new, more intimate and higher level with excitement, too. I was on the verge of chucking the whole thing.

◆ Everything slowed down physically, feeling like I'm in quicksand, digestion slow. The same emotional cycle, like the record that keeps replaying. Heavy feeling.

◆ I drew a picture of how I was feeling. It wasn't conscious, I just sort of started scribbling—there's something really sharp and pointy on the top, and the inside is just like a big scribble.

◆ I just had this feeling that the proving was a really important thing for me to do, in spite of the fact that I had these big exams to study for and I was going to go on vacation, and, in general, it felt like a really significant event for me to be participating in. And I did have the sensation while I've been on it that it wasn't at all what I expected and that maybe it was a very bad idea. I've had a lot of mixed feelings about it.

| Prover #15 • Female • 38 years old |

Day 0
- As I held the remedy in my hand, the immediate sensation was a sharp, expansive quality, and I had a vision of needles projecting out from my body and a soft greenish color, and an awareness of myself physically three feet out in front of me from the belly up, no sense of my pelvis or the ground at all. I was also slightly nauseated just holding the bottle, and I felt a tremulous vibration all over, like a high buzz you get with a lot of coffee, like a double espresso kind of buzz, everywhere. And immediately after that, my mind seemed to slip into almost a strange kind of stupor. I described it as being between asleep and awake, not really able to engage but not asleep. I put down the vial – and it immediately dissipated. Disconnected from body, a little sleepy.
- I took the remedy, and I immediately felt the same nausea, magnified 50 times, a hard nausea in the pit of the stomach. It lasted three or four hours. I also had a sense of having eaten something very pungent and stringent. And again, a hard time staying grounded. I couldn't find my pelvis. It was like I was floating up, but not in a nice sense, not like some of the other provings. They were a lot more fun. This was just sort of diffuse anxiety and not sure where I was in myself.

Day 1
- Light, buzzy and continuing difficulty keeping mind quiet. Fidgety. Generalized agitation, no specific anxiety. Intrigued by color/form—feel like I have more of an artist's eye.
- Unable to hold endurance for long run today.
- Appetite decreased.
- Bowels evacuated quickly—unusual.
- Bruised toenail suddenly drained.
- Flare of shingles left buttock—had been going away. Very warm.
- Sweating more than usual.

Day 2
- Anxiety dissipated—now more alertness. Feeling sensitive to energy—little wary.
- Awoke to cat licking himself outside my window at night.
- Dream: Huge goddess with a very huge mouth, huge, the size of the entire ashram, just huge. And Spiritual teacher was standing on her tongue, and he's laughing and motioning me inside, waving me inside this goddess. And I had a slight sense of hesitation, realizing she is the one who devours the universe and vomits it out again, and that this was what I was walking into. So it was again this sense of hesitancy and not quite sure of where I was going or what I was to do.
- Dream: Another dream that night of traveling through an old house, and a lot of sexual images with men, a lot of phallic symbols. Similar dreams occurred two other times. I was looking for a place to have sex. There was no romance in this at all. It was very much a sense of getting business done, of something that had to be completed, of almost intrigue, as I was working my way through the rooms of this house looking for men.

Day 3
- Dose two.
- Less anxiety this time. Keep thinking of cactus. Something green, spiny. Little jumpy—alert for danger in places I usually do not care. Hard to quiet mind for meditation.
- Still nausea and slight stomach upset for fifteen minutes.
- Right costosternal pain/ribs five through eight. Fascial tension.
- I re-took the remedy on day three and felt the nausea again as well as an increase in anxiety and agitation. I was alert for danger and in places that I usually do not care about. Watching the people out working on the scaffolding and having it occur to me they'd been doing that for a year, but I thought, god, somebody could fall. It was danger to others.
- There was a very increased sense of noise and irritability with any sound. Both noise and touch. But I was up doing something and someone was putting china away and the sound of the china was extremely agitating, like fingernails on a chalkboard, to the point where I almost said something, but I held myself back. Which is very unlike me.

Day 4
- Quieter—seem to have adjusted to remedy. Patients seem unusually demanding. Went to very deep place treating [another person] (osteopathically). Entire anatomy became tubes and line of light. Know that exercise would ameliorate greatly. Have not had any time to do it—very frustrating. Very irritated with noise this evening. Sound of dishes being moved around made me want to yell at the person doing it. Very surprising—realized it <u>had</u> to be proving symptom.
- Fatigued all day.
- Appetite increased for meat. Stomach upset after chocolate.

Day 5
- Strong meditation: Feeling everything as myself without intellectualization for brief moments. The building cracked—felt is as me. Not depersonalized—everything incredibly alive and connected by the energy inside. Very light feeling.
- Stomachache all morning. Gnawing pain epigastrium—slight nausea.
- Dream: Took bomb I had acquired over to friend's house who was a Vietnam vet. Bomb was not loaded—but I was excited that I had it and dismantled it to show everyone the nuclear portion. Feeling of battle excitement—precision of machinery—love of power. I was proud of this bomb that I'd built. And the whole dream had this sense of love of power, of excitement about battle, that I had an understanding of the intricacies involved in building this. I took it over to him, and I unscrewed the top so I could show him how I put this thing together. It was all intrigue and this sense of being on the edge, that this could go off at any time, that I knew how it worked. The feeling was pride and a sense of power over.

Day 6
- Continued irritability, more palatable now.
- Very thick leucorrhoea. Creamy white, minimal.
- Appetite increased in general. More thirsty for cold.

Day 7
◆ Feeling like I cannot possibly do all of the work in front of me. Hard to meditate—so much external need by people—difficulty calming down to sit. Much about paranoia, secrets in this state. Considering giving patient the proving as a remedy at some point.
◆ Up on roof finding ropes/harness replacements for men fixing roof. Concerned about their safety. Was coming off roof and 100-pound hatch hit me in the head as I came down ladder. Saw stars—loss of consciousness for a few seconds; held onto ladder so I would not fall. Then just wanted to go to my room alone to work with my pain. Went to room—suicidal call from patient. Had to do 72-hour suicide watch.
◆ The events in my life seemed to reflect my inner state as well. The most notable thing I had was a sense of an awareness of where this patient was at mentally, a sympathy to it and a concern about my own sanity in terms of that I could get into that state, I could sense the state she was in. And it was very similar to that initial feeling before I took the remedy, the in between asleep and awake.

She also believed herself very evolved—others jealous. It was very draining to be with her. I had a sense of her withdrawing, face collapsing. I am amazed at the fragility of the mind—the thin line between spiritual growth/insanity.

This was a delusional state where she believed she was going to marry her spiritual teacher, and this had been going on for a long time. She called me in the middle of the afternoon suddenly believing that she was going to be killed by him or that she'd been told by other teachers to kill herself. So she called me thinking that it was her last day alive and wanting me to know that she either had to kill herself or she would be killed. So when I walked into the house there was this lack of connection and, in my own self, a sense of an incredible drain on my energy just being around this situation. And I could feel myself getting into the space she was at. She was essentially completely disconnected from this reality and she was hearing voices, believing she was getting these high-frequency sounds. I'd try to talk with her, and she'd have me be quiet while she tried to listen to these voices. My feeling with it was being unable to connect with her. There was a huge void between us. As if my own mind was so frozen that I was having a hard time initiating what I should be doing appropriate to the situation, because I was feeling myself sort of drift into the place she was at. And at one point, she was describing this fear that she was about to be killed and I felt myself get afraid that she might decide that I needed to be killed. A striking comment was, "I've been liberated but it's a bad deal" and "they're evil, they're all evil." Those were the first words out of her mouth.
◆ The whole day was this compression of intensity, which has been the sense of this remedy. Feels like an accident waiting to happen, that's the quality.

Day 8
◆ Sense of life moving so fast it is out of control. Need for surrender at deeper level. Unable to write poetry—as if mind too tight for creativity to get through.
◆ Continue to be exhausted with caring for patient. Trying to get her parents here—keep her out of inpatient care. Sense of my own legal vulnerability—yet determined to do best thing for her.
◆ Severe left-sided shooting pain in spleen. Stronger today, actually noticed yesterday.

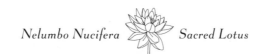

Nelumbo Nucifera   *Sacred Lotus*

Day 9
- Too busy with patients to exercise. Craving the outdoors—but also very sensitive to any stimuli.
- Patient will leave with parents very soon. Looking forward to be released from that responsibility.
- Bladder full, need to pee often.
- Dream: Phallic, large male—naked—unaware of face. Fascinated with size and erection. Very oral—sensual. Not transcendent feeling.

Day 10
- Still feeling more mundane than spiritual. Head foggy after wine tonight.
- Difficulty sleeping. No dreams.
- Sensitive to sunlight. Skin seems to burn easier.
- Much more perspiration, no odor. Especially under arms.

Day 11
- Dose three.
- Took third dose to see if it would help with hangover. Hangover felt much better immediately, but again noticed nausea—although less than first two doses.
- Again, extension—sharp agitation. Feeling mentally ambitious lately. Certain calculation that I am not used to.
- Like energy shooting out in yellow spikes. Overall sense hyper-vigilance, battle ready, like there is a great need in people that must be satisfied.

Day 12
- Irritable in a.m.—life seems overtaxing. Recurrent theme. Did have another strong meditation—more earthy than transcendent. Like a celebration of fullness. Also some concern I have somehow lost intensity of internal connection with the energy.
- Awaking fatigued. Very difficult to meditate in morning.
- Rectum/Stool: Stools soft, abundant: sick sweet smell.

Day 13
- Energy level still +6/10.
- Menses began this a.m. Frank blood without cramping.

Day 14
- Shaky with fatigue, feeling very externalized. Patients very needy; I am impatient, sense of overwhelm. Feel like going to beach and sleeping. Strong need for quiet and alone.
- Menses: More dark red clots than usual. Flow less, no cramping.
- Some white sediment in urine.
- Dream: Still having recurrent dream of phallus—not necessarily human. Sexual more than erotic, more about function. Some sense of intrigue, manipulation—<u>not</u> feeling.

Day 15
◆ Tried to lock sliding door at bed and breakfast this a.m.—lock broken. Did not like sense of leaving door unlocked even though on patio of second floor. Very excitable, but exhausted talking with N. Mind feels strong—but too <u>racy</u>. Went to Italian dinner—drank 1/2 bottle red wine with little effect. Hungry for meat. Then to jacuzzi until 11 p.m. Came back—opened bedroom door—saw mud tracks on floor, sliding door open. Sense of violation, concerned burglar still in house. Searched closets—called police instead of checking for myself like I would have ordinarily done. Heard the robber escape across the roof. Feel a little more paranoid, less strong than usual. Kept everyone on the porch while police searched, worried about gunfire. Sense of vulnerability—fragility of sanity and life.
◆ All my senses were very aware.

Day 16
◆ Feel the proving starting to dissipate. Realizing the manic quality, mentalizing, as it is changing back to my more usual state. Whew!
◆ Sense of deep fatigue after all of the recent events. Treatment from friend—needed to hold my hands over hers to show the amount of force needed to engage mechanism. Again, sense of deep tired.
◆ Appetite increased for past two days.
◆ Menses finished after four days—no cramping.
◆ Dream: Got to sleep about 1 a.m. last night. Another amorous dream; once again a business relationship thing. Sex without feeling—nonsensual/very unusual for me.
◆ Continuing to notice increased sweating under armpits.

Day 17
◆ Energy level beginning to improve. The high-pitched buzz of the remedy is dissipating.

Day 18
◆ Energy level improving.
◆ Some spleen pain in the a.m. Like a single finger poking into subcostal region on left. Broom handle. Had two other people in house, not on remedy, say the same thing.
◆ Constipated.

Day 19
◆ Continuing sense of intensity.
◆ External circumstance extremely busy.

Day 20
◆ Very antagonistic all day. Thank God the effect of this is decreasing—think I would have gotten into some fights. As it was—patients, attorneys, friends, angry around miscommunication and projection. Had hysterical quality to it.

Day 21
Proving meeting.
Overall sense of remedy:
◆ Mind: Stimulating with vibration high, intense—even more than coffee. Anxiety diffuse; Irritability; Tremulous all over; Mind alternating between sleep/wake state and racing with inability to concentrate; Lack of focus, ungrounded; Externally: Burglary, psychosis, paranoia in patient's family; External demands <u>very</u> high. Overwhelmed; Creativity dampened significantly; Overmentalized, manic state; Polarity: Mundane pulling at spiritual
◆ Dreams: Amorous/Sexual: men x3; Traveling through mazes/houses/intrigue x3; Building bomb: battle excitement/intrigue
◆ Physicals/Generals: Nausea; Splenic pain; Decrease in endurance; Increased underarm perspiration; Irritation with light, noises; Desire: Meat; Increased sense of hearing, kinesthetic sense;
◆ Meditation during this period this first week was difficult. It was as if I kept being pulled back to the sort of mundane world, that I was having a hard time focusing. My energy was completely out here and I couldn't get it down, centered deep.
◆ Overall for the mind, stimulating with intensity, high vibration, diffuse anxiety, irritability. Generalized body tremulousness. Mind alternating between sleep/wake state and racing with inability to concentrate. Lack of focus, ungrounded. And the external experiences of the burglar and of the psychosis and paranoia around that. Extremely high external demand in my life. With fatigue on my part, this quality of overwhelm. Creativity dampened significantly. Not able to stay up late at night and write like I do at times. And the physicals, the nausea, a spleen pain that happened probably the last week. It was like a single finger or a broom handle being stuck in my spleen, and would last all day and then dissipate, and then I'd wake up with it the next morning again. Decrease in endurance in physical activity. Significant increase in underarm perspiration. Extreme irritability with lights and noise. Desires: Meat increased. And increased sense of hearing and kinesthetic sense.

Prover #16 • Female • 50 years old

Day 2
◆ Headache persists, but less bothersome. Afternoon, slight headache.
◆ Energy really low—blame it on no coffee a.m.
◆ Nose runny, eyes watering a little.
◆ Almost diarrhea, gas. Had a spicy dinner.
◆ Ankles and wrists stiff this a.m. Shoulder, as usual. Afternoon, feet felt stiff.
◆ Sat down at work and felt very hot—just lasted ten seconds but very noticeable. Felt "hot" twice more.
◆ Tossed and turned a lot.
◆ Dream: I bought great tickets to a play, took my uncle, we sat down in row ten—but

it was behind a wall—we couldn't see the stage at all.
- I did lay flat on the floor in my living room in the middle of the day on day two, I think because I had no energy and I just had to lay down and stay down. But I blame that on the coffee.

Day 3
- IRS news—underpayment. That has me a little on edge.
- Tired in evening—no energy to do household chores.
- Runny nose early, then gone. Headache gone. Runny nose again after lunch.

Day 4
- Dose two.
- Still not up to par but feel generally good—optimistic.
- No headache today. Runny nose (but nose not feeling stuffy). Eyes watery (right side heavier).
- Appetite lighter than usual.
- Some urgency to pee.
- Shoulder sore.
- I didn't think I'd had any response to the medicine, so I took some more. On day four, I didn't have any headaches, but I continued to have my runny nose and my eyes were watering. I slept very soundly.
- Dream: I dreamt I was on a trapeze and all I could do was hang on and go back and forth while somebody else (male) was doing tricks. And all I could do was just hang on. And then I had another pretty spectacular one. Feeling was just hanging on and performing as good as I could but it wasn't very good.

Day 5
- Feel a lot of weight today—body, mind—generally feel I don't have enough time to get everything done.
- Nose not quite running but I sniffle frequently. Right ear seemed like it was running too, itchy, felt wet inside. Runny nose in a.m.
- Slept on right side all night.

Day 6
- Tired today. Low energy.
- Woke up in middle of night—all stuffed up on right side (never happened before—always left side for colds). Right ear feels like a cold, too.
- Feel like eating and drinking in p.m. Hungry for sugar and fat.
- Stiff ankles and feet.

Day 7
- Tense about all I want to get done.
- Energy high—paint fence, mow lawn, make sixty lefsa for family reunion.
- Right side of head plugged up, ear crusty.

Nelumbo Nucifera   *Sacred Lotus*

- Stool like a number of rocks.
- Hair oilier than usual.

Day 8
- Anxious about going to family reunion.
- Feel sick.
- Right side stuffed most of day. Ear actually popped; crusty stuff inside ear. Nose runny till about noon. Slight headache on right side.
- Not very hungry.
- Stool very loose at 7:00 a.m.
- Back achy; usual shoulder.
- Dream: I was flying to France but I just couldn't get to the airport on time. I lost my ticket, then I couldn't find the ticket counter when I did get to the airport. There was a gambling casino in front of the airport. It was like a maze to go through to get to the airport. So I ended up staying the night at an old friend's house, and she and her friend both were dressed in white paper that had been crinkled up to look like some kind of costume. And they had bleached this part of their hair shockingly white. And I don't know if I ever got to the airport. But it was a dream full of anxiety because I had to be somewhere and I couldn't get there. I felt like I was standing out on the edge somewhere watching something I didn't understand. And she looked ridiculous.

Day 9
- Up early, feel better.
- Energy—feeling like I have too much to do and not enough time.
- Still congested on right side but breathing is easier.
- Shoulder sore. Back stiff in a.m. Ankles and feet stiff in morning.

Day 10
- Calm, feel good.
- Good energy.
- Still clogged on right. No runny nose.
- Irritated hemorrhoids.
- Stiff in a.m. Shoulder sore as usual.
- Calm, sort of at peace. Felt really good. Could have been after the meditation retreat, too. Felt very good after that and not concerned about very much, just breathing good and feeling like I had no problems. From then on, continued good energy, congestion seemed to go away, I feel peaceful, pleasant, relaxed and feeling good. Congestion in my head still there.

Day 11
- Feel very good.
- High energy—up at 5:30—busy day.
- Head less clogged.
- Hungry for fruit.

Day 15
- Noticed when I sit for very long—on the porch reading—I'm very stiff when I get up.
- Woke up in middle of night with stuffed up right side of head.

Day 16
- Energy good.
- No congestion this morning.
- Shoulder, noticeably less pain today.

Day 20
- Peaceful, pleasant, relaxed.
- Feeling good.
- Congested on the right—just stays that way.
- Less stiff this a.m. Shoulder a bit better.

Day 21
- Feel great.
- High energy, up early, work in yard.
- Congested on right side during night. Fine in a.m.
- Shoulder painful.
- I took the medicine and quit drinking coffee. The first thing I noticed is that I was totally exhausted and had a terrible headache. My energy level was really, really low. I noticed my nose running and my eyes watering, and I'd been absolutely fine before that. I had all my normal symptoms, stiffness when I sit down too long, sore shoulder, and my sleep wasn't nearly as good as it usually is. I usually sleep solid and I was tossing and turning a lot. The headache seemed to go away slowly, and I thought my energy level was getting better. But actually, I noticed that it still wasn't up to par. Kind of knocked me out. And I don't think I pay close attention to how I feel generally or how my feelings might affect my relationships with other people, so I didn't record any of that in here. But I imagine, when my energy was low, I may have been irritable or anything else and I don't acknowledge that.
- I was overwhelmed about what I might need to be doing. Not enough time to get what I needed done, done. Like I had too much to do, I couldn't even figure out what to do first because there was too much. My coping skills were at their lowest.

GINSENG

American and Korean Ginseng Roots

GINSENG [GINS.]
American and Korean Ginseng Roots

Panax quinquefolius and *P. Ginseng*
Family: Araliaceae
Miasm: Tubercular

Ginseng ranks as the most highly regarded and sought after medicinal plant in the world. Known as the "gift of heaven" and reputed to be a veritable fountain of youth in ancient China, Ginseng inspired emperors to marshal powerful expeditions and engage in war to maintain control over its collection. Every Native North American tribe that had access to wild Ginseng used it medicinally and regarded it as having mystical properties in much the same manner as the Chinese. In North America, it made men's fortunes and shaped the early development of the American west. The impact of this renowned herb is still evidenced by the amount of modern research throughout the world exploring Ginseng's remarkable restorative powers.

Ginseng has a distinctive appearance. Its slender stalk, eight to thirty-six inches in height, divides into prongs with five oval-shaped serrated leaves at each tip. Each year one prong is added, developing between three and five prongs at full maturity. In winter, after the first heavy frost, the Ginseng plant sheds its stalk and lies dormant until spring when a new stem grows from a gnarled rhizome that lies above ground at the top of the root. At the stem's tip, leaves and a cluster of tiny yellow-white flowers appear, which later give way to small green kidney-shaped berries that ripen in the fall to a bright red. In late fall, Ginseng sheds the seeds for gravity to deliver down slope (**TRAVEL**) and the cycle begins again.

Of the Araliaceae family, Ginseng is native to China, Korea, Japan, the USSR, and North America. Most prized is the exceedingly rare wild Korean Ginseng that naturally thrives in remote hardwood forests on the mountains or hilly slopes of China, North Korea, and Eastern Siberia. There the summers are cool and moist and the winters enter a deep freeze. Its cousin, American Ginseng, is found throughout the eastern half of North America, especially around ash, maple, hickory, beech, and poplar trees. It avoids thick stands of oak or mountain laurel, making its home along the northern sides of bluffs and river cliffs. Companion plants, wild sarsaparilla, jack-in-the-pulpit, and golden seal are similar in form

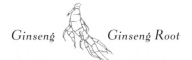

Ginseng   *Ginseng Root*

making the plant a challenge to find until fall when Ginseng begins to turn an opalescent yellow and the berries ripen. Neither variety does well in exposed sites, demanding the deep woodland canopy to protect it from intense wind, rain or sun. The roots of each variety are slightly different in shape and range from pale yellow to a brownish color with a slightly aromatic odor and bittersweet taste.

Touted as *the* prototype of adaptogens, a term coined by the famous Russian researcher, N.V. Lazarov, Ginseng helps the body "adapt" to any kind of stress (*Hobbs*). The first reference to Ginseng from the first century A.D. skillfully describes the root's adaptogenic effect: "It is used for repairing the five viscera, quieting the spirit, curbing the emotion, (**EMOTIONAL/INCAPABLE**) stopping agitation, removing noxious influences, brightening the eyes, enlightening the mind and increasing wisdom. (**FLOWING**) Continuous use leads one to longevity with light weight" (*Herbal Hall*). Over the past twenty to thirty years, these remarkable "adaptogenic" qualities have been confirmed by modern research. "Trials show that ginseng significantly improves the body's capacity to cope with hunger, extremes of temperature, and mental and emotional stress. Furthermore, ginseng produces a sedative effect when the body requires sleep" (*Herbal Remedies*).

Analysis of Ginseng's complex chemical compound has thus far isolated thirty ginsenosides or triterpenoid saponins. Resembling steroids at the molecular level, these chemicals are similar in structure to the body's own stress hormones. Researchers believe saponins are responsible for Ginseng's profound medicinal effects. The chief glycones are the ginsenosides Rb_1 (*panaxadiol saponin*) and Rg_1 (*panaxatriol saponin*). Notably, "Ginseng stored for 1200 years has the same saponin content as fresh ginseng" (*Grieve*).

Although similar in appearance, the effects of each type of Ginseng are distinctive, presumably due to varying amounts of Rb_1 and Rg_1. As a result, American Ginseng (*P. quinquefolius*) has "cooling" properties and the Korean Ginseng (*P. ginseng*) has "warming" properties. Terry Willard, Ph.D., describes the action of each ginsenoside:

> "Rb_1 group (highest in American ginseng) functions as a central nervous system depressant (anticonvulsant, analgesic, tranquilizing), hypotensive, anti-stress, antipsychotic, weak anti-inflammatory, antipyretic, facilitates small intestine motility, and increases liver cholesterol synthesis. Rg_1 group (highest in Korean ginseng); functions as a slight central nervous system stimulant, hypertensive, anti-fatigue, enhances mental acuity and intellectual performance, and anabolic (stimulates DNA, protein and lipid synthesis)."

Siberian Ginseng (*Eleutherococcus senticosus*), which is not of the genus Panex but still in the same family, has even more neutralizing and adaptogenic properties to combat generalized stress than either the American or Asian varieties. The founder of the Phytochemical Research Foundation, Jeremy Pettit writes:

> Scientists have long known that the pharmacological actions of individual ginsenosides may work in opposition to each other. For example, Rb_1 suppresses the central nervous system and Rg_1 stimulates it. This has been considered helpful in explaining the Ginseng's "adaptogenic" properties and its ability to balance bodily functions. (*86*)

Records in China show the use of *P. ginseng* as a medicine dating as far back as 2600 B.C. Recent archeological digs find the Chinese character for Ginseng carved on bones and tortoise shells, indicating its influence to be over 5,000 years old (*Red Cloud Ginseng*). Chinese physicians writing untold volumes on its properties extol its virtues. In 1711 Father Jartoux, a Jesuit priest allowed to study Ginseng in Manchuria, writes: "The root is chewed by the sick to recover health (if one is ill), and by the healthy to increase their vitality; it removes both mental and bodily fatigue, (**TIRED/EXHAUSTED**) cures pulmonary complaints, dissolves humors, and prolongs life to a ripe old age" (*Grieve*). The British doctors Smith and Stuart, working in China at the end of the 19th century, record:

> Ginseng, with the Chinese, is the medicine *par excellence,* the *dernier ressort* [last resort] when all other drugs fail . . . the Chinese describe cases in which the sick have been practically in *articulo mortis,* when upon the administration of ginseng they were sufficiently restored to transact final items of business. . . . It is prescribed in nearly every kind of disease of a severe character, with few exceptions. . . . (*Dharmananda*)

Not surprisingly, its Latin name, "*Panax*" is the root of panacea meaning, "all healing" or "cure-all." Christopher Hobbs in *The Ginsengs* explores the Chinese origin of its name, quoting Dr. Shiu Ying Hu, the renowned botanical scholar, ". . . the sound 'gin' stands for the Chinese word for 'man' and 'seng' is the equivalent of 'essence' . . . " (*12*). In fact the root, often split in two, resembles the hearty thighs of a strong man, bearing a similar shape to the potent mandrake root. Likewise, the Native Americans used the name *garantoquen* meaning "like a man" for this same plant (*Grieve*).

Chinese folklore claims: "Ginseng grows where a bolt of lightening strikes a clear spring, for the fusion of fire energy, water cohesiveness, and earth solidity produces a crystallized essence" (*Herbal Remedies*). Dr. Hu explains that according to conventional belief this crystallized essence in the form of a man "represents the

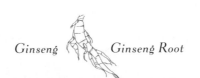
Ginseng   *Ginseng Root*

vital spirit of the earth that dwells in a root" (*Hobbs, 12*). In the Korean legend, "The Young Man and the Wild Ginseng," a devoted son and his wife, despite all their efforts, fail to nurse their ailing father back to health. They continue to care for him day and night as best they can, rising each dawn to pray for help. (**CALM/CAPABLE/DETERMINED**) Moved by their selfless devotion, the Mountain Spirit disguised as a monk, visits the young couple to make one last test of their devotion. Convinced of their genuineness, the Spirit sends them a one-thousand-year old wild Ginseng, in the form of their son. The broth made from his and their sacrifice restores the father to full health.

The restorative capacity of this root goes beyond folklore, reportedly acting in accordance with Hering's law. In *The Book of Ginseng* Harriman writes:

> According to the American counsel at Seoul in 1902, a single dose would cause a patient to lose consciousness for a period of time and undergo a few weeks of considerable discomfort as a result of skin eruptions, boils, and other afflictions. But soon thereafter "rejuvenation" commenced, whereupon the skin cleared and the body became healthy enough to resist disease for many years. (*49*)

Modern scientific literature overwhelmingly supports traditional claims regarding Ginseng's therapeutic benefits. Studies prove that Ginseng has a profoundly therapeutic effect on metabolic function, immunity, mood, mental activity, and physiological function at the most basic cellular level. (*Herbal Remedies*) Even the legendary status of Ginseng as an aphrodisiac is supported by research done on tissues and animals. An article published in the May 1995 issue of British Pharmacology concludes that: ". . . ginsenosides may be similar to Viagra, enhancing the effects of nitric oxide which relaxes artery walls and allows more blood flow into the penis" (*Jacobson*). However, Varro Tyler, Ph.D., Sc.D., professor emeritus of pharmacognosy at Purdue University, points out that a complex analysis of Ginseng may not be necessary to explain its effect on the libido, speculating that just feeling better in general may be enough to make one more interested sexually.

More substantively, large research studies have found Ginseng to be effective in lowering risk for cancer, significantly decreasing systolic blood pressure, decreasing muscle fatigue in athletes, improving pulmonary function, improving carotid and cerebral blood flow, and protecting people against the common cold. Three are worth noting, the first reported by Pettit is "a case-control study using a material dose on 4,000 subjects by Yun et al. [where] ginseng users had a statistically lower risk than non-users for cancer of the lip, oral cavity, pharynx, esophagus, stomach, colon, rectum, liver, pancreas, larynx, lung, and ovary" (*88*). The second is a 1990 study by Khuda-Bukhsh and Banik in India using potentized Ginseng in 200c doses. Healthy mice were subjected to whole-body irradiation at 100 and 200 rad respectively. One group received the Ginseng 200c before the x-ray and again after the x-ray in repeated doses. Both the Ginseng fed and control groups experienced structural changes in chromosomes of bone marrow cells. However, the Ginseng fed mice revealed a significant reduction in the frequency of aberrant chromosomes. The degree of difference was statistically significant at all intervals of measurement. Dr. Nikoli Gurovsky, head of Board of Space Medicine of Soviet Public Health Ministry, replicated this experiment using material substances. Two cosmonauts drank one cup of Siberian Ginseng daily while in space for 96 days. Upon return, their immunity levels and major glands and organs were comprehensively tested. Compared to their four colleagues who had not taken Ginseng, the results were striking. Those who took Ginseng had no adverse effects of the journey and the irradiation; those who went without Ginseng experienced depleted and weakened organs and seriously compromised immune systems (*Hobbs*).

Given these "miraculous" qualities it is not surprising that China coveted Ginseng's powers. Consequently, collecting it was both profitable and dangerous. Wild Korean Ginseng root, slow growing, thriving in remote regions, and a challenge to find, has always been regarded as the crème de la crème of all the Ginsengs. Reportedly the stress rings created each year as the plant pushes through the hardened forest floor increases the root's potency and hence desirability (*Huffman*). As one would expect, the emperors of ancient Asia held complete control over its collection, managing "imperial preserves that were kept free of the profanation of the vulgar herd" (*Harriman, 49*). Annually soldiers gathered it for the royal coffers. The Imperial family had sole access to the root, giving it occasionally to high officials when ordinary treatment was ineffective or their lives or ability to conduct business was at stake (*Dharmananda*). (**ENERGETIC/INDUSTRIOUS**) In addition, special friends of the court received it as a highly treasured gift. Attempts to control the forests where Ginseng thrived resulted in petty wars. Vicious bandits killed many of the Ginseng collectors to get the root. A red-bordered flag, (**RED**) laid next to the unfortunate victim, signified to other bandits that he had already been cleaned out. If he survived, the flag protected him from further attacks. Smuggling the root was punishable by death (*Herbal Remedies*).

Believing the plant to be "the manifestation of the spiritual phase of nature in material form" the Chinese considered its collection to be a mystical endeavor surrounded by many beliefs, folklore, and ceremonies (*Hobbs, 12*). A "Chinese myth . . . tells of villagers hearing a loud voice calling them from underneath a plant shaped like a man . . . [believing it to be] a manifestation of Tu Ching, the

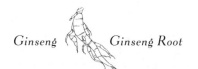

Ginseng   *Ginseng Root*

Spirit of the Ground, the Chinese went on spiritual quests to find ginseng, reciting an ancient chant before digging it" (*Herbal Remedies*). It was also believed that: "Ginseng spirits, appearing as children with red aprons, assisted and foiled many a ginseng seeker" (*Red Cloud Ginseng*). Tradition held that the root's power increased if dug up at midnight during a full moon and only revealed itself if the one searching was pure of heart. In Korea today, there are those known as *simmani* ("gatherer of wild ginseng") who dedicate their lives to roaming the deep valleys for this numinous plant.

The Native Americans also regarded the root as sacred, using it as a talisman for warriors, (**COURAGEOUS**) a love potion, and given to men to treat "old year's fire" (*Herbal Remedies*). While most tribes used the herbs to combat fatigue, stimulate appetite, and aid digestion, the Cherokee in particular "considered it one of their most sacred herbs and added it to many herbal formulas to make them more potent" (*Herbal Remedies*). When hunting for Ginseng, Cherokee priests would address the plant using the sacred term "Little Man, Most Powerful Magician." Seeing it as a:

> ... sentient being ... it is believed to be able to make itself invisible to those unworthy to gather it. In hunting it, the first three plants found are passed by. The fourth is taken, after a prayer that addresses the "Little Man" asking permission to take a small piece of its flesh. After digging it from the ground, a bead is placed in the hole as a payment to the plant spirit. (*Mooney*)

Even "Ginsengers," as they call themselves in Appalachia, treat Ginseng as if it had a will of its own. Mary Hufford in "American Ginseng and the Idea of the Commons" writes:

> Though in biological terms ginseng is properly flora, in the ginsenger's world it behaves like fauna. Ginseng is not merely "harvested," it is "hunted," and rare six-, seven-, and eight-prong specimens are coveted like twelve-point bucks . . ." It hides away from man with seeming intelligence," wrote Arthur Harding in a 1908 manual for diggers and cultivators."

Wild American Ginseng, discovered by westerners in the early 1700s, fetched an exorbitant price in the Asian market. Throughout the nineteenth century North American fortunes and political careers soared because of the demands made by the Chinese for wild Ginseng. However, flooding of the market, harvesting too early and too often, scarcity of the wild root as civilization pushed back the hardwood forests, and poor conservation all led to wildly fluctuating prices and eventual domestication of the root. Wild-crafted American Ginseng is almost extinct in this country because of indiscriminate harvesting in the 1960's when herbal medicine experienced a resurgence of popularity and the price was $600 per pound. Now, almost all Ginseng in North America is commercially planted and farmed.

Cultivation, for centuries the main source of Ginseng in Asian society, is an arduous process because the plant requires faithful replication of its woodsy environment. The most successful farms simply construct their Ginseng beds right in the core of the forest. Often these beds have guard towers built around them with lookouts on duty day and night to prevent the robbery of even a single valuable root. The tender root is transplanted three times during its growth period in order to maximize its strength of potency. Traditionally the harvest takes place at the full moon, a full seven years into its maturity. They say that no successful Ginseng will grow for the next ten years in those fields. Still, Koreans claim that they "have developed unique cultivation, treatment, and merchandising techniques to preserve the nation's honor as the home of the world's finest ginseng. Different locations of cultivation make for vastly different shapes, qualities, and medicinal powers. Hence, ginseng grown in other countries can hardly match Korean ginseng" (*Korean Culture*). (**CONFIDENT/ASSERTIVE**)

In spite of the predominance of cultivated Ginseng in the USA, hunting the wild root continues to be embedded in the culture and economy of the Appalachian Mountains. Hufford describes the high status accorded to ginseng in the counties of West Virginia. Interviewing many "ginsengers," Hufford shows that in an area of uncertain employment, people have relied on "the commons" to supply food for the table and far more:

> In the realm unfolded through ginseng stories and other tales of plying the woods, the commons becomes a proving ground on which attributes of courage, loyalty, belonging, stamina, wit, foolishness, stewardship, honesty, judgment, and luck are displayed and evaluated. (**SELF-WORTH/SELF-ACCEPTANCE**) Collective reflection on what it means to be a ginsenger gives rise to reflection on what in fact it means to be human. It is through such a process that the geographic commons nurtures a civic commons as a forum for consensus and dissent. (**COMMUNITY/CONNECTION**)

This sense of community and high status reverberates through the Asian culture with a similar tone:

> Older Chinese men will buy the most expensive pieces of root that they can afford. The root is sold in balsa-wood boxes, sometimes lined with lead to "preserve the

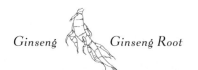

Ginseng   Ginseng Root

radiations emitting from the root." Inside, the root itself is carefully wrapped in silk or tissue paper. It will be taken home and nugget-sized pieces will be boiled in a little silver kettle designed specifically for the purpose. Or the root may be kept in brandy for years, the family eking out the precious liquid by taking it in little sips and offering a little to the most honored guests (*Herbal Remedies*).

Given Ginseng's reputation and influence, it was natural that homeopaths in the early nineteenth century turned their attention to this root. Believing the American and Korean varieties to be identical, the original proving combined the two. The initial proving was provocative but did not reflect the depth and scope of the plant's healing properties revealed through the scientific literature and its historical and cultural significance. A new proving appeared long overdue.

In this proving we used the same combination of American and Korean Ginseng, as had been used in the previous studies, but in this instance, what emerged from the journals was a remarkable series of polarities as illustrated below:

POSITIVE	NEGATIVE
Very high energy	Exhaustion
Calm	Wild
Capable/Do it myself	Unprepared/Helpless
Friendly/At ease	Outsider/Misunderstood
Peaceful/Centered	Labile
Patience/Tolerance	Irritablity
Assertive/Blunt	Over concern about the opinion of others
Flowing emotions	Tornado/Roller-coaster emotions
Lucid/Vivid ideas	Hallucinating thoughts
Safe	Fears attack/Calls 911
No fluster/No worry	Whirlwind
Job-well-done feeling	Guilty feelings
Chaos finds a pattern	Things go too fast
Optimism/All is possible	Hopeless

The key feature of this remedy proved to be its adaptogenic quality. The catalog of themes elicited from this proving reads like a generic list of basic healthy and unhealthy qualities for any human being. Many of the provers experienced both sides of these polarities during the course of the proving but in the end felt benefits reminiscent of the "panacea-like" effects of the herb.

The natural state of a human being is full vitality and flowing emotions. As we become exposed to more and more stresses, i.e. toxic environments, unbalanced workloads, and human interaction being replaced by technology, we become further and further removed from this natural state. Given the likelihood that this trend will continue for some time, Ginseng's central action to restore harmony and balance and increase vitality makes it an extremely useful homeopathic remedy for the 21st century.

Ginseng **Themes**

American and Korean Ginseng Roots

- *Calm/Capable/Determined*
- *Courageous*
- *Emotional/Incapable*

- *Self-acceptance/Self-worth*
- *Confident/Assertive*
- *Self-denigration*

- *Community/Connection*
- *Solitude/Alone*

- *Energetic/Industrious*
- *Flowing*
- *Tired/Exhausted*

- *Travel*

- *Red*

Calm/Capable/Determined

#1 . . . Can take on anything that comes along . . . Feel good—calm, capable, though many things on my mind. . . . Mind working well—logical when discussing/debating.

#7 Calm, relaxed. Nothing seems to bother me. Happy and very emotional and sensitive towards my children.

#1 Thinking clearly. Good perspective on my work—had to work with someone I don't like . . . Seem to be able to maintain my cool pretty much with ease. . . . Able to take appropriate action when things are a bit in turmoil.

#8 . . . I stayed up all night with my son, stroking his head, telling him I loved him, was worried for him but was completely calm. Wanted him to sleep in my bedroom so I could check on him. This was the end of my trip. . . .

#7 Mind positive—little things are not bothering me. Even after working night shift and not sleeping. My twenty-month-old threw cereal all over the floor and then squirted lotion all down the hallway and in the kitchen. I didn't really care. . . . Increase in patience and tolerance, more than usual. Calmer. The dog dug up the yard but I didn't yell.

#7 Dream: I was hiking/camping in the desert with a large group of people. It was very dusty and dry, and the whole landscape was a peach-orange color. I went into my tent and it was like walking into my bedroom at home. My baby was lying on the bed and there was a very large rattlesnake next to her. The next thing I did was try to grab the snake. Then someone else was trying to grab the snake's neck with a pole. I then stopped and told the snake that I would give her anything she wanted as long as she left and didn't harm my baby. The snake agreed. I was then outside in the desert somewhere. The snake was in front of me and she was huge. She was as big as me but with a bigger head. She had huge red eyes. I asked her what she wanted and she said, "Lipstick." So we discussed what shade would be best for her. She picked a lipstick out. I helped her put it on. She said, "Thanks," and left.

Ginseng   Ginseng Root

Courageous

#1 Dream: I was in an airplane—going down—however I was not afraid. Very unusual. Talked myself through it.

#4 Dream: . . . I had to climb a structure in the back corner of my yard to check on something. It was quite high. I pushed myself to do it. I was scared, especially coming down. But I did it and felt good about facing the fear successfully. I have fear of heights always.

#7 Dream: I lost my husband and my two baby girls. I couldn't find them. It felt like they were taken from me. While searching for them, I met a red-haired man who said to me, "I can help you, trust me," as he held out his hand. Then I was on a very high skinny plank that was over a raging ocean. The red-haired man was on a ledge below me and about twenty feet in front of me. He kept beckoning me to jump to him and to trust him. He kept saying, "Trust me, trust me." As I was jumping to him, I woke up.

#1 I am home and not very tired. This is unusual. While driving home I thought about staying out. The darkness was inviting. No fear. Can take on anything that comes along.

Emotional/Incapable

#8 . . . Visited my old therapist. She said it was like a black cloud over me, she has never seen me like this. People come up to me and tell me I look different, depressed.

#2 Mistakes in writing, evening at 9:30 p.m., at city council meeting. The worst were while someone was watching me (mistakes in writing are common for me, but not usually this bad). Mistakes in speaking when asked a question by councilmember. Couldn't say "homeowner," said "ho-nomer" twice, and couldn't get it correct.

#1 Don't seem to have patience this morning. Things annoy me. A woman that I know, when I asked how she'd been doing, decided to tell me all. I wanted to have my morning coffee in peace. . . . Essentially don't have patience for people. I am being unfriendly.

#3 C. and I did lots of "processing" in relationship. Very emotional. Both sobbing —"very easily to emotions." Shared with C. feelings of fear of true intimacy.

#1 While studying in the library felt unnerved—threatened when people walked behind me.

#3 Dream: Eating mushrooms, hallucinating, fear of "out of control."

#5 My life is about change and I'm scared—a new baby, a new job. I'm working two days a week 180 miles from where I live now.

#8 . . . This is what my son said about me at one point, "What's the matter with you? You are jumpy, you have attitudes. It's like how my friends describe their mothers when they have their period. You are cranky. You're a dickhead. It seems like you hate the world. Usually you are a very kind mom and willing to help us. Now we really have to need you. You're real moody." Because the emotions were just coming out, there was no control.

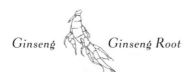

Ginseng   Ginseng Root

Self-acceptance/Self-worth

#1 I like the way I am handling myself, though. Seem to be able to maintain my cool pretty much with ease. . . . Very accepting of myself today.

#3 Tomorrow is my birthday—usual some small feeling of disappointment anticipated—none now, just really excited to simply experience the day!

#1 Gave afternoon cases away, a junkie on methadone, local sedation eye case—not worth my time. As I thought about it, decided I put too much into my life to give it away cheap. This includes working with disrespectful people.

#4 Dream: . . . I am thinking to myself that I am a beginning homeopath and I should make a disclaimer about my skills. But then I think, no, it doesn't matter. Just being with patients is a healing process—I could just lay my red shawl over them as they are lying down. There is not a goal in this healing process.

#5 Dream: . . . I get waylaid, and wind up in a fast food joint where I pee in the ice container in front of everyone. The manager tells me where the bathroom is afterwards. I'm supposed to feel embarrassed, but I don't.

#6 Dream: I was on a bus with a lot of people and we had just exercised. I was sweaty and cold, and badly wanted to change my shirt. I was afraid and ashamed to change my shirt in front of anyone (due to psoriasis on my chest) but eventually did because I was so uncomfortable (due to sweat). It ended up being no big deal. Most people hardly noticed it and my friend D., who was there, looked surprised and accepting. Then I felt healed and knew it would go away soon. Relieved!!

Confident/Assertive

#3 Very grounded—not as airy with grounding. Very efficient and productive. More confident with patients.

#4 Dream: Taking a test with other health professionals, such as chiropractors. . . . Others seemed worried about the test. I was aware that I didn't seem to be worried.

#6 . . . My car was running poorly and I brought it into the auto dealer, since it's still under warranty. After he patronized me and told me most newer cars run like that, I specifically stated, "There is something wrong with this car—please fix it." . . . When the car was finished the fellow at the shop was sheepish because the #1 spark plug was defective and partly off and not firing correctly. . . . Comfortably assertive.

#8 I studied for one hour before an exam, then put down the notes and didn't study anymore. Instead I called home, talked to the kids, showered. This is unusual for me not to study up to the very end. I sat down and took the test, and felt less anxious than usual.

#3 Stronger sense of self-confidence. . . . I can't believe how in my body I feel, so centered, confident and I feel like me. It's great.

#7 Bad weekend. Father injured himself and ended up at hospital. Battled with him at hospital. Had to take his wallet so he wouldn't leave. Put wallet down my pants. I told him to shut up and not mess with me. Had to treat him like he was two years old. Matter of fact about it, not emotional. Usually I am emotional. . . .

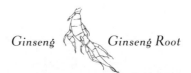

Ginseng   Ginseng Root

Self-denigration

#5 I feel a sense of heaviness in my chest—oppression. After taking the remedy, almost immediately I feel so sad—it's so unbearable. I feel like I can't do anything right and I'm all wrong.

#8 I was thinking that I was too weak not to raise my kids where there was an alternative school or where we had no television. Guilty feelings because son loves violence so much—listens to rap music, makes friends with kids only from the projects. Upset as I hear other son watching television, feeling like screaming but hold it in, feeling anxious, guilty and depressed.

#3 Dream: Someone didn't like me—big secret. I said to friend, "All that matters is the truth. I want to know what people think of me."

#5 I've been a bad boy and haven't written for the last ten days what "normal" is for me.

#3 My hands were not sensing, not able to palpate patient "mechanism." Feeling lost. "My God, what if I can't feel anymore . . . what will happen to me if I can't do my healing work?"

#6 Dream: My new friend and I were playing soccer with a bunch of kids and he passed me the ball and I passed it back. The pass itself was good but then I fell down. Could feel I did not have confidence in my abilities and when I did, I could do it and not fall down. Also remember feeling he might not think I was very good but I'd have to accept that possibility and keep on playing anyway. Did not feel overall very badly—just that I had to accept myself fully before someone else could accept me.

Community/Connection

#2 Some nice things happened today. My neighbor rototilled my weed patch, the new woman, who is pasturing the horse next door to me, came over to say hi, and M. (seven-year-old down the street) came and spent an hour in the evening while her parents were out.

#6 Emotionally grounded—more clear about myself, issues and relationships, ease with people, desire to help people. . . . Met new people and normally would be reticent but participated . . .

#3 Before, I had this anxiety about being with people—what would I say, how would the conversation flow, would I have to make "small talk" (which I hate and am not good at, at all). Now I feel quite comfortable, feel as if I could talk for long periods of time, just a simple sense of flow. . . . Overall, much more sociable, returning phone calls easier, happier to talk on phone to people and patients.

#6 . . . Visited with some people and have found it relatively easy to connect. Felt attracted to one fellow in particular and as it turned out, we developed a friendship and mutual attraction over the course of the weekend. . . .

#8 . . . shared my thoughts with the principal and the group . . . how I felt for the man who was concerned, and I said that I've studied homeopathy, and that there are a lot of brilliant doctors who really appreciate what children can learn by opening up their minds more, and they gave me a standing ovation! And the principal asked me if I would say what I said again so that he could tape it. The response from the group felt welcoming. I returned home feeling content and at peace and optimistic about connecting with the community. As I drove home I was blasting my radio in the car, and I was dancing, and I felt free and a part of something, and it was one of the most whole feelings I've had in a really long time.

#6 After the ride we visited at Alpine Lake and I talked awhile with my new friend and another fellow who was very funny and I instantly liked a lot. I have felt like I've made a few good friends on this trip.

#8 . . . it was a real sense of connecting with people, wanting to be with people.

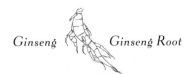

Ginseng   Ginseng Root

Solitude/Alone

#1 Spent the day alone, cleaning house, etc. I think I am better at being alone than I used to be. . . . Didn't want to be around people much. Though they were a pretty good bunch.

#5 A heavy emptiness abounds within my heart. Sighing doesn't seem to relieve it. I just want to be by myself.

#8 Woke at 2 a.m. feeling afraid and very alone. Worried. Fearful that I won't be able to live independently. Afraid won't be able to support self with a homeopathy practice. Wanting support. Wanting to work under the tutelage of a successful homeopath. Not satisfied with where I live, not satisfied with practice opportunities. Want to call someone for supportive, reassuring words.

#6 . . . I felt deep in my heart that I need to be true to myself even if it means being alone. . . .

#3 Dreams last night strong. With group of residents from SR, in hospital, but different hospital from "real one." I couldn't fit into the group. I wasn't willing to compromise my principles, but I wanted to be understood by these people. . . . Basic feelings—left out and misunderstood. I was angry in dream—angry that "they" couldn't see me for who I am.

#7 Dream: . . . My husband and I were trying to escape from someone or something. . . . We went to the train tracks to jump a freight train. My husband said, "Now are you ready? You are going to have to run!" I nodded my head yes as I looked at him. We got ready and the train approached, and then an old hobo appeared next to us and said, "Mind if I join you?" We said, "No." As we readied ourselves, the train came and my husband and the hobo started running. They jumped on the train. I was running and I kept missing the train by inches. Then the next thing I knew was that I was looking at the back of the train leaving me and I just stood there watching it go.

Energetic/Industrious

#1 . . . I feel very calm and put together, very coordinated, powerful, capable, feel larger, expanded. . . . Energy level seems high.

#3 Grounded, lots of energy, office manager stated, "You look different today."

#3 Lots of energy at office—highly motivated and efficient.

#6 Woke up feeling great and rested despite a cold night. Took my friend's dog for a quick jog up to the waterfall—it was a beautiful way to begin the day. Then we rode twenty-five miles up the pass once again—5,000 feet climb. It was tough but I felt strong and went up without any difficulty. I've been getting stronger each day and it feels great.

#1 I am home and not very tired. This is unusual. While driving home I thought about staying out. The darkness was inviting. No fear. Can take on anything that comes along.

#7 Thoughts are clearer. Happy. Lots of good energy. No lag time between 3:00–5:00 p.m. like I usually have.

#7 Energy remains high. I cleaned the rest of my house, including the ceilings and walls. Up until midnight cleaning. "Don't bother me, I'm cleaning." Similar to cleaning binge before going into labor. I had to clean <u>everything</u>. The whole house for three days.

#8 I don't drink any coffee at all before this test, no urge to. Usually I crave coffee before exams. This time my body had no problem being awake and alert.

Flowing

#3 . . . Now with remedy, definitely more of a flow. Dancing in the office. . . . Feel flow in body.

#2 Sensation as if [I am] moving through space to the left mostly, but also other directions; not like spinning or anything, a more linear movement. . . . Then I remembered that sensation of moving through space sideways as if something was pushing me but not with hands, maybe more like being blown by the wind. . . .

#3 . . . it's great to be able to express feelings as they come up. Supple—able to shift to new emotion without holding onto past feelings. It's been great for my relationship with C. Usually feelings come in discreet packages. Emotions with remedy flow into one another—in then out with dramatic changes. C. and I have worked through big issues with this remedy's help. (Curative)

#3 Very grounded, centered, much peace in body, but especially in mind. . . . Not as much minor anxious feelings. . . . Emotions flowing easily—one minute angry, then crying, then laughing—it's great!

#8 . . . I feel aware of a deeper harmony. . . .

#7 Calm, relaxed. Nothing seems to bother me. Happy and very emotional and sensitive towards my children.

#8 . . . As I drove home I was blasting my radio in the car, and I was dancing, and I felt free and a part of something, and it was one of the most whole feelings I've had in a really long time. . . .

Tired/Exhausted

#6 Woke up at 6:00 a.m. exhausted and felt like I was hit by a truck. Groggy and fatigued all morning.

#7 I felt tired today and lethargic. Sensation as if mind not connected to my body. Out of sorts. Felt in a haze, difficult to concentrate.

#1 . . . However, went running in the afternoon and had two beers at dinner—usually will only have one—and when I got home at 8 p.m. I was exhausted—went right to bed and slept through the night.

#8 There was so much emotion at the beginning, it was like a roller-coaster ride. The emotions were just here and there and everywhere. I've been through so much over the last few weeks and am exhausted emotionally. And that was phase one. And then it moved into phase two, which was much calmer and quieter, the exhaustion, it was the polar opposite. . . .

Travel

#2 Dream: Traveling with a group of people (students) we were sort of paired up like a buddy system for cooking and plane rides. We took many planes with overnight stops in between. People in the group left at different times on different planes, so there were always questions about scheduling, like what time are we leaving today? . . .

#3 Dream: Missed airplane, lots of anxiety. I knew plane was leaving at a certain time, then walked around airport (left baggage at arrival terminal) and lost track of time. Then total panic. Couldn't figure at what terminal (gate), connecting flight left from—asking for help, then wanted attendant to pick up baggage at arriving gate and drive baggage to new terminal while I ran to gate. Arriving Gate 28 and connecting Gate 88 (long way away). . . .

#3 . . . It was a bad traveling day—couldn't get out of Newark airport and I just got on any plane to Massachusetts—went to some town have never been to before—no way to get to Portland, and I said I was not going to accept this reality. Then ten minutes later a rental car opened up and became available. The two hour drive in pouring rain to B., don't know where I'm going, getting lost (that's very usual for me) and finally getting to motel at 2:00 a.m. and my bags are still in Portland. . . .

#6 I love to travel and experience adventures, especially in nature, and the mountains hold a specific fascination. The idea of riding through mountains in the fall with fresh air and beautiful scenery is exhilarating—I feel full of the love and wonder of nature and wish a natural disaster or force would whisk me away to an isolated mountain kingdom (with many trees and lakes), since this is not likely to happen, I can settle for an occasional adventure in these places.

#7 Dream: I was hiking/camping in the desert with a large group of people. It was very dusty and dry, and the whole landscape was a peach-orange color. . . .

#6 Once again woke up knowing we had a big mountain pass to climb. Slept fairly well in the cold. . . . Took a short run along a beautiful mountain stream to warm up.

Red

#7 Dream: ... While searching for them, I met a red-haired man who said to me, "I can help you, trust me," as he held out his hand.

#2 Dream: ... He was very friendly, muscular build, open, warm, red hair, not foreign but somehow Irish feeling.

#4 Dream: ... I could just lay my red shawl (given to me by my Guru) over them as they are lying down. There is not a goal in this healing process.

#7 Dream: ... She had huge red eyes. I asked her what she wanted and she said lipstick . . . . She picked a red lipstick out.

#6 Menses a little heavier than usual with small, dark red clots.

GINSENG RUBRICS...*Ginseng Root*

MIND	ABILITY, increased
ACTIVITY, increased
AFFECTIONATE
ANXIETY; conscience, of
  someone walks behind him
  studying, while; agg.
AUDACITY
AVERSION; newspaper or television news, to
  small talk, to
BITING; nails
CAPABLE
CAREFREE
CHARMED with description of beauties of nature
CHEERFUL
  happy, very emotional, sensitive
CHILDREN; desires to play with
COMFORT; sensation of
COMPANY; aversion to, agg.; presence of; people intolerable to her
  solitude, fond of
  desire for
CONCENTRATION; difficult
  in a haze
CONFIDENCE; feels capable
  increased
  self, in
CONTENTED
  flowing feeling, all is well
  self, with
CONTENTED; himself, with
CONTRADICTION; intolerant of
CONVERSATION; desire for
COURAGEOUS
DANCING with excitement
DARKNESS; desire for
DELUSIONS; imaginations
  at the edge of a rock
  body
    enlarged
    separated from
  expanded, he is
  great person, he is
  invulnerability, of
  large, he is
    while in shower
  out on a limb
  powerful, he is

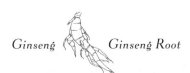

    separated
       outside his body
       world, from the, that he is
    slow motion, he is in
    superiority, of
    time; passes too slowly
DEPENDENT; refuses to be
DESIRES; cream to put on her body
    helpful, to be
    kingdom, isolated mountain, to be whisked to by a natural disaster or force
    play, to
    sex drive more in control
DETACHED
DISORGANIZED
DISTANCE; sees things from a
    watches people from a
DISTURBED, averse to being
DREAMS; airplane flight missed, ran to gate
    airplane going down, no fear
    angry, teeth pulled, at
    animals, of
       horse, nuzzling affectionately
       insects, wasps
          crunched in a ball by sister; surprised that she would do it
       pig
       snake; huge, near my baby
       snakes
    bus, travel on a
    calling the spirit of a patient over big choice
    child, children; about;
       lost, taken from her
    children, husband and children; lost
    climbing high structure, faced the fear successfully
    congressman
convent of isolated nuns
events; of the day
exams, not worried
father is missing
fearlessness
flood
    but not worried; feels blessed to be prepared for it
food; disgusting looking
friends; meeting, of, loving, caring feelings
    old, holistic healers
hallucinating, out of control
helpless and alone
houses with big windows and light
journey; difficulties, with
    making disgusting food
Kennedy flying airforce bomber
left out, she is
losing his family
    man, men; irresponsible, needs my car
       red-haired, says " trust me, I can help you?"

marathon, anxiety about finishing
misunderstood, she is
mushrooms, eating, hallucinating
pipes, opens, drains sludge to river
police, of
priest asks her if she is a mother
running; marathon
shame
   to have others see her psoriasis when changing her shirt
soccer, playing; fell down
stab, antagonist in the gut
teenagers; attempt to stab her
   vandalize yard
teeth, being pulled, needlessly
test
train
   jumping a freight train with hobo
   jumping from one to another
   left without her, watches it go
traveling
   on a plane
truth is all that matters
urinating, of; in front of everyone; not embarrassed
DUTY; cannot handle things anymore
EGOTISM
ELATED; riding bike through mountains
EMOTIONS
   changeable
      alternating laughter then tears
      labile, shifts without holding onto past
   flow easily into one another
   grounded
   happy, very emotional, sensitive
ENTHUSIASM
EXCITEMENT, excitable; amel.; pleasurable
EXPRESSING oneself; desires to be supportive but not a savior for others'
   problems
FASTIDIOUS
FEAR
   alone, of being
   animals, of; bears and lions while hiking
   attacked, of being, by animals while hiking
   behind him, when someone walks
FEARLESSNESS; can take on anything that comes along
FLATTERY; desires
FLIRTATIOUS, with women, then feels guilt
FRUSTRATION; with repertorizing
GOURMAND
HAPPY
   positive, little things don't bother
HAUGHTY
HOPEFULNESS
   IDEAS; abundant, clearness of mind

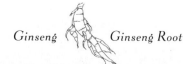

Ginseng   Ginseng Root

IMPATIENCE
   conversations, with
   people, with
   small talk, with
IMPORTANCE; feels his
INDIGNATION
   with disrespectful people
INDUSTRIOUS
   productive
   motivated, efficient
INSOLENCE, impertinence
   had to treat her father like a child
IRRITABILITY; eleven until twelve noon
   morning
   while being talked to
LEARNING; desire for
LOGICAL; while debating or discussing
LOVE
   children, of
   nature, of
MENTAL exertion; amel.
MISTAKES, makes;
   talking
      intend, what he does not
      when asked a question
   writing, in
      when watched
MOOD ALTERNATING
   changeable
      labile, shifts without holding onto past
   happy, very emotional, sensitive
MOTIVATED; EFFICIENT, SYNERGISTIC
OCCUPATION; amel.
OPTIMISM
PASSIONATE
PATIENCE
PERTINACITY
POWERFUL, feeling he is
RECOGNIZE; what is mine to do
RESPONSIBLE for everything, does not want to be
RESPONSIBILITY; unusual agg.
   wakes thinking of her
SELF-ACCEPTANCE, desire for
SELF-SUFFICIENT
SINGING; cheerful
SYMPATHETIC, compassionate
TALK, talking, talks; indisposed to, desire to be silent, taciturn; morning
TENSION
THOUGHTS; cannot collect
   distracted
   rapid
   rush, flow of
   tension in

       TRANQUILITY; grounded, centered
        responds to true inner core
        serenity, calmness; morning, on waking
       TRAVEL; desire to
        have experiences, to, and
       TRUTH; tells the plain; and shares feelings
       WEEPING; tearful mood, tendency
        alternating with laughter
       WORK; desire for mental
        fatigues
        motivated, efficient
        productive

HEAD PAIN GENERAL; eyes; knife-like, right inner canthi
        hunger; with
        morning; agg.
        walking; amel. while
       DULL;
        left sided, spreading to whole head
         hot drink amel.
         lying agg.
         with hunger
        occiput; 3:00 p.m.
         noise agg.
         stooping agg.
       LANCINATING; forehead; eye, right inner canthi
        forehead; morning; waking
       PULSATING; throbbing; afternoon, four p.m.
        throbbing; forehead
       TEMPLE; right, while reading

VERTIGO   MOVING; sensation, in space to the left

EYE   GLASSY appearance; chill, during
       PAIN; general; motion of eyes, on; agg.
       PHOTOPHOBIA

VISION   BLURRED; reading, while

NOSE   DISCHARGE; profuse; morning; rising, after
        profuse; morning; unable to swallow
       OBSTRUCTION; both sides
       PAIN; rawness; nostrils inside

EAR   ITCHING in; boring with finger; amel.
       NOISES in; humming

FACE   DRYNESS; lips
        thirst; with
       ERUPTIONS; acne
        chin
        nose

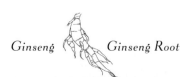

Ginseng   Ginseng Root

MOUTH	BITING; cheek, sleeping; when INFLAMMATION; gums ODOR, breath; offensive
THROAT	APTHAE PAIN; sore, bruised; right; canker sore, cold amel.
STOMACH	APPETITE; diminished NAUSEA; vomiting; without PAIN; general; morning; waking, on THIRST; gulps

ABDOMEN	ERUCTATIONS
	FLATULENCE; morning; rising, on and after
	   movement amel.
	NOISES; gurgling
	PAIN; general; inguinal region; right
	   aching; inguinal region; right
	   cramping, gripping

RECTUM	CONSTIPATION DIARRHEA HEMORRHOIDS running, onset after PAIN; general; stool; agg.; during
STOOL	ACRID; corrosive, excoriating ODOR; offensive SOFT THIN; liquid
URINE	ODOR; strong PROFUSE; increased
MALE	Sexual; desire; increased (British Journal of Homoeopathy)

FEMALE	HEAVINESS; uterus; menses, during
	LEUCORRHEA; brown
	MENSES; frequent, too early, too soon; three days too early
	   heavy and dark
	PAIN; cramping; menses; through day three
	   electric; vagina
	   sticking; vagina
	   stinging; vagina
	   stitching; vagina
	SEXUAL; desire; increased

LUNGS	PULMONARY; function increased
RESPIRATION	SNORING; night
COUGH	DAYTIME; agg.; night, and; expectoration, with

BACK PAIN;
    aching
        lumbar region
    boring; lumbar region, movement amel.
    general; dorsal region
    general; right
    sharp; cervical region

EXTREMITIES DRYNESS; hands
GENERAL; lower limbs; foot, left, plantar, movement amel.
PAIN
    aching
        elbow; left
            morning; bed, in
            weather, in wet
        shoulder; left
            morning; bed, in
    electric; tibia, right, intermittent
        knee; left
    sore; bruised; exertion, after
        joints
        upper limbs; joints of, wrist, right as if from overuse, up to forearm radial side
            right; motion agg.
SWELLING; leg

SLEEP BAD; coffee, after
DEEP
    night
LIGHT
NAP; refreshed after
POSITION; side, on; left
REFRESHING
SLEEPINESS; in morning
SLEEPLESSNESS; night
    night; middle part of night; in
UNREFRESHING
    morning
WAKING
    early, too
    every one to two hours
    feels as if truck hit him, on
    frequent
    groggy, fatigued, exhausted
    morning, toward; four a.m.; happy to be awake
    very difficult to; once awake feels fine

PERSPIRATION ANXIETY; during
FEELINGS; intense, with
GENERAL; in
NIGHT
TALKING; while

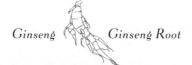

SKIN ERUPTIONS; psoriasis
ITCHING; tickling
  axilla, right sided
  chest, right sided
  like butterfly feet

GENERALITIES CANCER (Yun)
COLD; heat, vital, lack of
  bed, in; under covers
DEHYDRATED
ENERGY, abundant
  for cleaning whole house
  night
EVENING, sunset amel.
EXERTION, physical; amel.
  sluggish on starting, then much better
FOOD and drinks
  chocolate; desires
  flour tortilla; aversion to
  meat; desires
  salsa
  wine; agg.; overuse of
    desires
      dinner
      red
HEAT; flushes of; night
  throws covers off
HEATED; becoming
HYPERTENSION
LASSITUDE; tendency
  daytime
MOTION; amel.; rapid running, dancing
MUSCLE fatigue; athletes, in
PAIN; sore, bruised
RUNNING; amel.
SEXUAL; high drive
SMOKE, cigar does not taste good
STIFFNESS, rigidity; muscles
TRANQUILITY, general; physical
WARM; in bed under covers
WEAKNESS, enervation, exhaustion, prostration, infirmity; afternoon
  four p.m. to eight p.m.
    evening; agg.; eight p.m.
WEARINESS

JOURNALS ....*Ginseng*

EDITOR'S NOTE: *Punctuation, abbreviations, and individual stylistic nuances of the original journal entries have been preserved wherever possible.*

> **Prover #1 • Male • 42 years old**

Day 1
- I feel detached when watching other people—like an animal up in a tree. A separation, as though I'm not a part of them. I feel very calm and put together, very coordinated, powerful, capable, feel larger, expanded.
- In the morning while getting dressed—felt as if in slow motion. Sense of timing was distorted.
- I am home and not very tired. This is unusual. While driving home I thought about staying out. The darkness was inviting. No fear. Can take on anything that comes along.
- I think my appetite is decreased.
- Ate flour tortilla—didn't like it—usually do.
- Sex drive decreased, or more in control.
- Pain in right back, pain in left knee while driving car to work in morning. Like pains I have had in the past. No pains anywhere, feel great.
- Dream: Joseph Kennedy flying in his airforce bomber. I was watching pilot flying an airplane while being interviewed by news reporters. W.W. II pilot in uniform. The pilot says that life is full of "blown up photographs and pimps." Turned to girlfriend and said, "That is Joseph Kennedy, before he was killed."

Day 2
- Feel good—calm, capable, though many things on my mind.
- For quite awhile didn't feel as good as last night.
- Patient cancelled in morning—feel put out about it. Ruined my morning.
- Energy level seems high.
- Eyes a bit tired, as when I get upset. Sensitive to sunlight.
- Not hungry.
- Stool soft in morning—some cramping, gas.
- Bowel movement was acrid, irritating. Noticed I was irritated after my run, in the shower.
- Again, when the sun went down my energy level increased—felt uplifted at night. However, went running in the afternoon and had two beers at dinner—usually will only have one—and when I got home at 8 p.m. I was exhausted—went right to bed and slept through the night.

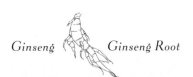

Ginseng   *Ginseng Root*

Day 3
- Feel a bit tired this morning, but not bad.
- Ran yesterday—it was hot. I'm probably a bit dehydrated.
- Have things on my mind but am handling them well.
- Energy level good. Not tired like yesterday.
- Was very warm during the night. Threw off covers—very unusual.
- It seems that my eyes are more sensitive to the sun.
- Headache today, like knife in right eye at inner canthus. Vision blurry today for reading.
- Woke up this morning with gas—but after moving around for a few minutes it was gone.
- Appetite decreased today.
- Slight coughing miasm with some expectoration.
- There has been no return of back or knee pain.
- Slept well. No dreams.
- Skin on hands dry. Probably not taking enough water after running.

Day 4
- Was awakened last night by storm, but still feel pretty well this morning.
- Mind working well—logical when discussing/debating.
- Feel good.
- Eyes feel better this morning (cloudy this a.m.).
- Seem to be having a problem with a hemorrhoid since running Saturday—haven't had that for some time, since five and one half years ago.
- No cough, small unit of sputum.

Day 5
- Thinking clearly. Good perspective on my work—had to work with someone I don't like—was able to maintain.
- Feeling of largeness when showering in the morning.
- Energy level good. Still appears to increase after sundown.
- I think that I bit the inside of my mouth when sleeping. I have done this before but not for some time. There is some soreness but no marks or redness.
- Appetite increased.
- Constipation and rectal pain—hemorrhoids recurring. Have not had to this extent before.
- Some left foot (plantar) pain like I have had in the past.

Day 6
- A bit irritable this morning. Someone from one of the hospitals started talking to me while I was having coffee and was very lengthy. I felt that I shouldn't have said hello in the first place.
- While studying in the library felt unnerved—threatened when people walked behind me.
- After-dinner cigar did not taste as good as usual.
- Rectal pain—hemorrhoids. Pain this morning with bowel movement which was hard stool—no blood.

- Rectal pain worse today. Stool offensive smelling.
- Left plantar pain, better after moving around.
- This morning while talking to C. at the auto dealership, I got sweaty—felt intense, not nervous. And after she left, I sat back and recuperated.

Day 7
- Irritable, but in good mood in morning. Have many worries this week.
- Felt better this afternoon from 4:00 p.m.
- Energy level decreased. Food and water make me feel better. Now energy level very good.
- Headache—right temple area while reading.
- Feel tense as day progresses.
- Appetite decreased earlier, then good.
- Rectal pain gone this morning following stool. As if it had never been there.
- Slept well. Felt refreshed in morning. Have been dreaming a lot about Hahnemann school—some have anxiety, and then don't. Some weird—out of place and time.
- Went to the zoo today. The Jaguar that I wanted to see was not being shown. I was very tired at times this afternoon, but now feel great. Again at night I feel very good.

Day 8
- Don't seem to have patience this morning. Things annoy me. A woman that I know, when I asked how she'd been doing, decided to tell me all. I wanted to have my morning coffee in peace.
- I think appetite is still decreased.

Day 9
- Felt good in the morning. There were some difficulties with a morning C-section. But I handled them well. Worked with someone disrespectful, but was able to do well working with him. Gave afternoon cases away, a junkie on methadone, local sedation eye case—not worth my time. As I thought about it, decided I put too much into my life to give it away cheap. This includes working with disrespectful people. When the money was good, I still didn't like it much. But the money was good. Now, forget it. I still enjoy working with my patients—enjoyed the C-section patient—like helping people through things. But the nurses, surgeons, accountants—I've had enough of. It makes rather stressful work unbearable.
- I like the way I am handling myself, though. Seem to be able to maintain my cool pretty much with ease. It is my experience with these remedies, at least initially, when taken—first one to two weeks.
- Bowel and rectal symptoms have not returned.
- Saw my homeopathy patient, T., and enjoyed the hour very much. I think she is doing very well—though she thinks she is not doing as well as she would like. She is having headaches almost every day—11 a.m. onset—and wants them cured.

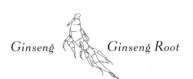

Ginseng   Ginseng Root

Day 10
- Was tired this morning. Feel rushed. Have much to do for school and review T.'s case. She called at 7:30 a.m. to tell me she has some eruptions on the palms of her hands—vesicular as before but not ulnar. If the headache does not return today, I might hold off treating. I am enjoying my studies in homeopathy—but get frustrated repertorizing—don't know very much materia medica. Saw *Unstrung Heroes* last night and the movie stayed with me this morning.
- Had a very good run this morning. Feel good from it. I was sluggish when I started but felt great when I got into it and since then.

Day 11
- Have much on my mind today—though doing well.
- Supervised a young anesthesiologist at Arrowhead. It's amazing what experience brings to the operating room. And did not care to bring attention to myself I realized as I was writing this up.
- Lips dry and getting chapped—I think it's the time of year—dry air.
- Dream: I was in an airplane—going down—however I was not afraid. Very unusual. Talked myself through it.
- Talked to T.—told her to take Sulphur (headache returned). Read that it was the chronic of Aconite, and I have given her Aconite for the acute fright/panic attacks scenario. Other symptoms make sense here.

Day 12
- Essentially don't have patience for people. I am being unfriendly. Went out to dinner with K. Sat next to the owner's husband at the bar where I ate dinner and didn't talk to him much. He doesn't have much to say and I didn't feel much like small talk. Irritable in the afternoon at the bank. The money didn't come in this month (because of my surgery, I was off for three weeks). And I have been tense. However, I believe this remedy has helped me get through this month better.
- I still have the feeling of being larger—more powerful. And also of watching people from a distance—not being part of the picture, as if I'm not really one of them.
- Have had some bad groin pains today and yesterday. They come and go suddenly—right groin. I've never had this before. If I was a woman, I would think it was an ovary acting up—deep pain, ache, but not bowel.

Day 13
- Today I was having my morning coffee. The people in the coffee shop are not who I like to be around in the morning. Dull people. Nobody I would care to talk to. I feel much more at home having my morning coffee downtown.
- Spent the day alone, cleaning house, etc. I think I am better at being alone than I used to be.
- I am getting more hemorrhoid trouble when I run. This hasn't really been a problem since minor hemorrhoid surgery two years ago. Now, returning symptoms.
- Groin pain is gone. I went running this morning—good run, beautiful day.

- Slept well last night—no dreams. Wonder if I will have some more of the airplane dreams.

Day 14
- Very tired. Energy level increased mid-afternoon, and in the evening I was more awake.
- Hemorrhoids are the same.
- Low backache from mopping floors on Saturday.

Day 15
- Able to take appropriate action when things are a bit in turmoil. One step at a time. I have been enjoying my work. Have had some difficult cases to do with surgeons of questionable quality.
- I am reminded of my basic laziness and ongoing fight against it.
- A fellow student from language class—female—is interested in me. We talked after class for a long time in the parking lot—it was sensual and very nice. I could have been hers pretty easily, I think. I know. And I feel some guilt because of K.
- Low backache this morning, better movement.

Day 16
- Very accepting of myself today. Had an enjoyable time this morning with S.
- My patience with people is short-fused, but I get over it easy and go on to being nice to people.

Day 18
- Having a difficult time with ex-wife. Haven't talked with my daughter in over a month—I feel used by them and I'm tired of it.
- Have been doing well with my work—enjoying it very much, enjoying the patients.
- Still have hemorrhoid pain, though decreased.
- Slept well. No dreams that I can remember.
- Have not been as interested in the news as usual. Perhaps this feeling of separateness that I have been experiencing has something to do with this.

Day 19
- A bit on edge this morning. Slept poorly, and feel there is much to do for school this weekend. But once I get to work, feel better.
- Still have feeling of largeness and separateness when I think about it—call it to my attention at times to see if it is still there—like it. It gives me a feeling of invulnerability—superiority. I think it's the invulnerability that I like about it.
- Have not been running because of hemorrhoids.
- Slept poorly. Drank coffee at dinner—woke up at 3:30 a.m. and couldn't go back to sleep.
- Met K. at bar after work last night—didn't want to be around people much. Though they were a pretty good bunch.

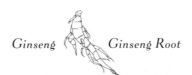

Prover #2 • Female • 42 years old

Day 1
◆ Tickling sensation inside right ear canal—boring with finger temporarily relieved. Short duration of symptom.
◆ Sensation as if moving through space to the left mostly, but also other directions; not like spinning or anything, a more linear movement—lasted probably less than a minute.
◆ Suddenly more chilly even though I'm in bed under down.
◆ Abdomen—audible gurgling.
◆ Tickling sensations mostly right-sided on chest and axilla and arm, like just the tiniest hairs or butterfly feet are walking first in one place, then in another. Almost enough to make you scratch.

Day 2
◆ 1:30 a.m. had been dreaming, subjects changing, jumping from one to another—couldn't remember. Urinated small amount. Too warm, removed some covers.
◆ Dream: Traveling with a group of people (students) we were sort of paired up like a buddy system for cooking and plane rides. We took many planes with overnight stops in between. People in the group left at different times on different planes, so there were always questions about scheduling, like what time are we leaving today? I was sitting at a small crowded table preparing our lunch of crackers, spread with either tuna or liverwurst. The tuna didn't look too good and the liverwurst looked like it had been rolled in cat fur. I was sort of disgusted but I also knew we had been eating it for days. I wondered if it was supposed to be this way since it was something I never ate before. I made some comments about it to see the others' reactions but I got no response. I sort of shrugged at it the best I could, and hoped we wouldn't get sick. (I ate tuna.) Then I was in an apartment with my sister, whom I asked about the plane schedule, 5:30 or 6:00 p.m., so we had plenty of time. I got into bed but a large wasp was flying around being enough of a nuisance that I asked my sister to see if she could get rid of it since she was still up and about. To my surprise, she grabbed it out of mid-air with a pillowcase covering her hand, rolled the pillowcase up in a ball, crunching the wasp. I never thought she would do that.
◆ Nose more stuffed than usual, both sides.
◆ Last night while trying to go to sleep (after 1:30 a.m.) a dull, sort of electric, localized pain, intense, on my shin bone about four inches below knee. Irregularly intermittent at short intervals, then gone for moments, then recur (right knee).
◆ 10:00 a.m. electric stitching, sticking, stinging pain from opening of vagina, up a short ways. The pattern of the pain resembled the knee pain from last night.
◆ Right wrist sore (began while gardening), worse rotating, worse bending it in any direction, like the tendons are sore from overuse. This seemed unusual since I had only been working a short time and had worked much longer the day before with no ill effects. One muscle is sore from the wrist all the way up my forearm on the radial side.
◆ Menstrual cramps started again, which is unusual for day three, although they didn't last long or get severe (afternoon). Bleeding seemed to start up more also.

◆ Mistakes in writing, evening at 9:30 p.m., at city council meeting. The worst were while someone was watching me (mistakes in writing are common for me, but not usually this bad). Mistakes in speaking when asked a question by councilmember. Couldn't say "homeowner," said "ho-nomer" twice, and couldn't get it correct. Doodling on my note pad at the meeting—overlapping vortexes in different directions.

Summary of day: When I first tried to describe that tickling sensation on my chest (after I first took the remedy) I couldn't, so I left it out of my notes. But the next morning that butterfly thing came to my mind and I kept thinking of butterflies. Then, when I went into the sun room to warm up there was a small orange, black-and-white butterfly right outside the window where I was sitting. Then I remember N. saying it would be a gentle remedy. Then I remembered that sensation of moving through space sideways as if something was pushing me but not with hands, maybe more like being blown by the wind. Then the dream of traveling by flight with all the stops and eating in between flights and with a buddy, could be like migration or something. So either I'm onto something or I'm theorizing. I can't say that I felt any deep effect on the emotional level. I seemed to react to things as usual.

Day 3
◆ I had dreams last night, one in particular, but I can't remember it. It wasn't a nightmare or anything exciting or action-packed. I only remember that there were people and maybe they were sitting at desks in school or something like that.
◆ If there's any food desire at all since taking the remedy it would be for sweets.
◆ Energy level is lower today than yesterday, but I don't feel this kind of fluctuation is unusual for me.

Day 4
◆ Dream: My father was sick and nowhere to be found. He had been missing from our home for several days. We didn't know if he had moved out or gotten an apartment, or if he had committed suicide, or what. I'm the one who mentioned suicide to my mother, who hadn't thought about it that way. It seemed he was depressed from his illness. It was like he would show up any minute and the puzzle would be solved, but also it had been enough time that I was beginning to be concerned. This wasn't an emotion-packed dream—I just remember mostly "the sense" that someone is missing and wanting to discuss the possibilities.
◆ Dream: I barely remember, about a horse sticking his nose in my hand—a gesture of affection—nuzzling.
◆ Awoke at 2:30 a.m. (by the cat wanting out), couldn't go back to sleep, thoughts of things that should be done before snow comes. Then a headache, dull, occipital, mostly left-sided, spreading to whole head. Felt like blood congestion as well. Better walking around, worse lying, with hunger.
◆ 3:30 a.m. got up, ate something and drank a hot drink with alcohol in it. Headache better, slept till morning and dreamt as above.

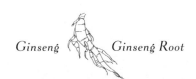

Ginseng   Ginseng Root

♦ Afternoon headache at 3:00 p.m. while working in garden, dull, occipital, vague, spreading over head, worse stooping with head low, worse noise, worse fumes (rototiller operating near me).
♦ Some nice things happened today. My neighbor rototilled my weed patch, the new woman who is pasturing the horse next door to me came over to say hi, and M. (seven-year-old down the street) came and spent an hour in the evening while her parents were out. I felt guilty talking on the phone while she was here.

Day 5
♦ Dream: I was at the orthodontist and it was closing time, but different teeth kept breaking and cracking off so that no one could leave till they were fixed. Since it was after hours, everyone was more casual and I went into a room that was full of animals. Some in cages, some loose. People knew the dentist had a soft heart for animals, so they would bring strays, etc., to him. There was something flirtatious going on between us. Everyone was tired and wanted to go, but it was taking a long time to get all my teeth fixed. (The next part seems like a different dream but there is a tooth in it also.) I had a nice green VW Bug that I had my sandals, jacket, two loaves of French bread and my video camera in. It was parked outside. This man who was a character, actually quite a lush, from the movie I saw last night was going to need my car, and I wasn't really sure I wanted to loan it to him. I knew he wasn't very responsible and I told him to be sure and lock it wherever he left it. I took all my stuff out and piled it on the sidewalk. He had a tooth of mine that had been pulled and was quite fresh with tissue left on it. He wanted to give it to me as a token of affection or something. I said I wasn't sure I even wanted to look at it, much less handle it. He gave it to me anyway, and we examined it a bit together.

I would be surprised if this dream had anything to do with the remedy. I have a long history of dreams about teeth, especially when I've had braces as a young adult now. Also, dreams with animals in cages or rooms is common.

Prover #3 • Female • 34 years old

Day 1
♦ First day of menses.
♦ Slept great. No change. No anxiety dreams—awoke 4:00 a.m. and took puppy outside to pee. Happy to be awake. Went back to sleep, slept well—rested.
♦ Awoke with stomachache. Big change. Still sore throat.
♦ Dream: With friends in community, loving, caring feeling towards one another.
♦ Dream: In house with friends, big flood happening—people awaiting water to come into house, expecting water and not worried about flooding. I was glad we lived in a kind of boat house. Same feeling of lucky, blessed and prepared (for flood).
♦ Grounded, lots of energy, office manager stated, "You look different today."

- After work very emotional—cried with C. Feelings of remedy to speak the truth, to share my feelings. Feels great to cry—cleansing. Easy to tear. Big change. Shared with C. feelings of fear of true intimacy. Feeling overwhelmed with work (not new).
- Menses heavy, darker blood.
- Less anxiety overall.

Day 3
- Tomorrow is my birthday!!! So excited!!!
- Just came back from African dance class—lots of energy.
- Interesting changes. Have felt core immobility, specifically around social interaction and kind of "stop and go" feeling. Now with remedy, definitely more of a flow. Dancing in the office, able to move with patients' emotions easier. Feel flow in body.
- Definitely craving chocolate more.
- Face breaking out.
- Much bigger appetite.
- Numbness < first three toes with dancing—not totally unusual.
- Increased biting fingernails.
- Lots of energy at office—highly motivated and efficient.
- Tomorrow is my birthday—usual some small feeling of disappointment anticipated—none now, just really excited to simply experience the day!
- Right knee pain.
- Throat pain again—old.
- Stronger sense of self-confidence.
- E.'s comments: softer face, change with hair.
- Overall decreased level of anxiety, relationship with C. much more synergistic.

Day 4
- Dream: Missed airplane, lots of anxiety. I knew plane was leaving at a certain time, then walked around airport (left baggage at arrival terminal) and lost track of time. Then total panic. Couldn't figure at what terminal (gate) connecting flight left from—asking for help then wanted attendant to pick up baggage at arriving gate and drive baggage to new terminal while I ran to gate. Arriving Gate 28 and connecting Gate 88 (long way away). Very clear dreams, I was going to miss flight with friends. Main themes—alone, anxiety, helplessness.
- Dream: Someone didn't like me—big secret. I said to friend, "All that matters is the truth." "I want to know what people think of me." It is my reflection—he (friend) was telling me a big secret of what people thought of me. He had shame. I wanted the truth.
- Great day . . . <u>flow</u>!!
- Ate another chocolate cake.
- Upper thoracic pains.

Day 7
- I love this remedy.
- No stomachache since started remedy—a miracle. (Curative.)

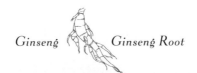

Ginseng   *Ginseng Root*

- Dreams—about friends, high school reunion, running a marathon, anxiety about not being able to finish, but friends were there to support me. Vivid dreaming—called in the spirit of a patient, talked. Very clear understanding of some "big choice" that was going to take place with next treatment.
- Craving chocolate (big!)
- Lots of burping.
- Biting fingernails.
- Very grounded—not as airy with grounding. [Curative.]
- Very efficient and productive.
- More confident with patients.
- Temperature—hot.
- Menses—shorter than usual, four days.
- Burning and numb feeling (old).
- Perspiration—more smelly (usually sweat with odor).
- Increased appetite.
- Fears: while hiking, fear of being attacked by bears and lions (mountain lions), looking over shoulder.
- Increased desire for indulgence—wine and food. Drank two glasses of wine (Friday) with slight headache in morning Saturday. Then two glasses of wine again Saturday at Highlands Inn. Ate a very indulgent dinner at Highlands Inn for birthday dinner—slight (only) stomachache in the morning.
- Very emotionally liable—it's great to be able to express feelings as they come up. Supple—able to shift to new emotion without holding onto past feelings. It's been great for my relationship with C. Usually feelings come in discrete packages. Emotions with remedy flow into one another—in then out with dramatic changes. C. and I have worked through big issues with this remedy's help.

Day 11
- I still love this remedy.
- Very grounded, centered, much peace in body, but especially in mind. Emotions flow easily. Not as much minor anxious feelings. [Curative.]
- Much more restless, but I feel as though I am responding to my true inner core. I would visually not want to go to the bathroom on airplanes, secondary to bothering other people. But now I move in ways I want to move—I'm not so stiff and my conversations are much more flowing with people.
- C. loves this remedy for me.
- Love babies. Made a new friend, two years old, today. She really bonded with me within minutes. We had fun playing while the "adults" had dinner.
- I'm in Maine today at a conference—great to be with friends. I'm so centered—it's great.
- Yesterday, great fear of being alone. It was a bad traveling day—couldn't get out of Newark airport and I just got on any plane to Massachusetts—went to some town have never been to before—no way to get to Portland, and I said I was not going to accept this reality. Then ten minutes later a rental car opened up and became available. The two

hour drive in pouring rain to Bittford, don't know where I'm going, getting lost (that's very usual for me) and finally get to motel at 2:00 a.m. and my bags are still in Portland. So very determined, capable, but I was really scared. 1:00–2:00 a.m., nobody up and I didn't know where I was going.
- Dizziness.
- Delusions out on a limb, edge of rock, fear of heights.
- Tinnitus left ear, irritated by constant low humming noises.
- I like drinking wine! One glass this evening—I can't believe how in my body I feel, so centered, confident and I feel like <u>me</u>. It's great. Maybe I should just do proving and forget constitutional.
- Still no stomachaches in morning. I have had stomachaches in morning for seven or eight years—without relief or any idea why, except <u>anxiety</u>.
- Stool—thin and looser, not diarrhea.
- Two nights ago woke in morning with copious mucous, almost unable to swallow all of mucous. In morning, decreased energy but recovered quickly.
- Halitosis (not new) worse.
- Sweating at night (new) especially neck.
- Before, I had this anxiety about being with people—what would I say, how would the conversation flow, would I have to make "small talk" (which I hate and am not good at, at all). Now I feel quite comfortable, feel as if I could talk for long periods of time, just a simple sense of flow.
- I still <u>love</u> my time by myself, though I don't create much of it in my life. I seem to have an "obligation" to be with people—but it's not what I really love to do.
- Swelling of legs - both, L > R, (old, but worse now).
- Right knee still hurting (old).
- Thoracic complex restricted with pain.
- Left diaphragm restricted.
- Love drinking water (old), makes everything better.
- Don't seem to be as addicted to lotion, though used to be that lotion on my hands made me feel so much better.

Day 12
- Dreams last night strong. With group of residents from SR, in hospital, but different hospital from "real one." I couldn't fit in to the group. I wasn't willing to compromise my principles, but I wanted to be understood by these people. One resident in particular, B., somehow I would also provoke. One time she rang the emergency button and the police started to come. I went outside the hospital and then got on the payphone (I think I was trying to act non-suspicious). I wasn't really scared because I knew I just wasn't being understood. I wasn't really guilty—it actually is B. who is overstimulated with life and over-sensitive. During the dream I was calling B. Aconite (hahaha). I was having teeth problems and going to a "traditional dentist." He recommended pulling my left upper first and second molars—he did. They were very big and I was walking around with them in my hands. I was scared and angry. Scared that I had been permanently damaged with a sphenoid strain pattern in my cranium, and

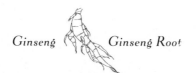

angry at "traditional" medicine because I found out my teeth did not need to be pulled. One tooth was curved and the dentist didn't know that before he pulled it. Once pulled, he said that there was no way he could have known it didn't need to be pulled. I could feel a big space in my upper left maxilla. I thought I would go see D. and he could put a bridge in and I would see E. in combo with D.
- Basic feelings—left out and misunderstood. I was angry in dream—angry that "they" couldn't see me for who I am.

Day 14
- I woke C. and I did lots of "processing" in relationship. Very emotional. Both sobbing—"very easily to emotions."

Day 16
- Lots has happened.
- Dream: Eating mushrooms, hallucinating, fear of "out of control."
- This morning—first time stomachache since proving began.
- Awoke with lethargic feeling—thought maybe remedy burned out—re-took remedy.
- Today—anxiety and fear.
- My hands were not sensing, not able to palpate patient "mechanism." Feeling lost. "My God, what if I can't feel anymore? What will happen to me if I can't do my healing work?"
- Body feels sluggish—tired.
- Apthous ulcer, right upper gum.
- Gingivitis lower right.
- Tinnitus, both.
- Urine and vaginal smell—"concentrated smell."
- Craving meats (strange for me!).
- My cat of five years hasn't come home in four days—lots of sadness—also a feeling of trust of the universe.
- Sleeping soundly through night. Much sweating.
- Overall, much more sociable, returning phone calls easier, happier to talk on phone to people and patients.
- Overall, very, very hot. Usually I have to wear pajamas to bed, now no clothes—too hot!
- Emotions flowing easily—one minute angry, then crying, then laughing—it's great!
- C. says, "You seem much more centered with this remedy," and "You don't care much about your diet" (eating chocolate, sweets, dairy).

> **Prover #4 • Female • 46 years old**

Day 1
- Dream: In middle of night. Convent of isolated nuns—floating as individuals on little individual boats which are not literal looking (actual people had not seen)—getting support and inspiration. Floating on a lake (a small body of water, but borders not defined). My patient K. is there.
- No physical symptoms.
- Emotions: feeling very discouraged and anxious about several homeopathic patients I don't know what to do with—all patients I've had for some time. A real low point. This emotion pre-dates the remedy. I hadn't been feeling too good for past ten days—menses had been five days late. Emotions had been building. This night, I talk to a good friend, cry afterwards briefly, then begin to come out of it.

Day 2
- Dream: Middle of night. I went to meet a woman who was hosting a visiting Catholic priest who had come to say Mass. It was a bright, sunny, crisp fall-type morning. He was very friendly, muscular build, open, warm, red hair, not foreign but somehow Irish feeling. We are walking along—three or four of us—to Mass. He is saying that he wants to find out about his family background—he thinks it may be in coal (mining). He asks me, "Are you a mother?" "Yes," I say. My thoughts, "Yes, I'm a mother—I'm other things too, but it's not important to bring it up. What is his image of me—it doesn't matter." I am quiet and observing in the setting.

Day 3
- I notice that I'm sleeping better—sleeping all through the night. This has not been my pattern in the past few months for the most part.
- Dream: Taking a test with other health professionals, such as chiropractors. We were walking around a long block. It was winter—very grey sky and slushy snow. Others seemed worried about the test. I was aware that I didn't seem to be worried.
- Dream: An image of hugging my elderly aunt, whom I felt I had neglected. I am reassuring her.
- Dose two at bedtime.

Day 4
- Dream: Walking by a large city house that I have some relationship to. An image of L., snakes and a pig. First L. and then he is surrounded by snakes crawling around him. I am mildly alarmed. Then the pig appears and the snakes fade. Not much emotional reaction to the dream.
- Gradually over the week I have come out of the discouragement—taken control to take some pressure off myself and nurture myself with a massage. Becoming quite hopeful and centered again. Better each day.

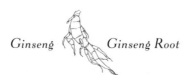

Day 5
- I spoke with my niece the night before—she has just moved to college in California, and I'm concerned about her.
- Dream: My husband and I have gone to visit her. My husband wants to study at her liberal arts program—he liked it. A congressman from Michigan and his wife are behind us. The congressman feels the same as my husband. We are sharing a hotel room with them and their two kids. It's crowded. Then my husband's mother, grandmother and other relatives appear at the door. They've all come to visit my niece.
- I make a yoga retreat this day.

Day 6
- I take another dose (third) today.
- No dreams remembered.
- My son wakes me up—he is ill at 5:00 a.m.
- I am still sleeping through the night quite well.

Day 8
- Slept all through the night.
- Dream: About woman friend. We had been living together, but then got separate houses. Sharing with each other our places, with which we were very pleased. Both were older, two-story homes with big windows facing the south, letting in a lot of light. I had to climb a structure in the back corner of my yard to check on something. It was quite high. I pushed myself to do it. I was scared, especially coming down. But I did it and felt good about facing the fear successfully. I have fear of heights always.

Day 12
- Dream: I am with a group of people interested in holistic medicine—some in homeopathy. Some are old acquaintances from 25 years ago—political days (though none I specifically remember in my non-dream state). I am thinking to myself that I am a beginning homeopath and I should make a disclaimer about my skills. But then I think, no, it doesn't matter. Just being with patients is a healing process—I could just lay my red shawl (given to me by my Guru) over them as they are lying down. There is not a goal in this healing process.

Day 13
- Continuing to sleep well—all night.
- Today (after awake about an hour) at first I felt kind of stiff waking up—especially in upper body. I was outdoors in damp night for party yesterday. After being awake an hour, the generalized stiffness was gone, but I felt an aching pain in my left shoulder and elbow all day. It was almost gone by 7 p.m. tonight. Now it is 10 p.m.—my left arm feels a little achy writing this, but no pain when I stop. Never remember this type of symptom before.

Prover #5 • Male • 39 years old

Day 1
♦ I've been a bad boy and haven't written for the last ten days what "normal" is for me. My life is about change and I'm scared—a new baby, a new job. I'm working two days a week 180 miles from where I live now.

♦ Dream: Asking Dr. M. what to do about a patient given Nux vomica 200C that worked for three days and stopped working. Should I go up in potency and repeat or give in low potency daily? He says give it once in low potency daily. He goes out to eat and I'm supposed to meet him, but I get waylaid, and wind up in a fast food joint where I pee in the ice container in front of everyone. The manager tells me where the bathroom is afterwards. I'm supposed to feel embarrassed, but I don't.

♦ Dream: At a chemical factory where I walk up to the top floor and open a pipe that drains sludgy oil into a river—I feel eerie during this dream. I'm supposed to do this and I have no choice.

♦ Lately, I've had neck pain—sharp—that stops me. I've been doing a lot of reading in the car and my left eye hurts when I move it.

Day 3
♦ Three doses today.

♦ I feel a sense of heaviness in my chest—oppression. After taking the remedy, almost immediately I feel so sad—it's so unbearable. I feel like I can't do anything right and I'm all wrong. A heavy emptiness abounds within my heart. Sighing doesn't seem to relieve it. I just want to be by myself.

Prover #6 • Female • 45 years old

Day 1
♦ Took a dose of remedy last night and this morning.

♦ Feel normal, fine, no real change.

♦ A little tired since did not sleep well last night, but it's been a great day. Have had amazingly interesting homeopathic cases the past two days. People I feel I can help and can't wait to go home and study their cases.

♦ A rainbow is out right now—a good omen. Also, we have been planning a trip to Hawaii for a year (next spring break) and was able to make final reservations today!! We also purchased a family hot tub today (a second model but wonderful no matter). My son loves the hot tub. We don't have much money but live frugally so I'm not too worried and the clinic is thriving.

♦ No real physical symptoms. Hamstrings are chronically tight so it has bothered me to sit awhile.

♦ Later in day, 9:00—10:00 a.m. symptoms began. Mild headache, fatigue, malaise. Do not feel well, feel tired. Took ten minute nap at lunch. Did not feel well all day.

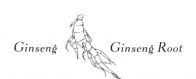

Exhausted by 6:00 or 7:00 p.m.—had to rest but a lot of work to do at home plus two cases. Fell asleep at 10:00 p.m.

◆ Sleep—frequent waking and light sleep after taking the remedy. Woke up thinking about all that I have to do at work. Feel pressured these days due to amount of responsibility. Dream continued—essentially the dream represented the pending relationship with the fellow who I feel is in love with me and not vice versa and I have reservations.

Day 2
◆ Took another dose of remedy last night and this morning.
◆ Sleep horribly—waking every one to two hours. No real dreams, just light, unrestful sleep.
◆ Woke up at 6:00 a.m. exhausted and felt like I was hit by a truck. Groggy and fatigued all morning. Felt better after I took a nap at lunch.
◆ Also mild headache in the morning.
◆ Sleep helped these things.
◆ Decided against taking any more doses of the remedy because it is difficult to function and I'm scheduled for this major bike ride this weekend in the High Sierras which I've wanted to do for a month or so with some friends.
◆ Backache and headache are gone later in the day and energy seems to be coming back.
◆ Appetite and thirst are normal.
◆ Bowel function normal.
◆ Skin psoriasis is a little improved in past week.

Day 3
◆ Woke up in a good mood and emotions felt back to normal. Energy pretty good. Would like a little more sleep but so much to do for the office and at home (son and dog) before I leave town for three days (to High Sierras).
◆ I love to travel and experience adventures, especially in nature, and the mountains hold a specific fascination. The idea of riding through mountains in the fall with fresh air and beautiful scenery is exhilarating—I feel full of the love and wonder of nature and wish a natural disaster or force would whisk me away to an isolated mountain kingdom (with many trees and lakes), since this is not likely to happen, I can settle for an occasional adventure in these places.
◆ I am surprised at how good I feel because my work partner and I decided against including the new potential partner in our practice. What it makes me realize is how draining it can be to have a close friend totally absorbed in their pity or their pain. Even though we can help each other, it seems like we get more from life and others when we are positive and hopeful. This is the first time in my life I am not a bleeding heart or savior, and I feel it is better to be supportive but not necessarily to rescue. This person will just need more rescuers as time goes on, and it may help if he's forced to look at himself now. At any rate, we have to communicate to him this week that we've decided not to join forces and I feel badly for his pain.
◆ Energy—fairly good. Need more sleep since I haven't caught up from the two nights of poor sleep when I took the remedy. My energy patterns vary. Recently fatigue at

12:30–1:00 pm and again at 4:30–5:00 pm. A lot of this is related to stress at work when people call a lot and I'm pretty busy between my regularly scheduled patients.
- No real change in nose or sinus. Mouth, teeth, throat are fine.
- Good appetite and digestion.
- Attended Feldenkrais class last night. I like that it seems to balance hips and legs.
- Sleep—great. Did not remember dreams but I think I had a few. My dreams are about events of the day and people.
- Psoriasis seems a little better.
- One good thing is that I have a lot of enthusiasm and energy for my homeopathy cases and did two children from the same family this morning. We had a wonderful visit. I felt like I could really help and connected with the mother, who can be a bit introverted and standoffish.
- After a big rush, ended up on the airplane and studied for awhile. I felt extremely sleepy, so slept for an hour and a half in the airport between planes.
- My friend D. picked me up at 6:00 p.m. and we had a fun reunion. We picked up a woman who was going on the trip, a massage therapist, and we hit it off immediately. We all talked for three and one half hours while we rode to the site where the bike ride began—a town in the Sierras. Even though we could not see well (it was night and dark with a half moon) the essence of the mountains was definitely present. We met some friendly people and headed to bed. I was exhausted and fell immediately to sleep.
- Dream: I was on a bus with a lot of people and we had just exercised. I was sweaty and cold, and badly wanted to change my shirt. I was afraid and ashamed to change my shirt in front of anyone (due to psoriasis on my chest) but eventually did because I was so uncomfortable (due to sweat). It ended up being no big deal. Most people hardly noticed it and my friend D., who was there, looked surprised and accepting. Then I felt healed and knew it would go away soon. Relieved!!

Day 4
- Due to the immense physical strain of biking a mountain pass and going sixty-five miles, nothing really sticks out other than I had good spirits and felt a little fatigue since we did not fall asleep until after midnight. We had to bike up a very long difficult set of hills—thirty miles—and sang songs and helped each other stay upbeat. I met a lot of very nice people and enjoyed the day. That night was beautiful but cold. We ate a lot of salad and lentils and fell asleep early—by 10:00 p.m.—after sitting around the campfire. I can honestly say I noticed no change.
- D. said I snored last night. My nose is a little stuffy.
- I felt a little constipated but was able to have a bowel movement each morning after a short run and relaxation. We were a little dehydrated and did not eat regularly, so felt that was responsible.
- Appetite—whatever I could eat that was not meat or dairy.
- Urinary delay, which I attribute to pressure of bike seat all day. My crotch was sore and it is not the remedy but the bike seat.
- Cold last night but camped at thirty degrees.

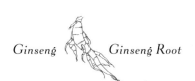

Ginseng Ginseng Root

Day 5

♦ Once again woke up knowing we had a big mountain pass to climb. Slept fairly well in the cold. No real dreams. Took a short run along a beautiful mountain stream to warm up. Visited with some people and have found it relatively easy to connect. Felt attracted to one fellow in particular and as it turned out, we developed a friendship and mutual attraction over the course of the weekend. Unfortunately, he is married, so I nixed any additional ideas, but nonetheless enjoyed meeting him and talking awhile. He has a son near my son's age and loves children.

♦ No real symptoms. Once again a little constipated, but that resolved after short run.

♦ Appetite pretty good. Eating for energy. We climbed over 4,500 feet by bicycle to 8,500 feet! The downhill ride was fun. Ended up camping near a hot spring and the water felt great. Spent the evening by the campfire and enjoyed all the company (including my new male acquaintance). This new situation helped me realize I had no real attraction physically for my friend D. and I made a promise to myself to be true to that and not get involved physically—it would create a muddle and I'd lose a close friend.

♦ Vulva still a little sore and some urinary delay, but I attribute this to cycling.

♦ Dream: My new friend and I were playing soccer with a bunch of kids and he passed me the ball and I passed it back. The pass itself was good but then I fell down. Could feel I did not have confidence in my abilities and when I did, I could do it and not fall down. Also remember feeling he might not think I was very good but I'd have to accept that possibility and keep on playing anyway. Did not feel overall very badly—just that I had to accept myself fully before someone else could accept me.

♦ Oddly enough had no dreams of cycling or concern regarding having to perform above my ability. I've accepted the fact that I can say no and quit if it hurts my knees too much. My knees have been holding up reasonably well.

Day 6

♦ Woke up feeling great and rested despite a cold night. Took my friend's dog for a quick jog up to the waterfall—it was a beautiful way to begin the day. Then we rode twenty-five miles up the pass once again—5,000 feet climb. It was tough but I felt strong and went up without any difficulty. I've been getting stronger each day and it feels great.

♦ After the ride we visited at Alpine Lake and I talked awhile with my new friend and another fellow who was very funny and I instantly liked a lot. I have felt like I've made a few good friends on this trip. We spoke of working in the Third World and of our travel adventures. Laughed a lot. I felt so good and glad that I've been able to ride a fair amount without any real difficulty.

♦ We drove back and D. and I had a nice heart-to-heart talk. We have kind of avoided talking about our lack of intimacy, but I think we'll eventually get to it since we have an honest relationship.

♦ We then had to drive to the airport and our other friend came along (the massage therapist), and we had a wonderful conversation about healing and high intensity people, and analyzed the weekend. It was interesting to see how we each had our own perspective on the situation and we've learned a lot from each other. Felt like she will become a good friend.

◆ No other changes. Appetite good after cycling a lot. Energy fine. Looking forward to sleep tonight.

Day 7
◆ The day was very hectic—actually the entire week was. So much work to do. I was very tired by noon and by 10:00 p.m.
◆ My work partner and I made the painful decision not to include the new potential person, and we had to discuss this with him. I dreaded this. I hate to hurt people in any way.
◆ I felt good about my short trip—like I'd accomplished something.
◆ Went to a friend's birthday party Monday night and danced and it was fun.
◆ Sleep was fair. Still toss and turn more than usual.
◆ On the positive side—so many people have had colds or genito-urinary symptoms, and I've been fine.

Days 8–11
◆ Once again there is so much to do—especially at work. I'm trying to be conscientious about my homeopathy cases but find I want two to three more hours in the day to spend on them. There's so much to consider. One of my main issues in life is learning not to be overwhelmed. This stems back from grade school and I've never been balanced in this department. I either go whole hog and become obsessed, or figure I'll never be good enough and do a half attempt at something.
◆ A friend did massage—deep tissue on my neck and shoulders after work and it was a healing experience for us both. We spoke for awhile regarding our relationships and understood all of the personal compromises we make—some of which are personally harmful. I felt deep in my heart that I need to be true to myself even if it means being alone. It is too painful to live in a situation where there is poor or little communication or where values are dramatically different.
◆ After a full day of work (Day 11), went to Feldenkrais class. I enjoy it a lot even if it is a bit slow. I hope to be able to use these tools every day—more conscious awareness of movement. Even though I'm reasonable at sports, I'm a little clumsy and not very graceful or flexible.
◆ Wednesday night I slept poorly—restless and woke up two or three times with trouble falling back asleep.

Day 12
◆ Even though I had most of the day off work, it was full of chores and catching up. My car was running poorly and I brought it into the auto dealer, since it's still under warranty. After he patronized me and told me most newer cars run like that, I specifically stated, "There is something wrong with this car—please fix it." I spent the rest of the day on bicycle, which is fine. A little tired though (pre-menstrual symptom). When the car was finished the fellow at the shop was sheepish because the #1 spark plug was defective and partly off and not firing correctly. At last the car is ok, but I can understand women's frustration at being treated as mindless beings.

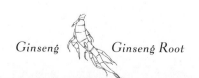

◆ Went to a party at a girlfriend's—we had fun but I miss guys. One of my friends has breast cancer so I listened to her for awhile. It is overwhelming to consider your body could harbor a terminal disease and one day, that's it. I've consistently noticed the role that stress plays in the development of cancer. Oddly enough I have no real fear of cancer, just normal things like rats and snakes.

Day 13
◆ Before my period I generally am fatigued (but can function ok, sleep restlessly for three to four nights) and have an increased appetite. My mental and emotional state is fine, however. I don't feel depressed or anxious or irritable. The only difference is maybe feeling overwhelmed, like how can I get all of this done. After a busy day at work and finding out there was enough money in our account to cover expenses and being really excited by it (less pressure), had a family of friends over. They are not close friends—more or less acquaintances—our kids play sports together. I was filming the teenage daughter for my homeopathy presentation. I've always been interested and enjoy children and teenagers. We went off into a guest room and did the case and it was most enjoyable.
◆ Also felt my nose (inside nares) very raw, especially on the left. Constantly felt like putting salve on it. A little nasal congestion—maybe the first signs of a cold, but do not feel ill.
◆ Relieved that the case went well on film and now on to other homework this weekend. Friday night did not sleep great but was able to fall back asleep. No dreams remembered.
◆ Crave chocolate a little—common before menses. No other changes.

Day 14
◆ Felt fine. No real change. Glad to have weekend to catch up on things.
◆ Meeting with a friend/patient to make plans for Community Project. She had big emotional upset with the program this year and needed to talk so spent time with her.
◆ Dog and I went for a nice run on the river.
◆ Had diarrhea two times, and stomach a little queasy (a lot of people had symptoms at work this week—assume it's viral).
◆ Also nose still burning inside, both a little stuffy too, crusty nostrils.
◆ A little tired.
◆ Menses began three days early and I'm never early (effect of remedy?).
◆ Got a lot of chores done and felt good. Exercised a little in afternoon and had an ok talk with some buddies.
◆ Interviewed my son and it was interesting. He is very funny. I wonder what he's thinking sometimes. We played *Risk* and I realized we need to share those things a little more.
◆ Felt very exhausted and heavy uterus, kind of cramping. Wanted to lie down and get warm. Enjoyed the full moon outside, though.
◆ Slept better. Always after first day of menses, I feel pensive.
◆ A friend came by at 9:30 and wanted consultation. So I went out with him for an hour for a glass of wine and just talked and realized he wanted more than friendship. So I asked to go home. Ended ok.

Day 15
- Woke up feeling fine. Glad my period started. Will make coming week easier at work.
- Strong desire to travel and have experiences.
- Appetite a little decreased.
- Major diarrhea this morning—really loose, brown. No pain or cramps.
- More fatigue than usual with my period at 8:00 p.m. Spirits are fine but I don't like feeling heavy in the uterus. Also, if I eat the food feels heavy and stomach is upset.
- Menses a little heavier than usual with small, dark red clots.
- Sore throat, right-sided, began at 4:00 p.m. after short hike with the kids and a friend. Better cold.

Day 16
- I was exhausted, especially in the evening and night (after 7:00 p.m.), which is unusual for me. It made keeping a journal difficult.
- Sleep disrupted, waking two to three times a night.
- Canker core on back of tongue, right-sided (new symptom). It's lasted more than one week. I don't think I actually had a sore throat, just the canker sore.
- Still had nasal obstruction, lots of crusting in nose.
- Urinary symptoms, even at night. Still in good mood.
- Do not crave sweets, and sometimes do with flow.
- More tired than usual from exercise (running and working out). But feel better after.
- Things good at work and home, just wish I had more energy to do homework and cases.
- Back ached a bit.

Summary:
- Emotionally grounded—more clear about myself, issues and relationships, ease with people, desire to help people.
- Comfortably assertive.
- Met new people and normally would be reticent but participated—felt ok in general.
- Desire for travel and play.
- Insomnia—slept lightly. Woke up two to three times a night.
- Fatigue in evening and early morning on waking.
- Menses, heavy uterus, lasted two days a little heavier.
- Sore throat with myalgia and had an apthous stomatitis gingivitis, front of mouth.
- Stools loose three days.
- Nose crusting.
- Backache.
- Relationship—more grounded.
- What is mine to do.

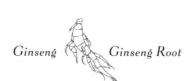

Ginseng　　Ginseng Root

Prover #7 • Female • 30 years old

Day 1
- Took remedy at 7:00 a.m. Held remedy before and felt tingling in my hand. Felt like little electrical shocks.
- Did not feel any different or any symptoms during day. Started feeling symptoms while working night shift that night. So I started journal at that point.
- Generally speaking it takes a lot to get me angry and I'm not so irritable. But after giving birth the second time, I went through a definite irritable, touchy phase. During remedy I felt returned to original non-irritable phase.
- I had difficulty getting my thoughts organized and the thoughts were flowing very fast. Faster than I could write them down.

Day 2
- Mind positive—little things are not bothering me. Even after working night shift and not sleeping. My twenty-month-old threw cereal all over the floor and then squirted lotion all down the hallway and in the kitchen. I didn't really care.
- Thoughts are clearer. Happy. Lots of good energy. No lag time between 3:00–5:00 p.m. like I usually have.
- Feel good after working out and/or walking. Chilly in morning around 8:00 a.m.
- Very thirsty for water—room temperature. Drink in gulps.
- Desired salsa and chocolate.
- High sex drive. Bummer husband is at work.
- Urinating frequent—large amounts.
- Legs and arms are extremely itchy—scratch until they bleed. After scratching, small bumps appear around each follicle. Worse at night, worse scratching, worse thinking about it (old symptom, past three weeks).
- Sleep on left side, I usually sleep on right side. Could not remember any dreams at this point.
- Yesterday usual itchy rash, but didn't scratch last night.

Day 3
- I felt tired today and lethargic. Sensation as if mind not connected to my body. Out of sorts. Felt in a haze, difficult to concentrate.
- Energy level low.
- Sleep on left side, could not remember dreams.

Day 4
- Mind returned to baseline—no longer lethargic. Felt connected again, my mind and body. Increase in patience and tolerance, more than usual. Calmer. The dog dug up the yard but I didn't yell.
- Energy level is at my normal level.
- Thirst remains increased.
- No specific cravings today.

- I broke out with a couple of pimples on my nose and chin.
- Sex drive remains high.
- Urinating frequently, large amounts. Drinking more water.
- Haven't been able to remember dreams.

Day 5
- Everything remains unchanged from day before.
- Husband came home. Relaxing of sexual desire.

Day 6
- Remain patient and tolerant.
- Energy level is at a "normal" level for me. Until 4:00 p.m., then I felt very lethargic until 8:00 p.m., when I got another burst of energy.
- Sex drive remains high.
- Small amount of mucous discharge—beige in color. I tend to not have any mucous at all.
- I slept more deeply than I have been.
- Dream: I lost my husband and my two baby girls. I couldn't find them. It felt like they were taken from me. While searching for them, I met a red-haired man who said to me, "I can help you, trust me," as he held out his hand. Then I was on a very high skinny plank that was over a raging ocean. The red-haired man was on a ledge below me and about twenty feet in front of me. He kept beckoning me to jump to him and to trust him. He kept saying, "Trust me, trust me." As I was jumping to him, I woke up.
- I woke up with a sharp, splitting headache that went right across my forehead. It only lasted for five to ten minutes, then disappeared.

Day 7
- Felt good all day. Happy. Patience and tolerance remain high.
- Energy level good all day, no drop offs and no highs.
- Appetite decreased. I did not feel like eating all day. So I didn't, until dinner. Couldn't turn down dinner.
- Sex drive remains high.
- Slept deep.
- Dream: Took place in late 1800s. I could tell by the way we were dressed and the scenery. My husband and I were trying to escape from someone or something. We were running away from a small town along a narrow country road lined with tall wheat fields. We went to the train tracks to jump a freight train. My husband said, "Now are you ready? You are going to have to run!" I nodded my head yes as I looked at him. We got ready and the train approached, and then an old hobo appeared next to us and said, "Mind if I join you?" We said, "No." As we readied ourselves, the train came and my husband and the hobo started running. They jumped on the train. I was running and I kept missing the train by inches. The next thing I knew was that I was looking at the back of the train leaving me, and I just stood there watching it go.
- Bad weekend. Father injured himself and ended up at hospital. Battled with him at hospital. Had to take his wallet, so he wouldn't leave. Put wallet down my pants. I told him

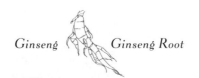

to shut up and not mess with me. Had to treat him like he was two years old. Matter of fact about it, not emotional. Usually I am emotional. We ended up going to another hospital. The way they treated him was pathetic. Later on I got mad and called chairman of the board of the hospital and told him what happened. Normally I would not have done that.

Day 8
- When confronting a situation I stopped and thought about it first, and I thought about what I would say before just opening up my mouth and letting it all pour out as I usually do. Not real emotional.
- Husband did something irritating and instead of bursting out, I thought about what I said.
- Appetite remains poor. Continue to drink lots of water.

Day 9
- Dream: I was hiking/camping in the desert with a large group of people. It was very dusty and dry, and the whole landscape was a peach-orange color. I went into my tent and it was like walking into my bedroom at home. My baby was lying on the bed and there was a very large rattlesnake next to her. The next thing I did was try to grab the snake. Then someone else was trying to grab the snake's neck with a pole. I then stopped and told the snake that I would give her anything she wanted as long as she left and didn't harm my baby. The snake agreed. I was then outside in the desert somewhere. The snake was in front of me and she was huge. She was as big as me but with a bigger head. She had huge red eyes. I asked her what she wanted and she said, "lipstick." So we discussed what shade would be best for her. She picked a red lipstick out. I helped her put it on. She said, "Thanks," and left.

Day 10
- Irritable today. Upset because I had to keep picking up after him. I would clear then he would mess it up. At night I was much less irritable, I felt calm.
- 11:00 a.m.–12:00 in morning. Threw a hissy fit. Yelled, then I was fine.
- Low energy from 11:00 a.m.–1:00 p.m.
- I went and exercised, then felt better.
- Decreased appetite.

Day 11
- Happy. I feel good. Very tolerant and patient. I'm in no hurry to do anything. I'm calm, it's nice.
- Lots of energy. I had to clean. I cleaned all of the baseboards and windows in the house. I tore apart the whole house and cleaned.
- Decreased appetite. Nothing sounds good. Yuck.
- Deep sleep. I could not remember any dreams.

Day 12
- Energy remains high. I cleaned the rest of my house, including the ceilings and walls.

Up until midnight cleaning. "Don't bother me, I'm cleaning." Similar to cleaning binge before going into labor. I had to clean <u>everything</u>. The whole house for three days.
- Appetite remains decreased.
- Deep sleep, no dreams. Had difficulty getting out of bed. But once I was up, I felt great.

Day 13
- Calm, relaxed. Nothing seems to bother me. Happy and very emotional and sensitive towards my children.
- Energy high but steady. Still feel the need to clean and stayed up late scrubbing the floor on my hands and knees.
- I could not remember any dreams. Slept deep, but felt like a truck hit me when I woke up. Very difficult to wake up. But once awake, I felt fine.

Day 14
- I felt a little disorganized and foggy. I couldn't quite put my feet on the ground.
- Energy level good in the morning, but dropped off at around 4:00 p.m. and then stayed low the rest of the evening.
- At around 4:00 p.m. I got a headache, a dull throb in the middle of my forehead. My eyes were glassy, I was flushed but had the chills. I was nauseated but no vomiting. I had diarrhea. My body was sore like I had been working out, especially my neck, lower back and legs.

Day 15
- Sex drive—none. Too busy cleaning.
- Calm, relaxed, not irritable.
- Morning lethargic, "What was that truck that just hit me?" Once up, ok.
- General energy level is ok, but more to the low side. I still feel sick. Headache is gone but stomach is still nauseated and diarrhea remains. Muscle soreness is gone.
- I slept from 1:00–3:00 p.m. and felt better when I woke up.
- Thought of food is disgusting. I'm not the type that usually throws up.
- Dream: A group of about ten teenagers was walking by my house. They started to vandalize my yard. I came out of the house and said, "Hey, what do you think you're doing?" They stopped, then turned and started to attack me like they were going to kill me. Luckily the doors to my house were locked and my children were inside. I ran and climbed up my apricot tree. Attempting to escape. They continued to throw things at me and try to stab me. I yelled to my dog, "H., help!" She said, "Can I stay inside every night?" I said, "Yes!" So she jumped the fence and started to attack my attackers, along with another dog. This gave me enough time to jump out of the tree and run inside. Once inside I called 911. They told me that it would take forty-five minutes for them to respond and that I would just have to wait. Then I called San Francisco 911 and they told me that they were too busy to help me. So, then I called the fire department and told them I had a raging fire. They told me to put it out myself and that I should have a fire extinguisher handy at all times. Then my two brothers showed up. I had to go

outside to help them get inside. While outside, the gang leader attacked me. I was near my husband's truck and he had a hatchet and a couple of knives in the truck. I grabbed them. I threw the hatchet at the leader and he caught it. Then he looked at me and said, "You're messin' with the wrong guy!" He threw the hatchet at me and it skimmed my head. Then I turned to run, but he caught me. I still had the knives and he didn't know it. So I reached behind myself and stabbed him right in the gut, pulling the knife up as I did it. After I killed him, the crowd broke out into a frenzy, and my brothers and I barely made it back into the house with the two dogs. Once inside the house I tried to keep the kids out of sight so no one could see them. Meanwhile, one of my brothers decided he could talk this out with these people. So he invited them inside to talk. My other brother and I kept saying, "What's the matter with you? Are you crazy?!" He said, "Trust me, I'll handle this." When I looked into the living room, they were all sitting there very civilized, drinking coffee while they talked. I went into the living room and said, "I'm the one that killed your brother." They looked at me and said, "Oh well, he probably deserved it anyway." Then they got up and left.

Day 16
- Remained calm, no change.
- I feel much better today. Energy level still a little low, but on the upswing.
- Slept a little in the afternoon, and when I woke up I felt completely recovered.
- Stomach nauseated in the morning, but by 3:00–4:00 p.m., no nausea.
- Diarrhea today.

Prover #8 • Female • 42 years old

Introduction: My emotions were so intense this entire month and there was no theme to them. It was this, and then it was that, and some incredibly intense emotional situations happened to me. My son tried drugs for the first time and had a bad reaction. I had many, many vivid dreams every single night and was exhausted because I had to write about them every morning. I usually wake up at 6:30 a.m. and get my kids ready for school, but now I had to wake up two hours earlier because it took me two hours to write down all my dreams. Visited my old therapist. She said it was like a black cloud over me, she has never seen me like this. People came up to me and told me I look different, depressed.

It was an exhausting experience, just the writing, the technical aspect of participating in the proving. As a matter of fact, it was just a couple of days into taking the remedy that I wished I'd had a proving supervisor. That I could have just woken up today and said, "This is what happened today." It was a lot of dreaming, a lot. And a lot of dreams about past experiences, resolving past conflicts with people. It was difficult for me to write in the journal because there were so many dreams about people in the past. And if I'd just write, "Susan said this," it didn't quite make sense if no one knew the context of who these people were.

Day 1

♦ I had a very vivid dream regarding my ex-husband. I've never gotten over that experience. This happened 14 years ago when I got divorced, and when I left my ex-husband I had told him that all I wanted was for him one day to say he was sorry about what happened. And that never happened, and I hoped it would happen. And shortly after taking the remedy, it was one of the first two days, I had a very clear dream.

♦ Dream: I saw him (my ex-husband), and he was coming to me with this black velvet cloth, and on this cloth was a beautiful shimmering diamond, and I looked at it. I don't think he said anything to me, but I knew, as he gave it to me, that the diamond symbolized a tear, which symbolized "I'm sorry."

Day 2

♦ Woke at 2 a.m. feeling afraid and very alone. Worried. Fearful that I won't be able to live independently. Afraid won't be able to support self with a homeopathy practice. Wanting support. Wanting to work under the tutelage of a successful homeopath. Not satisfied with where I live, not satisfied with practice opportunities. Want to call someone for supportive, reassuring words.

Day 3

♦ I was thinking that I was too weak not to raise my kids where there was an alternative school or where we had no television. Guilty feelings because son loves violence so much —listens to rap music, makes friends with kids only from the projects. Upset as I hear other son watching television, feeling like screaming but hold it in, feeling anxious, guilty and depressed.

Day 4

♦ I had arranged a trip to go up to the town that we had lived in before. For many years now I hadn't been comfortable where I'm living, and someone told me that people in this town want a homeopath. And I contacted an old friend of mine who had lived with me in that town, and she said, "You're not going to believe this, I just got a job offer from someone in that town!" So I then contacted a lot of people from my past who are still living there. And I planned this trip to go back, and my kids wanted to go with me.

We were all set to go, and then just before we were leaving, I went into my house. And my older son (who wasn't going to be coming with us) was as white as a ghost. And he said to me, "Mom, I'm just laying down in my room, I'm a little sick." And I said to him, "You don't look good, what's going on?" I followed him into his room and I said, "Something's going on, you've got to tell me everything that's happening now." And he told me that he had tried pot. He's fourteen years old. And he said, "Mommy, I'm really afraid that it was mixed with heroin." So I was scared.

Ever since my kids were little, since I raised them as a single mom their whole lives, I've always enjoyed my kids getting older and more independent. Because it always made it easier. But as I sat there terrified as to what was going to happen with him, it brought me back to this place of: "I don't want you to grow up." This is my little baby who has made a choice for himself, and I was very frightened. And just like N. said, I

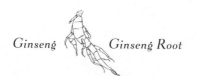

Ginseng   Ginseng Root

didn't want to take him to a hospital because I didn't know what they'd do with him in a hospital, and I thought, "I'll call up the doctors in this class." And N.'s phone number wasn't on the sheet, and I called S. and got a recording, and nobody was home. And so I called P. And in all the time that it took me to get through to someone, I decided to give him cannabis, because he kept saying that he was bigger than everybody in the house. He said, "I can't stop growing, Mom, I'm just getting bigger and bigger." And his face was white and he was completely dry-mouthed. And I wanted to help, and I called people. And then P. called me back and we stayed on the phone for awhile talking about what was happening.

My son was taking ice cubes and rubbing them on his body and he kept saying, "I'm so hot, I'm so hot." And he just kept going into the kitchen and taking ice cubes and rubbing them on his body. And I was completely calm. I stayed up all night with my son, stroking his head, telling him I loved him, was worried for him but was completely calm. Wanted him to sleep in my bedroom so I could check on him. This was the end of my trip. And, it was like a switch from the tumultuousness of the beginning of the remedy to more of a calm.

Day 8
♦ In the past many, many years, since my divorce, my focus has been on how in the world am I going to get a degree to learn homeopathy, practice homeopathy. It's been focused on work one zillion percent. And getting the degree, and getting the ability to finally attend Hahnemann was this thing that was going to take forever and ever. And I was plugging away at it, and all of a sudden it was as though someone scooped my brain out and had taken all of those occupational concerns and put them in the garbage, and just had me deal with people. So it was a period of patients cancelling, and my being happy that they did, and my rearranging my work schedule so it is much less than it usually is. My not being concerned with finances at all, not spending a penny on anything because I just figured I'm not going to be working much. And it was a real sense of connecting with people, wanting to be with people.

Day 9
♦ I hardly ever drink. I was drinking every evening at the beginning, and then I started to drink while I was working during the day, and then, for the proving I wanted to continue with it and see where it went, but for my patients' sake, I stopped. But there was definitely a big desire. Rose wines, pink wines. Desire for glass of wine at 10:00 a.m. And I also wanted to have lunch. I ate chocolates and then had lunch. There was really no holding me, you want wine, go have wine. 10:00 a.m.? It's ok.
♦ Dream: In a restaurant a man was crying and sobbing and ranting to his family about a painful experience that had happened to him with his family, and he was misunderstood.

Day 10
♦ As a part of this shift, one of the biggest things that's bothered me since I've moved to where I'm living now is, I used to teach in a Waldorf school, and when I got divorced I left that town and my kids have been attending public school. And I have felt guilty

from that day on, that my kids went to a regular old public school, and the work that they did came from boring dittos. I'd go to a PTA meeting, and they only serve the kids chocolate milk in school, and I'd raise my hand innocently and say, "Why don't we serve non-chocolate milk?" And these very aggressive women told me, "Because chocolate milk is made with skim milk and it's low-fat and we don't want our children fat." Well, I never went back to any PTA meetings because I figured I didn't fit in. And for ten years I've felt like I haven't fit in.

While I was on this remedy I went to a meeting at the high school, my son is now in the high school, and I sat in the back, expecting to not be a part of the "in clique" of moms in my area, and the principal shows a movie on finding the pattern in the chaos of nature. And from allowing things to be what they are, and allowing the chaos to happen, you can find a pattern which expresses the diversity of the whole and makes us evolve. Now this is a public school. And all I could think of was, "I feel a part of this for the first time in ten years!" I feel like, maybe I can fit in to this town. The people in the room were saying that they were so excited that the principal had shown this movie. My jaw was dropping. And this one gentleman raised his hand and said, "I'm just concerned that the children will not get into the colleges if we allow this to happen in the school." And the principal responded so eloquently, it was beautiful. It was magnificent. He assured this gentleman, who has true concerns about his children getting into good colleges, how if we change the way public schools are run, it really will move in a more positive direction.

Anyway, I felt so good that I raised my hand and shared my thoughts with the principal and the group. This was the first time since the chocolate milk PTA meeting, and I said how I felt for the man who was concerned, and I said that I've studied homeopathy, and that there are a lot of brilliant doctors who really appreciate what children can learn by opening up their minds more, and they gave me a standing ovation! And the principal asked me if I would say what I said again so that he could tape it. The response from the group felt welcoming. I returned home feeling content and at peace and optimistic about connecting with the community. As I drove home I was blasting my radio in the car, and I was dancing, and I felt free and a part of something, and it was one of the most whole feelings I've had in a really long time. That happened on this remedy.

Day 12
◆ A lot of things that I have wanted for myself and my kids I haven't brought into my life because I knew it would make waves. Like I was aware of the softer aspect of my personality. An example, when I moved into my parents house, I was a vegetarian, my kids were vegetarians. My mother would always offer them meat at the table, "Why don't you try it, why don't you try it?" And I realized that it was healthier for my kids to eat the meat and have a peaceful dinner table than for me to make a stink about the fact that it was important for me to have a vegetarian diet. And I had originally lived in a house without a television and I loved that, the peaceful home we had. And when we moved in with my parents they had a television. And I realized that my constantly saying, "I don't want you guys to watch television," was causing more disharmony than helping them.

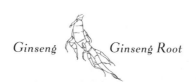

Ginseng   Ginseng Root

Day 21
- I studied for one hour before an exam, then put down the notes and didn't study anymore. Instead I called home, talked to the kids, showered. This is unusual for me not to study up to the very end. I sat down and took the test, and felt less anxious than usual.
- I didn't drink any coffee at all before this test, no urge to. Usually I crave coffee before exams. This time my body had no problem being awake and alert.

Summary of Proving:
- I had physical symptoms I hardly ever have. I was nauseous a lot during the remedy and I felt it right in the epigastrium, it was very specific. I had a lot of throat symptoms and I thought I was going to come down with strep, and then I thought it was going to be the flu. And I never got anything, but it was real burning, that eventually moved into a difficulty breathing because it was so painful.
- I woke up one day with my hands clasped at my chest, and my forearms felt real heavy and thick.
- My kids knew that I was doing this proving, and I told them that at the end of the month I'd ask them about it. This is what my son said about me at one point, "What's the matter with you? You are jumpy, you have attitudes. It's like how my friends describe their mothers when they have their period. You are cranky. You're a dickhead. It seems like you hate the world. Usually you are a very kind mom and willing to help us. Now we really have to need you. You're real moody." Because the emotions were just coming out, there was no control.
- There were so much emotion at the beginning, it was like a roller-coaster ride. The emotions were just here and there and everywhere. I've been through so much over the last few weeks and I am exhausted emotionally. And that was phase one. And then it moved into phase two, which was much calmer and quieter, the exhaustion, it was the polar opposite. And that's how different it was. I feel aware of a deeper harmony. And I'm still in that.

MANDRAGORA OFFICINARUM
Mandrake Root

MANDRAGORA OFFICINARUM [MAND.]
Mandrake Root

Mandragora officinarum
Family: *Solanaceae*
Miasm: *Leprosy*

*E*lusive and magical, Mandragora has been, since ancient times, the most sought after and mysterious of all esoteric herbs. Its many names reveal some of the dark qualities attributed to it: devil's apples or Satan's apple, lust apples of the fool, magic root, apples of the genie, Satan's testicles, dog's apple, devil's candle, "the herb of life and death," and "little man of the gallows."

Yet, it is extolled in the Song of Solomon: "Let us get up early to the vineyards; let us see if the vines flourish, whether the tender grape appear, and the pomegranates bud forth; there will I give thee my love. The mandrakes give forth a fragrance, and at our gates are all manner of pleasant fruits, new and old, which I have laid up for thee, O my beloved" (*7:12-13*).

The mandrake, a plant indigenous to the Mediterranean, is a member of the Solanaceae family. Almost stemless, it has a large, brown root that grows three to four feet into the ground, often divided into two long branches in a convincing imitation of the human body. The root acts as a very powerful emetic and purgative. The fruit is large, globular, and yellow, emitting an apple-like scent, which is both aromatic and poisonous. James Duke in *Herbs of the Bible* says of it: "The fruit, eaten in quantity, produces dizziness, delirium and may cause insanity" (*159*). (**MENTAL ILLNESS**) The whitish-purple, bell-shaped flowers are about three to four inches high. The large dark green leaves, which have a disgusting, fetid odor, initially stand erect and then lay along the ground.

The main alkaloid in mandrake is hyoscyamine, while atropine and scopolamine are also present. These are all potent anticholinergics. Skin reddening, dryness of the mouth, tachyarrhythmias, mydriasis, accommodation disorders, heat build-up caused by suppression of perspiration, micturition disorders, and constipation can occur. Poisonings lead at first to somnolence, then to central excitation with restlessness, hallucinations, delirium, and manic episodes followed by exhaustion and sleep (*PDR*). Large doses can cause respiratory failure and death.

The rich, multi-ethnic history and folklore reveal the provocative and pernicious effects of the mandrake when used as a narcotic, anesthetic, hallucinogenic, aphrodisiac, hypnotic, trance mediator, and poison.

The temple physicians of ancient Greece used Mandragora as a sacred sedative, practicing their art of healing in temple-like hospitals, located in beautiful settings near streams and mountains. (**WATER**) (**MOUNTAINS**) By the use of medicinal herbs, ointments, and massage, they would create in their patients a peaceful and relaxed mental state in which to heal. The "infernal trinity" of hyoscyamus, belladonna, and mandrake were their main healing herbs.
(**MEDICINE/HOSPITALS/TESTS**)

Pliny, Galen, and Lucian, all mention the mandrake's ability to induce a state of insensibility to external impressions when cutting or cauterizing. Isidorus is quoted as saying: "A wine of the bark of the root is given to those about to undergo operation that being asleep they may feel no pain" (*Catholic Encyclopedia*). According to Thomas Cisterciensis, a twelfth century monk, contemplatives used this state as part of their spiritual discipline:

> The mandragora is a plant which effects such a deep sleep that one can cut a person and he feels not the pain. For the mandragora symbolizes striving in contemplation. Its reverie allows a person to fall into a sleep of such delicious sweetness that he no longer feels any of the cutting which his earthly enemies inflict upon him, and he no longer cares about any earthly thing. For his soul has now closed off its senses from all that is external—it lies in the benevolent sleep of the internal. (*Rätsch, 139*)
> (**NUMB/NO EMOTION**)

A similar soothing, trance-like effect was probably the goal of many female healers, who used the mandrake and other medicinal herbs for childbirth, tending to the ill, making potions and charms, and rituals worshipping the earth goddess. As paranoia and suspicion increased about these pre-Christian healing arts, these herbalists were accused of riding on broomsticks to Black Sabbaths, where they supposedly had sexual relations with the devil himself. "Although most accused witches seem to have confessed to flying only as a result of being tortured, some appear to have actually believed they were flying." A number of written accounts from the fifteenth and sixteenth centuries refer to the use of unguents and ointments which allow a witch to fly. These unguents, largely made up of mandrake, belladonna, and hyoscyamus, rich with hallucinogenic alkaloids, "promoted a sense of flying and the ability to convene with the spiritual world . . . extending the normal boundaries of human experience"
(**OTHERWORLDLY**)

> Andrés Laguna, a sixteenth-century physician practicing in Lorraine, described the discovery of a witch's jar "half filled with a certain green unguent . . . with which they were anointing themselves: whose odor was so heavy and offensive that it showed that it was composed of herbs cold and soporiferous to the ultimate degree, which are hemlock, nightshade, henbane, and mandrake." Laguna obtained a canister full of this ointment and used it to carry out an experiment . . . He anointed this woman from head to toe, whereupon "she suddenly slept such a sound sleep, with her eyes open like a rabbit (she also fittingly looked like a boiled hare), that I could not imagine how to wake her." When Laguna finally managed to get her up, she had been sleeping for thirty-six hours. She complained: "Why do you wake me at such an inopportune time? I was surrounded by all the pleasures and delights of the world." (*Harris, 218-219*)

Ironically, in the tenth century the Canon Episcopi states that people who believe witches can fly through the night are heretics, but by the fifteenth century that canon was reversed and it became a heretical offense to deny that witches could transport themselves in body and in spirit. In *Herbs of the Bible* James A. Duke states: "As late as 1630 in Hamburg, Germany, three women were executed for possession of mandrake root, supposed 'evidence' that they were involved in witchcraft" (*161*). (**HARASSED/PERSECUTED**) In the same vein, "the little man of the gallows" legend, believed that: "the plant [mandrake] grew under the gallows where a man of virtue had been wrongly hanged" (*141*).

In *Plants of Love,* Rätsch gives us remarkable stories about the gathering of the mandrake root:

> In Rumania, (**EXOTIC PLACES**) a mandrake can only be removed from the ground when certain customs and taboos are respected; these include sexual virginity, cleanliness, and concealment. It should only be excavated without the knowledge of anyone else; (**CONCEALMENT**) it should be done far away from the village and in seclusion. Pairs of women (**WOMEN**) and girls, their hair loose, (**HAIR**) must first dance naked around the mandrake. The two females caress and embrace one another during the wild dance . . . while they dance they sing (**MUSIC**) or recite the following words:
>
>> Mandrake, good mother
>> marry me in this month,
>> if not in this one,
>> then in the next,
>> but make it so that I no longer
>> remain a girl.

He continues:

> The most favorable time to harvest mandrake is during the full moon between Easter and Ascension Day. . . . The plant is addressed as . . . 'Very honorable Empress Mandrake, I honor you with bread, with salt, and bow to you. Give me your clothes, cleanse me, purify me, free me of all magic. Make it so that I remain clean and thus radiate like washed and sieved silver, like the Mother of God, who brought me into the world.' (*142*) (**AWARENESS/SPIRITUALITY**)

The magician Agrippa (1486-1563) recounts the Jewish legend surrounding the mandrake root's excavation as described by the first century historian Josephus [*Wars of the Jews, book vii, cap. vi*]:

> It is namely of a fire-red color (**RED**) and gives off a glow at night, but . . . it is very difficult to obtain, for it avoids the hands and eyes of one who reaches for it and does not stand still until it is sprinkled with the urine of a menstruating woman. But even then, the root cannot be ripped out without danger, for it instantaneously greets the person who pulls it out with death if he is not protected by an amulet of the same root. (**FEAR**) For this reason, those who do not possess such an amulet must dig up the earth around it in a circle, tie a dog to it with a rope then leave immediately. Struggling to free itself, the dog pulls out the root and then dies in the place of his master. Now anyone can take the root in his hands without danger. (*138*)

Each legend Rätsch cites warns that if the mandrake "is not harvested according to . . . [certain] rules, its magical properties will turn against the person who pulled it from the earth" (*141*). (**ASSERTIVE**) Likewise, the root has the power to bless the one who excavates it properly. In Grimm's *German Tales* we read: "If he now questions the mandrake, he [it] will answer, revealing future and secret things concerning his welfare and prosperity" (*142*). (**OTHERWORLDLY**) (**COMMUNICATION**)

People in various parts of the world today still use and sell the mandrake root. In *The Fascinating World of the Nightshades* Charles B. Heiser, Jr. says: "In China mandrake root is still regarded as a powerful medicine, and reportedly, there are still 'artists' there who make a business of reshaping roots into a human form" (*136*).

In German-speaking areas mandrake roots serve as *atzmanns*:

> An atzmann may be carved from a genuine or false mandrake root, or may be formed from clay, wax, gruel, menstrual blood, head and pubic hair, and sometimes even from feces. The figure is given a human shape and is intended to represent the beloved

man or woman, or the rival man or woman. Whatever happens to the atzmann is said to also happen to the person that it represents. If the atzmann is loved, then its likeness will love its possessor. If it is tortured with nails or fire, then its likeness is also tortured or killed. (*Rätsch, 142*) (**VIOLENCE/TORTURE**)

These darker themes haunt the mandrake's history. The "hand of glory," derived from the French *'main de glorie'* or *'mandrogore'* and related to the legend of the mandrake, was a tool of the burglars' trade. This magical torch, believed to render the victim motionless, mirrored the narcotic effect of the mandrake. Formulas and instructions for making the hand of glory were in *Petit Albert*, supposedly written by Albertus Magnus, a great medieval scholar and magician, under another name. In it the reader is instructed to: "Take the hand of one who has been hanged, or strangled, dry it. . . . When thoroughly dry, sprinkle the hand with salt and a number of other ingredients . . . and wrap it in a coffin-pall. Then make a taper of virgin wax, anoint it with various fantastic oils and fats. Fix the taper between the fingers of the dried hand. The light of the taper will paralyze completely the faculties both mental and physical of everybody who comes within its influence" (*Williams*). (**DEFORMITY/PROSTHESIS**) Use of this tool went on into the nineteenth century (*Rudgley, 163*).

Richard Miller refers to Porta's *Natural Magick* [1658]: "A potion containing henbane, mandrake, stramonium, and belladonna was drunk to make a man act like a beast" (*103*). "In one hallucination, [called] lycanthropy, the person imagines himself turning into a wolf" (*Duke, 161*). (**ANIMALS**) Other hallucinations illustrate a profound sense of derangement, fear of impending death, and loss of memory. (**FORGETTING**) M. Grieve cites the sixteenth century herbalist William Turner: " 'They that smell too much of the apples become dum. . . If taken out of measure, by and by sleep ensueth and a great lousing of the streyngthe with a forgetfulness' "(*3*).

Grieve also notes: "In small doses it was employed by the Ancients in maniacal cases" (*2*). (**MENTAL ILLNESS**) Shakespeare uses the popular beliefs surrounding the mandrake root for dramatic purposes in many of his plays: "What with loathsome smells / And shrieks like mandrakes torn out of the earth / That living mortals, hearing them, run mad" (*Romeo and Juliet, 4.3*); and "have we eaten on the insane root that takes the reason prisoner" *(Macbeth, 1.3)*?

William Emboden writes in his book *Narcotic Plants*:

> The mandrake, having a root about a foot in length and sometimes branched so as to suggest the body of a man, would, of course, be the herb without equal. . . . If the root

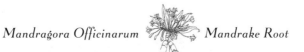

Mandragora Officinarum   *Mandrake Root*

did not conform to the shape of a man or a woman, it would be carved by charlatans to take on such an aspect. When the market was low, these same quacks would seek a surrogate, such as *Bryonia dioica*, and sell it to the unsuspecting victim. (**CONCEALMENT**) (**CHEATED/RIPPED OFF**) It was not uncommon to drill small holes over the surface of such a root and implant millet seeds. The root was then buried until the grains sprouted, after which time the whole thing was dried and had the aspect of a hairy little man. Both male and female forms were carved, and some of the females were shown to have children in their arms.... For the childless woman it was said that these roots used as talismans or amulets could overcome barrenness. (*10*)

People of antiquity knew the mandrake to be a love charm, intoxicant, and stimulant to sexual desire. "In homes, during this time, small oil lamps burned before the desiccated roots of mandrakes" (*Emboden 11*). In the Old Testament, Rachel "lends" her husband for a night, in exchange for "love apples" meant to cure her infertility (*Gen. 30:14-20*). The Greeks believed the satyrs used it in their revelries, and Rätsch writes: "In ancient Egypt the mandrake was considered an aphrodisiac and an erotic symbol . . . (**SEXUALITY**) often depicted as a gift of love between a man and a woman" (*Rätsch, 138*).

A wine made with mandrake, attributed with very inebriating and aphrodisiac powers, enjoyed great popularity. (**INTOXICATION**) The Papyrus of Ebers, the oldest of all the world's collections of medicinal recipes that has been preserved, contains a number of references concerning the use of mandrake. One recipe recommends a decoction made from mandrake fruit, milk, honey, 'herbs of the fields,' and wine. (*136*)

To this day, the cult of the mandrake lives on in Romania, where it "is considered an erotic plant and love agent . . . [possessing] magical properties for increasing . . . love (fertility) and prosperity" (*142*).

Mandragora stands out as the most complex, confusing, and fascinating substance of all my provings. It took four dedicated homeopaths a full year of intense work to study this proving and delineate the themes and rubrics. The historical, botanical, medical, and folklore research began only after the completion of that work. Unlike most of the other substances proved in this book, we in the U.S. have little experience with Mandragora, pharmacologically or with the mythologies surrounding it. We were pleased to discover through this research the strong congruence between the provings and the plant, its history and folklore. I cite many experts in the field in order to provide avenues for continued research and to broaden our general understanding of this multifaceted substance.

Mandragora Themes
Mandrake Root

- *Confusion/Forgetting*
- *Mental Illness*
- *Communication/No Communication*
- *Intoxication*
- *Numbness/No Emotion*
- *Organized/Disorganized*
- *Violence/Torture*
- *Fear/Fearlessness in the Presence of Danger*
- *Harassed/Persecuted*
- *Cheated/Ripped Off*
- *Assertive*
- *Sex*
- *Animals*
- *Medicine/Hospitals/Tests*
- *Deformity/Prosthesis*
- *Mechanical Failure*
- *Otherworldly*
- *Awareness/Spirituality*
- *Women*
- *Hair/Wig/Appearance*
- *Colors, Especially Red*
- *Concealment*
- *Water*
- *Mountains/Rocks*
- *Travel/Vehicles*
- *Gatherings*
- *Music/Singing*
- *Exotic Places*

Confusion/Forgetting

#10 My mind is really unfocused and it has been like this for weeks. Whenever I talk about this I totally lose it. I feel like I'm having a nervous breakdown. I can't think clearly. I can't focus. I really haven't attributed this to the remedy. My life for the last year has been really stressful.

#1 Thoughts are scattered. Difficulty focusing, worse in the evening. . . . Driving home at night through the fog, reminded me of the "cobweb" of fogginess of my mind.

#10 . . . The main thing is I haven't been able to think clearly or transfer my thoughts to paper. I haven't been able to write in my journal. My daughter helped me transcribe the bits of paper that I wrote on.

#9 . . . Forgot remedy in Phoenix. Forgot to call N. . . . Poor sense of time. Lost track of it. Late getting ready for evening out, really rushed. . . . Difficulty remembering names of places, evening.

#10 I've been forgetful. I can't remember names of people, things people told me. My scenario is my house: getting up and getting ready doesn't take a rocket scientist to get going in the morning. If I didn't get the umbrella immediately I would forget. All of a sudden I would be in the bedroom unable to remember what I was doing.

#9 Forgot to pack overnight clothes, general personal care items. Not even a book. Follow up on several small details.

#8 Experienced difficulty with remembering people's names. Thought that was funny. . . . Thoughts were fuzzy. Hard to concentrate at work. Had strong desire to go take my constitutional remedy to "feel normal."

#2 Dream: . . . Dreamt I must write that this was about female energy. In the dream I get a card and write this down. . . . When I wake up I am relieved that I wrote it down and then I realize that I didn't write it.

Mandragora Officinarum   *Mandrake Root*

#6 Dream: Traveling with a large group to a campground. We have boats and kids, many people I do not know. Lots of confusion. My children are there and receive gifts from their dad. I have to hide them. Other children are winning contests. All are confused. Mixed in all this is meeting new people, all with children. I am just floating around in this chaos. Relaxed and happy.

#10 Last day of five week course with twelve- and thirteen-year-olds. Found course difficult and seems chaotic in our classes. I have usually loved working with teens —never so frustrating.

Mental Illness

#1 Again woke up early, about 5:45 a.m. Was lying in bed when telephone rang at 6:15 a.m. It was my youngest brother, who recently had sent me an angry letter falsely accusing me of intentionally breaking his sofa (when I visited him) and of arrogantly lecturing to him. . . . He seemed manic. That was very upsetting. He said, "Let's call a truce." He went on with pressured speech, was hyper-verbal. Was talking inappropriately about his patients. About sexually coming on to him but afraid he would be sued. I had to be careful what to say because he would feel attacked.

#2 Dream: . . . in the house with other women, my sister and niece. She is anorexic and manic depressive.

#4 Energy unusual, friend wondering if I may be bipolar.

#8 . . . Cried . . . ended when I found all these pictures of my brother (he committed suicide when he was 18 years old) that I had never seen.

#10 My mind is really unfocused and it has been like this for weeks. Whenever I talk about this I totally lose it. I feel like I'm having a nervous breakdown. I can't think clearly. I can't focus. . . .

#10 One day I was home alone all day. That afternoon I had a dark heavy feeling. Depressed and dark and heavy. I thought to myself, "This is why people commit suicide." I wasn't hopeless, the feeling was just there. That was the only day I felt that feeling I had when my husband died. I had a depression on top of everything. . . . Did not feel suicidal but afraid of feeling that way. . . . I'm ready to see a psychiatrist. . . .

#10 Dream: . . . Her sister E. (who is schizophrenic) was there.

#10 <u>Huge mood swings.</u>

Mandragora Officinarum *Mandrake Root*

Communication/No Communication

#6 Dream: In a car with the H. family. It isn't the right car, but they won't listen. I know it is not right but am frustrated because I cannot get that across.

#11 . . . A man approached us and started a conversation with me. I couldn't follow a thing he was saying.

#12 . . . There was a wedding. I was trying to convey a message to the groom to look down at his tie or something without really coming out and saying it (while he was getting his picture taken). He wasn't really getting it, which was a cause of mirth.

Intoxication

#2 Feel dizzy, almost intoxicated. My eyes see very clearly.

#11 Dream: I was totally stoned (which I don't do). . . . I couldn't focus. . . . Being stoned, I felt unsure about my ability to drive well.

#7 Dream: . . . They were smoking cigarettes or marijuana. . . . I had a sick feeling.

#8 Dream: . . . There was a brewery there, passing out free beer. Beer was very thirst-quenching—it tasted different than regular beer. This was a perfect tasting brew. It was made from this special water and it had plant juices mixed in.

#8 Dream: . . . The table next to us has four white people who were very rowdy and seemed drunk. . . . The four of us were sipping some wine.

#10 Dream: Went to a party with friends. . . . I came down in morning to find that people had overdone it. C., my ex, was very hung over and had been throwing up. . . . Then I am with same friends driving—the police are chasing us. . . . I took his stash (of what?) and stuffed it in a cupboard.

#11 . . . Suggested I take Sabadilla. I went in search. Turned my house upside down. Felt like a drug addict looking for a fix.

#11 Dream: The principal of my daughter's high school called to tell me she had been noticed being "under the influence" (of drugs) at school, and she was failing classes.

#10 Dream: . . . We went into a store to buy tequila—there were about 50 brands.

Numbness/No Emotion

#1 Perhaps more emotionally distant. I felt less connected, empathic, than is my norm while speaking with brother on telephone. . . . Emotional flattening. Shallow feeling. I usually love riding my bicycle. I didn't have my usual joy. Felt "I've got to get there." Functional. . . . I'm usually so in tune with my kids even when we're not in the same room. Son went upstairs to get dressed. He started to cry out. Normally I would have been there right away but I felt detached. Daughter got there first. Normally I would have felt the pain and been upset by it.

#10 Felt lack of excitement at news of my daughter being pregnant again—<u>NOT</u> natural response for me. . . . My daughter also said she felt I had been very detached in recent weeks. It seems that I did not care about her. I was not aware of this. . . .

#1 Dream: A reptile—perhaps a crocodile? I am the crocodile? A man has had his arm eaten by the crocodile, yet I am not horrified. Somehow he deserved it. I felt an emotional distance. Not really caring. Later I thought that was strange that I felt that he deserved it. An aggressive feeling.

#9 Dream: Friend L. wrote a play (saw movie *Beloved* last night, the play is very much like the movie). It is her first play. Someone saw her script and wanted to produce it in a small theater. . . . I plan to attend and in order for me to do so I need to have an epidural (I don't know why). Then I have to get myself there with paralyzed legs. Because my legs are so numb I have difficulty, through traffic, etc.

#10 Dream: . . . Someone has stuffed toilet paper into the vent on the floor. There is also a wad of paper on the wall that has feces on it. I am not grossed out, have seen it before.

#10 Dream: Scene in Laundromat. I was doing laundry and drying clothes in small drying compartments (not real dryers). I heard what sounded like a gunshot in another aisle. Three men were nudging each other like boxers in a ring. Feeling: not upset, just wondering what to do. I sensed that one of them had been shot by the other two. I could not run and was trying to figure out what to do. Climb in a washer and hide? Were they going to kill everyone there?

#12 Dream: . . . I was driving it next to the curb, and my passenger told me I almost ran over a baby that was lying on the curb. I said, "That's the way it goes in this city."

#6 Loss of sense of taste. Things are bland. Even candy isn't sweet.

Organized/Disorganized

#2 . . . Very efficient, good concentration, etc. (better than usual).

#3 Doing things that are waiting for months to be done . . . don't waste my time . . . very quick, clear thinking.

#8 Felt organized and clear-headed at work.

#9 Felt efficient, confident, not rushed. Very busy.

#10 . . . When I've been home I've had to be really organized and am easily disorganized. I've had to take care of the piles. I spent an afternoon cleaning out my closet. I don't do that sort of thing. All the blouses on one side, all the dresses on the other. I had many pressing things to do. I did the same thing with my pantry, and that was so unlike me.

#8 . . . Rearranged furniture and cleaned.

#12 Dream: . . . I was plotting my income growth, trying to see how I could have enough for retirement.

#1 . . . High energy but ungathered.

#1 Dream: I signed up for a class on flying an airplane. . . . It didn't seem very organized. I was very apprehensive, feared we would crash, that I would die, that I would never see my kids again. . . . The plane seemed to be flying very unevenly, accelerating then decelerating, leaving puffs of black smoke behind it, and flying too close to ground. It seemed we would get entangled in the branches of the trees.

#10 Dream: I was working at teaching hospital with my old medical staff. I got a page from Dr. B. asking if I was still going to come talk to them—the surgeons. I felt anxious that I hadn't remembered and was not prepared. I couldn't find his pager number and no one seemed to have it. I asked many, many people. I finally found a woman who had the number and she had done some kind of a security check on me to work at the facility.

#4 Awoke this morning very lost. Flitted around one thing to another in my office, no motivation, no direction.

#9 . . . We had to grab a quick breakfast rather than have a leisurely one. Had to give my order three times. Given the wrong change, moved three times to find comfortable place to sit. Just settled, busboy came by to sweep around us/under foot. I wanted to scream at him or push him away.

#10 . . . On Thursday I tried to pay attention to the dynamics and I think whenever there is chaos or disorganization I get really anxious. I think that is what I responded to in these kids. It drives me crazy to be with them.

#9 Dream: . . . I am throwing things together trying to find something I can wear that is suitable. The men arrive and I am caught not dressed, the bed unmade, the room strewn with clothes.

#10 Dream: . . . I was in the mountains . . . lots of snow. . . . I have flip-flops on, I am very disorganized but not worried about it. Not even after a train ran over one of my flip-flops.

#9 Forgot to pack overnight clothes, general personal care items. Not even a book.

#10 . . . I reached classmate who confirmed that proving meeting time had been changed. Felt that I <u>HAD</u> to be there. Made numerous calls to change my flight—would arrive at Hahnemann at 4:00 a.m. Made other calls regarding: my class, dog sitter, etc. Missed plane by five minutes. No other flights would get me there.

#11 . . . I went in search. Turned my house upside down. (Felt like a drug addict looking for a fix.)

Violence/Torture

#1 Dream: I'm in an apartment on the top floor of a building. I hear a gunshot, maybe a cry. . . . But he, too, suddenly has to disappear because of danger (guns?), and I can't follow.

#2 Dream: My sister and others . . . are to go to a meeting/training with the main teacher. The training has some title like "Aggression, Force, and Violence Necessary in the Future." She attends this and comes back and tells me that they were all trained to give torture and if necessary kill people—as the future was likely to become so dangerous and we would all be threatened. They were shown how to fix electrodes in people and give shocks—and other really horrible things.

#11 Dream: An older black woman and her companion were walking down the hall in an institution—she was sweet and kind. Then these two people who were wanting to escape encountered them. They had knives and were going to kill her. So she said, "Ok, stab me." One of the people threw a knife in her chest which hit but didn't really penetrate and then she knew she had a chance and started running. She had been so brave even though she was so frightened.

#10 Dream: Scene in a boxing ring. One fighter received heavy blow and was stunned, wobbly, tried to fight it, his body could not—his brain? He went down on one knee and fell on to the mat. I was thinking what a brutal sport it is that we take so much pleasure in watching such insult to someone.

#4 Dream: . . . Finishing a dinner in someone's home and being led downstairs to den where the couple had set up a little theatre where they showed slides of fetuses/babies who had been aborted and buried, founded by this group of Right-to-Lifers. Slides showed frontal views of bodies curled into balls with heads bowed into knees, armed folded at sides, fists. . . . Purpose was to show the tragedy, all these babies unearthed. I was noticing that this couple had lots of weapons showcased, collection of handguns and machine guns, antiques. Feeling was that I was trapped by conservatives, no debate or arguing of any points being made, just observing and making mental notes.

#10 Dream: Working at hospital, patient angry with me. Followed me to the basement... don't know what happened. I shot him and thought he was dead.

Mandragora Officinarum   *Mandrake Root*

There was a lot of bleeding from the head wound. I was calm, started to call security and realized he was still alive. He asked why I had shot him.

#11 I've been on my own for the last two days and doing fine. But when my poor husband came home, I became snappy and irritable. I felt as though I could bite him. He actually put out his arm in jest (as we were both acknowledging my odd mood) and I really had a strong impulse to bite him hard!

#11 Dream: . . . Then we were in the back of the building; there was this dark foreboding pond. These black men were being thrown into it in these sacks. If they could work themselves loose and swim out then they were free; otherwise they were dead. We saw one die and one live. Awful.

Fear/Fearlessness in the Presence of Danger

#1 Dream: . . . old military cargo type planes . . . I was very apprehensive, feared we would crash, that I would die, that I would never see my kids again. It took off unexpectedly while I was in the airplane lavatory. I ran back to where the seats were, holding onto the seat backs to keep myself from falling. . . . I was really scared.

#11 Dream: . . . we were walking away from a high seacoast and realized we were going to get hit by a huge wave. I was terrified we were going to get dragged in. We ran. It hit but we were ok. But another one was coming. I was afraid it would take my husband. Woke up scared.

#6 Dream: My youngest son is riding with me in a car, I keep having to ask him to step on the brake because my hands are full. Even though I knew it was dangerous.

#7 Dream: . . . I see suspicious headlights driving on the property. I feel someone is trespassing with bad intentions. I realize my mother is alone in the house and may be in danger. I go off to investigate the possible intruder. Feeling of possible threat.

#7 Dream: Frightening. My daughter ran out of her bedroom and said someone was trying to come in the window and get her. I went in and saw a shadow and the dream ended. The feeling was fear and having to meet the danger.

#9 Dream: . . . A wild mountain cat the size of a small dog is in the room with a couple of other pets and a few children and some adults. I am very distressed. I want someone to take the wild mountain cat out of the room before it hurts or attacks someone. It is menacing. Some woman walks by and casually pets it thinking it is domestic. I think the children are in danger.

#10 Dream: I was cross-country skiing up to top of mountain. . . . Then I was surrounded by lions. I had to lie motionless to hide—very afraid and worried about people behind me on the trail.

#11 Dream: . . . I was being driven in a car by a short Mexican man and his wife and a friend of mine. They were all engaged in a conversation. The driver was controlling the car from the back seat. He was so short I wondered how he could see. His wife was in the front seat. I guess she didn't know how to drive. He was driving so fast through all this busy crazy traffic. I kept watching these almost fatal accidents.

#10 Dream: Scene in laundromat. I was doing laundry in and drying clothes in small drying compartments (not real dryers). I heard what sounded like a gunshot in another aisle. Three men were nudging each other like boxers in a ring. Feeling: not upset, just wondering what to do. I sensed that one of them had been shot by the other two. I could not run and was trying to figure out what to do. Climb in a washer and hide? Were they going to kill everyone there?

#5 Dream: About going fast. I was driving with my sister in a car on this big bridge/hill. Went down really fast. She was scared and I was exhilarated.

#11 . . . I was crossing a bridge. This woman was there with a board over a gorge and she tipped the board so that I fell into the gorge. Awareness of falling knowing that I was going to die. No fear but wishing that I wasn't going to die. Empathy with the woman who had killed me.

#2 Dream: Driving in a car with my kids. I don't know if I'm driving or someone else, but whatever it's really dangerous driving. Squeezing between two trucks going really fast, and fast around corners. I'm more disturbed than scared. We go to a seaside holiday place on the Mediterranean. We all go straight into the sea. It's night and the sea is very dark and quite warm. We all get pulled out quite far by a current. I shout to the children, "Be careful, it's a strong current," but with none of the fear that I would expect to have. . . . Not feeling fear in the dreams where normally I would do so.

#8 Dream: I was eating with some friends and these sharks kept swimming around us—like dogs begging for food. Everything was blue—no fear of sharks and remember thinking one of them had lost a tooth. In reality I do not like sharks at all!

#2 Dreams of scary situations but I am not really scared. A kind of lack of emotion in a way. Maybe it is more low key. I felt a balanced state. Funny spiritual thing with fear and danger, but being ok.

Harassed/Persecuted

#1 At the Health Center where I work, I was asked to re-do a form explaining need for granting medical leave for a student with chronic fatigue. On the form I had written "see attached progress note." I was told that this was insufficient and that the student had not signed a release. I asked for the chart and easily found the medical release note (and plenty of documentation). I felt harassed.

#1 Dream: . . . I notice that people are taking my *Science News* . . . using them for a project I'm not invited to participate in. I grab them (like a child who takes back his toys) and bring them back to my room. . . . The feeling was . . . exclusion from the group, falsely accused.

#1 I put an ad in a local paper as a homeopath. I got a call from someone who accused me of advertising that I was selling health insurance. I couldn't believe it. . . . I was so shaken I went and looked in a newspaper at my ad. Fortunately it still said homeopathy!

#4 One very irate mom, not interested in my reassurance that her child had only a virus. Couple of callers angry at me this weekend, unwarranted, very unusual.

#7 . . . Feeling persecuted, put down, not cared for.

#8 Dream: . . . a very pricey and stuffy restaurant. The four of us and the four rowdy people were "plants" to see if this restaurant discriminated against people of color. . . . the restaurant manager was clearly perturbed by the rowdy ones and hovered around us. . . . He was overly attentive and did not give us time to enjoy the food.

Cheated/Ripped Off

#3 There was a situation where I promised a friend I would buy them a camera. I went to Fisherman's Wharf—an earlier time there I was cheated. This time I was determined not to do it again. This guy gave me a hard sell. At the moment of paying, he tried to raise the price!

#7 My wife took my daughter to the orthopedic doctor today. . . . He literally spent two minutes with her, and decided to cast her arm without explaining anything to my wife. . . .The bill will probably be $300–$400. I feel resentful that being a practitioner of acupuncture and homeopathy, I have to work a full day to earn what this doctor makes in five minutes. . . . Even though the state has put me through vigorous requirements to be licensed . . . health insurance coverage for my services is extremely minimal. This makes it difficult to earn a decent living. The feeling is anger, resentment, ripped off.

#5 Dream: . . . I stood in a line to buy a swimsuit for $100. . . . I put on the swimsuit and the salesgirl told me it was $300. I felt they were ripping me off, so I punched her, gave $100 and wore the swimsuit as I left the store.

#7 . . . Today was an unpleasant day. . . . Two patients did not show up for their appointment. Two patients called at the last moment to re-schedule their appointments. . . . I was angry with my Maker—I was cursing God. I try to do the right thing always, I do my best work—why should I have to put up with this bullshit.

#5 Dream: I go to have a pedicure and they make me stand in a machine that takes a picture of your body. Then they scan it, three different outputs, and want me to pay $75 to read each evaluation. I am so mad, so indignant. I keep saying, "Just do the pedicure!" Finally I leave in disgust.

Assertive

#11 Dream: There was gravel in the hallway. I asked the janitor if I could have his broom and dustpan. He said it was against the rules. I grabbed it from him saying, "Don't be ridiculous, someone is going to slip and get hurt."

#1 Dream: . . . I notice that people are taking my *Science News* (a subscription magazine), using them for a project I'm not invited to participate in. I grab them (like a child who takes back his toys) and bring them back to my room.

#2 More assertive in circumstances with a particular person I can be wimpy with. I said, "No, this is what I want." Then I noticed that usually I am self-apologetic. A voice says, "You don't have to be like that." My voice dropped and I felt I was stopping a habitual attitude. I was more assertive with patients, reassuring them that they would be better.

#1 Brought my new used car to mechanic to fix horn. He had said beforehand that he could work with the extended warranty. But when I came to pick up the car they said they hadn't received pre-authorization, implied that I may have to pay. Wouldn't let me drive away until they were sure they were going to receive payment from insurance. I became angry and said, "I feel like you're holding me hostage." They relented and gave me the key.

#6 Dream: I was at a spiritual gathering where each person was going to say something important. One friend was not allowed to speak. I insisted she be allowed to speak.

#12 . . . Waking dream: Someone was asserting the tire shop had or hadn't done something to the tires with a block of iron containing chlorine. We were supposed to have a group protest.

#3 Jehovah people ring on my door. I can tell them very clearly and at the beginning that I respect them and I am not interested. Incredible, normally I would need a lot more time to tell them diplomatically that I am not interested. . . . More impatient, more assertive.

Sex

#9 Dream: . . . There is an older man. . . . He has suggested to me that we will be lovers. . . . There are also two younger men living in the house . . . sleeping in the same bed, yet act more like brothers. They are involved in some playful seduction with me. The older man knows about it . . . he has secrets of love making I have not yet been introduced to. . . . I am considering whether I want to have sex with him to get in his good graces or if I just want to have sex with him or not.

#5 Dream: . . . My husband came up to me and said, "No sex." I said ok, turned away, and left. He chased after me, grabbed me, and kissed me. We decide to have a "high school" relationship and just make out. That made me feel really good. That's all I wanted anyway—to be hugged and kissed.

#1 . . . Was talking inappropriately about his patients. About sexually coming on to them but afraid he would be sued.

#10 Dream: . . . Young girl with me . . . Not sure if I was a man or a woman, or who this girl was. I made love to her, kissing and fondling her. I was experiencing both sides. Wondering whether to use a condom, but then it was over and I was holding a capillary tube that said the test was negative—I wasn't pregnant. I wondered if she was a prostitute.

#2 Dreams: . . . Robin Williams was there pretending to be a woman. . . . Dreamt I must write that this was about female energy.

#12 Dream: . . . A nurse was . . . helping me breathe oxygen or something. After a while I noticed her hand was on my genitals. As attention shifted there, she started literally beating me off. Each time she would whip it, a little bit of semen would leak out, spraying over my face and everything. We were interrupted by a man . . .

#11 Dream: A mysterious woman, beautiful, tall very unusual looking was having an affair.

Animals

#10 Dream: Scene—beautiful red, roan-colored horses in a valley running, then swimming. My horse was white with a black trimmed mane . . . swam up to where I was sitting . . . was very loving, nudging me. I was tempted to jump on its back, but instead I dove deep into the water to see if it would dive also. We played for a while. It was a powerful swimmer and would retrieve objects that I threw.

#1 My dog and cat and I seem more connected. I'm more empathic with them (served them dinner before I scavenged food for myself).

#11 We have raccoon problems like crazy. Just had a fish-and-game trapper here. Gonna trap 'dem coons! Set the trap, and in fifteen minutes we caught our first raccoon. I can hear all the other raccoons sounding with each other. Poor things.

#2 Wakened at 3:00 a.m. by one of the kittens. He wants to play, and we stay up for two hours.

#12 Dream: . . . A sheep crosses the road, just narrowly missing getting hit by a car. There are three or four dead sheep lying next to the embankment.

#10 . . . [My daughter] also shared how out of character it was for me to bring a stray dog home, but I acted like it was not unusual. My voice sounded so sweet when I'd talk about Dog. I am now struck by how Dog has followed me everywhere in house—constantly nudging my hand.

#8 Resting quietly in bed about 9:30 p.m. while reading and all animals in bed with me (except birds)—heard garbage can fall over again! Went out and yelled at the dog in the garbage. "Dog" stood up and looked at me. It was a black bear with white spot on its chest! Then another larger black bear appeared. Then a third little bear came up to the bigger ones. I ran inside and felt really 'blown away'. It felt totally surreal. Watched the three bears from my window with my cat. All the animals were completely quiet. I called the Sheriff's Department and wanted to know if someone could just drive by and scare the bears. No one could. The bears finally left.

#7 Dream: I caught an Orca (whale) and it was tied to a rope. The whale took off and was spinning . . .

#9 Dream: . . . I then find myself back at the theater parlor. A wild mountain cat the size of a small dog is in the room with a couple of other pets and a few children and some adults.

Mandragora Officinarum   Mandrake Root

#8 . . . Just wanted to stay in bed with my two dogs and two cats. Had moved the birdcage with my two birds right by my bed. I wanted them to be close to me. Felt like I wanted all my animals around me. They seemed to like that. Animals were more affectionate and clinging to me. I liked it. . . . Did not go to Halloween Party. Felt like I did not want to socialize with people. Rather be home with my animals. Felt a distance with people.

#10 Dream: Scene from an old house we used to live in. . . I was out in the wooden addition, pulled up planks on floor and saw a huge snake. I tried to reach for his tail and he snapped at me. Then I realized that he was in water. A much larger snake with orange and red on its neck appeared, and it changed into a large shaggy cat or pig or sheep-like creature—not sure which. I was not afraid. It climbed out of the water and went to the back of the room. We opened the back door and let it out—then shooed it away. It seemed like a cat then. Another one climbed out, my younger brother put it out the same way. I ran outside and looked across the property as these creatures moved slowly eastward.

#7 Dream: I was treating a patient and told him about the proving. He fell into a deep sleep. He had a dream that his sheep were in danger. He is a police officer. He felt like a shepherd that needed to protect his sheep.

#8 My cat woke me up meowing and meowing like crazy. This was so unusual—as she is a very quiet kitty. She just wanted me to pet her and give her attention.

#1 Dream: A reptile—perhaps a crocodile? I am the crocodile? A man has had his arm eaten by the crocodile, yet I am not horrified. Somehow he deserved it.

#10 Dream: Me standing with back to mirror; I get a glimpse of my face. Am I wearing a mask of a wolf?

#8 Dream: Mice everywhere, cute little mice with big heads and little bodies. Mice had an awful lot of teeth. I did not want to kill the tiny mice—had to gently sweep them into newspaper in order to carry them out. It was spring outside. One mouse hid inside my bed and I could not get him.

#11 Got home from the coast to find our fish bowl half empty, with the two fish gone. I presume eaten by either a cat or raccoon. Very upsetting.

#10 Dream: . . . I was surrounded by lions. I had to lie motionless to hide—very afraid and worried about people behind me on the trail.

Medicine/Hospitals/Tests

#12 Dream: . . .This gave her a chill that presumably led to her death. Then I was in a kind of field hospital with lots of little white tents. A nurse was putting camphor around my mouth and nose, and helping me breathe oxygen or something. . . .

#10 Dream: I was working at teaching hospital with my old medical staff. I got a page from Dr. B. asking if I was still going to come talk to them—the surgeons. . .

#10 Dream: I am medical personnel waiting for a patient. There are three to four people assisting a young man. Everyone seems to be having great difficulty. I approach and grabbed his right arm. I pulled off his prosthesis and saw a stump. He had a motorcycle accident some years earlier. I was living in a small town. A call came for all medical personnel to report for emergency. I was with EMS.

#10 Dream: . . . Wondering whether to use a condom, but then it was over and I was holding a capillary tube that said the test was negative—I wasn't pregnant.

#9 Dream: . . . I plan to attend and in order for me to do so I need to have an epidural. . .

Mandragora Officinarum   *Mandrake Root*

Deformity/Prosthesis

#9 Dream: Friend L. wrote a play. . . . I plan to attend and in order for me to do so I need to have an epidural (I don't know why). Then I have to get myself there with paralyzed legs. . . . I am attempting to make my way to the chair to sit when I realize I am the only person who has had an epidural to come to the play. I am confused. I thought we would all have one.

#11 Dream: . . . my good friend came in the room. I looked up at him and he seemed so tall. He was maybe fifteen feet tall. Very strange. Such distortions.

#8 . . . Instantly I glanced at my friend R. and he was covered with feathers and a beak and I was repulsed.

#10 Dream: I was in a bathroom and had two babies' heads, only the heads, and sensed that I had done something wrong by not creating whole babies, so I stuck the heads in my bag.

#1 Dream: Genital mutilation.

#9 Dream: . . . A patient and her family are somewhere in the house, she has delivered. . . . the midwife exposes the fact that she has eleven toes on one foot and something like eight on the other. They are web toes and small extra digits. The meaning of this has to do with something about babies being born with anomalies and how they can be accepted. Her family did not know until this time that she had abnormal toes.

#8 Dream: . . . I went to check on my male friend. . . . He was lying down and I pulled his arm—it came off—it was made of wax. The whole body was wax. I was upset and started to cry. . . . His spirit had just left his body temporarily.

#11 Dream: Some people put together a Christmas scene in their backyard using two very tiny deer. They were alive, real and eight inches tall. They just sat there and watched us as we walked by. I was charmed and amazed.

#10 Dream: I am medical personnel waiting for a patient. . . . I approach and grabbed his right arm. I pulled off his prosthesis and saw a stump. He had a motorcycle accident some years earlier.

#9 Dream: A woman has a small restaurant and Bed & Breakfast in Point Richmond. . . . She is behind a high half-door. I can only see her head and shoulders. She has big hair. . . . she comes from behind the counter/half-door and she is a tiny, dwarf-like person.

Mechanical Failure

#1 Brought my new used car to mechanic to fix horn.

#4 Computer pointer failure, had to turn off computer to reboot without saving info, lost important letters and seven days of proving journal. Spent rest of day trying to reconstruct data.

#5 I just realized in the past few days four major things that went wrong in the office after I took the remedy.

#5 There was a plumbing water leak today in the office. Soaked the carpet. Had to turn the water off for the whole building.

#5 . . . We had to eventually evacuate our building in the afternoon due to an ammonia leak from a chemical tank.

#8 Video machine broke—tape got stuck in it.

#8 Computer completely messed up. Frustrated as can't check and answer e-mails.

#10 I bought batteries for my smoke alarm and for my remote control for my car. None of the batteries have lasted more than a day.

#10 Dream: Cast iron pan melted that I was washing while doing the dishes . . . .

#10 Endless computer problems—spent hours on phone with computer technical service.

#12 Dream: . . . She has trouble using the boss's phone; there seems to be a key missing.

#12 Waking dream: Seem to be having trouble logging in to a website.

Otherworldly

#8 Spent afternoon looking through my father's pictures and mementos. Cried . . . ended when I found all these pictures of my brother (he committed suicide when he was eighteen years old) that I had never seen. Later made the connection of the "wax-man" in my dream with my brother. The feeling was he is not coming back tonight but I will see him again. Theme of spirit-world going back and forth.

#11 Dream: A mysterious woman, beautiful, tall, very unusual looking, was having an affair. Later I saw her with few clothes on and she was short. Maybe four feet tall. Her body was odd, almost non-human. I couldn't believe my eyes. It was as if something was off but I couldn't place it.

#8 I ran inside and felt totally "blown away." It felt totally surreal.

#10 Dream: . . . I woke up feeling that I was traveling within my own body???

#8 . . . Felt like I was in a bardo state—a state of nothingness and luminosity. Got home. Listened to a tape of *Tibetan Book of the Dead*.

#11 Dream: There was a knowingness that the world as we know it was coming to an end. We knew we had to stock up on water and essentials.

#8 Overall I felt like I didn't want to be here. I'd rather be on the other side because it is prettier, nicer and more fun.

#8 Dream: . . . I remember thinking we had crossed into the astral world and that was why the colors were so rich . . .

Awareness/Spirituality

#2 Dream: . . . All night I am aware of being at a spiritual retreat, and with people who are aware and guiding.

#10 Dream: Woke at 1:30 a.m. with vivid picture of an altar-like setting with candles burning. The thought was, "Oh this is what this remedy is about—Spirituality??"

#4 Today I feel more centered—I am more aware about a lot of things: about the bigger picture of the world, the universe, how all is one, about life, about friends surrounding me, about their worries, about their friendships, my life, my inner voice, my ego which is in my way, my path, my mission, my fragility and vulnerability, my body.

#3 Went to a presentation about Yogananda and the Self-Realization Fellowship. Inspiring. . . . Energetic, empowered, open minded—more spiritual, meditation. . . . It was a very inspiring day, powerful women speaking about spirituality . . .

#2 . . . as though I had been meditating all night. . . . as though I had been meditating with awareness and deep well-being. . . . Feeling of deep well-being.

#4 . . . I woke up with the dream of an oil lamp that was given to me and I was going to use it at a spiritual talk. It would be private at her table. I never got to see the speaker. Yesterday I opened a catalog and saw the lamp of my dream.

#4 Dream: I was at a spiritual gathering . . .

Women

#2 Dreams: Large public lavatory with six toilets of stainless steel all were blocked with tampons, and there was blood all over the floor. Robin Williams was there pretending to be a woman. I kept flushing and was embarrassed trying to get the blockage down. Dreamt I must write that this was about female energy. In the dream I get a card and write this down. The dream continues in the house with other women, my sister and niece.

#9 Dream: A midwife's family home. She has a birthing room in her house.

#3 Dream: . . . I am with a woman friend. She is lesbian, she is very lovely and caring to me. . . . It is my mother's house; it seems to be closed in the front. . . . She told me she was there. . . . A group of girls appear; they are looking at some flowers outside of the house. Peaceful feeling. Now the house is open, my mother is there.

#4 Dream: Interviewing old ladies each in her own home, all with Southern drawls, just matter-of-fact info about themselves.

#5 Dream: I played peacemaker for the girls in the office at a hotel room.

#12 Dream: . . . Best part was returning home and seeing my daughter. . . . Before that, I had been to a family reunion where they started talking about a matriarch of the family, named Mary, saying she had been "flexible," implying she may have had one or more affairs.

#6 Dream: About grandmother. . . . She is peaceful and I am. I never dreamed about her before. She has been dead for ten years.

#8 Dream: . . . I went outside and this very nice older lady who was dressed in Victorian style (blue dress with lace collar) talked to me.

#10 Dream: Young girl with me at a house I did not recognize. Not sure if I was a man or a woman or who this girl was. I made love to her, kissing and fondling her.

#10 . . . My daughter also said she felt I had been very detached in recent weeks. It seems that I did not care about her. I was not aware of this.

#11 Dream: An older black woman and her companion were walking down the hall in an institution—she was sweet and kind.

Hair/Wig/Appearance

#2 Dream: . . . There is a party planned—I don't much want to go, but it is part of the retreat. I wear a bright, pink, long dress, and a wig all different shades of pink. My own hair is tumbled in a high ponytail of dark chestnut ringlets around the top of the wig. I think it looks weird but am aware it's just my vanity and it doesn't matter. The same situation recurs with the variation that my hair is short (and no wig). I remember getting it cut but am surprised he cut it so short. Again I am a bit upset but feel "never mind, it's just an aspect of my body."

#5 Dream: Going to a friend's house to get my haircut. My hair is bright red. It's a big party and a lot of my friends are there. All are drinking beer and smoking. Everyone is getting their hair done. A new male hairdresser cuts mine.

#6 Dream: . . . We are driving along, I am rinsing the soap out of my hair. . .

#10 Dream: I stop at a shop late at night. A woman is putting on makeup. I look in the mirror and I have face powder, red lipstick and black eye makeup. It is very unnatural. The blush-on is not spread out evenly so I take one of her brushes and decide to steal it, except it is very long, a couple of feet. I stick it down the front of my dress, but it sticks out so I try to conceal it with my coat. At some point I decide this is silly to be doing this and I put the brush back down on the counter.

Colors, Especially Red

#3 Image of a white bird

#6 Dream: . . . House just painted. The color and feel of the house was peaceful, cheerful, light and pastel colors.

#8 Dream: . . . I remember thinking we had crossed into the astral world and that was why the colors were so rich . . .

#8 Dream: . . . Everything was blue.

#11 Dream: . . . art work on the ground . . . with that bright red paint. It's almost an orange/red.

#10 Dream: Scene—beautiful red, roan-colored horses in a valley running, then swimming.

#8 Dream: . . . The man and I went out and bought a motorcycle—a red Honda Gold Wing.

#10 Dream: . . . I look in the mirror and I have face powder, red lipstick, and black eye makeup.

#10 Dream: . . . A much larger snake with orange and red on its neck appeared . . .

#8 Dream: . . . We then were driving through red rock like in Sedona, Arizona.

Concealment

#8 Dream: . . . The four of us and the four rowdy people were "plants" to see if this restaurant discriminated against people of color.

#10 Dream: . . . the police are chasing us. All of a sudden E. took off, so the cops chased him. I took his stash (of what?) and stuffed it in a cupboard.

#10 Dream: I was in a bathroom and had two babies' heads, only the heads, and sensed that I had done something wrong by not creating whole babies, so I stuck the heads in my bag.

#10 Dream: . . . so I take one of her brushes and decide to steal it, except it is very long, a couple of feet. I stick it down the front of my dress, but it sticks out so I try to conceal it with my coat. At some point I decide this is silly to be doing this and I put the brush back down on the counter.

#11 Dream: Me standing with back to mirror. I get a glimpse of my face. Am I wearing a mask of a wolf?

#10 Dream . . . I could not run and was trying to figure out what to do. Climb in a washer and hide?

#11 Dream: I was on an island. It was geologically made up of a volcano maybe or some raised land. The inside was hollow. There were a couple of secret ladder/shutes that can get you down quickly.

Water

#10 Dream: Scene—beautiful red, roan-colored horses in a valley running, then swimming. My horse was white with a black trimmed mane . . . swam up to where I was sitting . . . was very loving nudging me. I was tempted to jump on its back, but instead I dove deep into the water to see if it would dive also. We played for a while. It was a powerful swimmer and would retrieve objects that I threw. I was diving deep into the water, taking my granddaughter down with me to touch the bottom of the lake. She had learned to hold her breath. I remembered that we would both swim around and quickly burst up out of the water.

#2 Dream: . . . We go to a seaside holiday place on the Mediterranean. We all go straight into the sea. It's night and the sea is very dark and quite warm.

#10 Dream: Small village somewhere with a lake. We were at the beach. At first just the three of us, my daughter as a little girl, her dad, T., and my brother K. I walked out into the water, which was very shallow. I was quite far out but still able to walk.

#3 Dream: . . . I look outside, the sea is surrounding the house and there is a little boat moving in the waves. I go outside and ride on the boat. It is my mother's house, it seems to be closed in the front. I look from the boat to see if she is there or if a window, a door is open. Why is all closed? She told me she was there. The wind and the waves move the little boat from one side to the other of the house. Suddenly the sea is gone.

#4 Dream: . . . More impressive were the fountains, natural ponds with waterfalls, well-designed.

#5 There was a plumbing water leak today in the office. Soaked the carpet. Had to turn the water off for the whole building.

#8 Dream: Friend was visiting walking down trail to waterfall and it was beautiful. . . . Then the trail ended at a beautiful lake. I remember asking if this was the Amazon? No it wasn't. I was really happy then because there was my sailboat that I have wanted. Woke up. Felt good. Felt peaceful.

#5 Work was good today. But an air/water syringe leaked water—probably a washer.

#8 Dream: I was ice-skating in Holland. I enjoyed the gliding motion on the ice—felt free.

#10 Another dream: Camped at beautiful spot at water's edge.

#10 Dream: Vivid dream of flooding city—colonial city? I was navigating my way through—some streets not deep water.

#11 Dream: . . . Then we were walking away from a high seacoast and realized we were going to get hit by a huge wave. I was terrified we were going to get dragged in. We ran. It hit but we were ok. But another one was coming.

Mountains/Rocks

#4 ... The view of the mountains with a nearby storm was inspiring.

#8 When going home it was dark and the mountain pass is very curvy. I was having a hard time gauging my speed and was a little afraid to drive—felt like I was going to go off the road.

#10 ... Driving up a mountain, came to the first site which was literally an acre of concrete. I could not believe that someone would think this was how it was supposed to be... what was this place for??? I tried to picture us in our lawn chairs and tents. I could see myself sitting at a small table studying.

#10 Dream: I was cross-country skiing up to top of mountain. . . . I came to a place where everything in the trail became slushy and turned to water. I had to maneuver myself up and over boulders and trees.

#11 Dream: I was on an island. It was geologically made up of a volcano maybe or some raised land. The inside was hollow. There were a couple of secret ladder/shutes that can get you down quickly.

#2 Dream: I am in some sort of retreat situation, and there is a progression of places we are suggested to go to—certain rocks and caves. I keep being told by the staff of the retreat it is Vedanta—this word again and again. I follow the route, sit on the bare rocks, go in the caves. One is a long horizontal split on the top portion on the rock. I lie in it, aware of my breathing, lying like the reclining Buddha.

#10 Dream: With W. (best friend)—plans to go to Hawaii. She had carved army scenes from a green rock of marble.

#8 Dream: ... We then were driving through red rock, like in Sedona, Arizona.

Travel/Vehicles

#12 Dream: Lots of traveling around, returning home or to a family reunion. Best part was returning home and seeing my daughter. I had such a peaceful feeling. . . . Lots of driving. I traded cars with my ex, or somehow got her old car. . . . We were on a ship or plane with some Tibetans.

#10 Dream: . . . By the time I got there the Africans were getting on their boat. We realized that they had taken our ice chest by mistake, so I yelled at the boat to stop. I realized that the men were packed into the boat, like slaves, all lying down to fit in the hull. Yet they all seemed happy and said they were going home. I wished them a happy voyage.

#6 Dream: My youngest son is riding with me in a car. I keep having to ask him to step on the brake because my hands are full. Even though I knew it was dangerous. . . .

#11 Dream: I had done something wrong and I was being asked to leave the country. At first I thought about how exciting that would be to start a whole new life. New surroundings, friends, lovers, jobs. I was quickly being driven in a car by a short Mexican man and his wife and a friend of mine. They were all engaged in a conversation. The driver was controlling the car from the back seat. He was so short I wondered how he could see. His wife was in the front seat. I guess she didn't know how to drive. He was driving so fast through all this busy crazy traffic. I kept watching these almost fatal accidents. I searched in my purse and was glad to see that I had my passport. Then I remembered that I wouldn't see my kids again. Felt really sad.

#10 Dream: I had to helicopter into someplace to go for a hike. I saw this "vehicle" that we were going to use for a river trip. It looked like a giant suitcase. I thought to myself, "How cool—that the rafts can fit in here."

#2 Dream: I am on Thai Air going to Thailand. We fly really low—through city streets—and then along the canals of Venice. . . . It takes off again—along a little street—and I see it heading toward a building, then the sails of a galleon (ship). . . .

#10 Dream: I was driving late at night, tired, started to exit the freeway, next thing I remember, I am walking and have no idea where my car is. Did I wreck?

Or is it parked on an exit ramp? It is the middle of the night. I call someone to see if he will drive me to find my car.

#6 Dream: Traveling with a large group to a campground. We have boats and kids, many people I do not know. Lots of confusion.

#10 Dream: . . . traveling with friends and a trailer to a place to camp. Driving up a mountain . . .

#10 Dream: This dream seemed to last a long time, mountain trek. I was in the mountains with W., going to hike into a camp, lots of snow. Going to take a long time. . . . I have flip-flops on, I am very disorganized but not worried about it. Not even after a train ran over one of my flip-flops.

#3 Dream: . . . I look outside, the sea is surrounding the house and there is a little boat moving in the waves. I go outside and ride on the boat.

#5 Dream: About going fast. I was driving with my sister in a car on this big bridge/hill. Went down really fast. She was scared and I was exhilarated. Missed the exit and ended up in a corn field. Then I was getting on a carnival ride. It was going fast too.

#10 Dream: The earth was covered white, snow and ice. I was driving a large four-wheel drive vehicle and maneuvered the bad roads. I am not sure who was with me.

#2 Dream: Driving in a car with my kids. I don't know if I'm driving or someone else, but it's really dangerous driving. Squeezing between two trucks going really fast, and fast around corners. I'm more disturbed than scared. . . . Dream: Of a train journey. In the dream I think, "This proving has a lot of travel images."

#6 Dream: In a car with the H. family. It isn't the right car, but they won't listen. I know it is not right but am frustrated because I cannot get that across.

#10 Dream: I am driving down a windy road with a huge patch of ice coming up. At the bottom is the driveway of a family I grew up with. There is a little girl on a bike, I tell her to get out of the way because I was afraid I was going to slide into her.

#1 Dream: I signed up for a class on flying an airplane. I was at a rural community college-type campus with some old military cargo-type planes lying around.

#10 Dream: Traveling in huge snowstorm. Two cars with friends and family into the mountains somewhere.

#10 Dream: I was cross-country skiing up to top of mountain. It felt good to be exerting myself so effortlessly. . . . I woke up feeling that I was traveling within my own body???

#11 My brother called to offer us a round-trip ticket to anywhere British Airways flies, which is almost anywhere. That was pretty exciting! We're thinking of Bali.

#11 Dream: Buses everywhere. I was trying to find my daughter on one of them, feeling a little panicky. Then I heard/saw her in my mind's eye as though we were psychically linked (which we are often).

#10 Dream: Camped at beautiful spot at waters' edge. Have pulled rafts up on shore. I wonder in my dream why I keep dreaming of rafting.

#11 Dream: Motorbikes and wine.

Gatherings

#4 Dreams of retreats. . . . Banquet of food spread. We all slept in the same room. I was seeking privacy. In the retreat it was taken for granted that there was no privacy. It was ok because the other people were interesting.

#6 Dream: Traveling with a large group to a campground. We have boats and kids, many people I do not know.

#10 Dream: I was at some kind of gathering outside—wedding??

Music/Singing

#2 Singing all morning. Made up songs. Singing, whistling and humming. Very unusual. Normally I don't like playing music.

#5 Really felt sad this morning. Put on some music while working on a patient and started to weep. Felt better after that.

#7 Just before I arrived back home from traveling, late in the evening, I was listening to the radio in my car. An extremely beautiful rendition of the old Byrds' song (Turn! Turn! Turn!—There is a season, turn, turn, turn. . .) began to play. I had an overwhelming sense of grief and began to weep. I had to pull over for a few minutes to let the emotion out. I thought, "What a painful world we are passing through. Everything that we cling to, must leave us."

#2 I am definitely appreciating and wanting music, which is unusual.

Exotic Places

#2 Dream: . . . a seaside holiday place on the Mediterranean.

#3 Dream: In a nice Italian villa . . .

#8 Dream: I was ice-skating in Holland.

#11 Dream: Husband and I were on the coast of Italy.

#10 Dream: Vivid dream of flooding city—colonial city?

#8 Dream: I was at homeopathy class, but it was in a resort place. Actually we were in the Swiss Alps and were skiing between classes.

#2 Dream: I am on Thai Air going to Thailand. We fly really low—through city streets—and then along the canals of Venice.

#11 My brother called to offer us a round-trip ticket to anywhere British Airways flies, which is almost anywhere. That was pretty exciting! We're thinking of Bali.

#10 Dream: Shopping with my daughter someplace like Mexico.

#8 Dream: . . . We then were driving through red rock, like in Sedona, Arizona. . . . Then the trail ended at a beautiful lake. I remember asking if this was the Amazon?

#10 Dream: With W. (best friend)—plans to go to Hawaii.

#10 Dream: Pyramid Lake scene . . .

MANDRAGORA RUBRICS .... Mandragora Root

MIND   AILMENTS from;
    alcoholism, dipsomania
    ambition, deceived
    anger, vexation, suppressed
    disappointment
    frustration, disappointment
ANGER
    irascibility, agg.
    irascibility, tendency
ANIMAL, consciousness
ANSWER, answering, answers; reflects long
ANXIETY
    chest, in, heart, region of
    children, about his
ANXIETY OF CONSCIENCE; leaving animals, for
AUDACITY
    usually self apologetic
AWARENESS heightened
BED; desires to remain in
BITING
    husband, impulse to
    nails
BROODING
CALMNESS
CHEERFULNESS; gaiety, happiness, tendency
    friends, with
CLAIRVOYANT
COMPANY; desire for
    desire for, evening
    desire to sleep with pets in bed
CONCENTRATION; active, engaged in work, very efficient
    difficult
        evening, agg.
        nice weather, from
        working, while
CONFIDING
CONFUSION of mind
    concentrate, on attempting to
    electronic equipment previously working fails
CONSOLATION, amel.
CRUELTY
CURSE, God, desire to
DANGER, protecting others in
DEATH, thoughts of

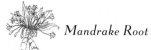

DELUSIONS; imaginations
  alone
  altars and candles
  animals, bird, sees white
  animal, she is
    of, birds, friend covered with feathers and beak
  causes electronic equipment to fail
  cheated, ripped off
  failure, of best effort
  fat, she is
  forsaken, beloved by parents, wife, friends, feels is not being
  light, incorporeal, immaterial, he is
  lost, confused in time and space
  machines break
  neglected
  persecuted, he is
  religious
  reproached unfairly by society
  squirrel, she is
  struggle, must
  time, passes too quickly
  ugly, is
  unloved, uncared for
  wrong, everything is going
  wrote down a dream which she did not
DESIRES; drugs, recreation
DREAMS
  abscess, on heel, from high heel shoes
  accidents
    fatal
    running over people, unconcerned
  accusations
  adolescence, of, chaperoning
  airplanes
    with fear of crashing
    of, flying in without fear
    of, flying upside down
  amorous
  anger, angry, employees, towards
  angry, indignation over an overcharge at a store, punches salesclerk
  animals
    bird, she was, looking down on herself
    cats
    crocodiles
    dinosaurs
    deer, tiny
    dog
      not understanding command
    grasshoppers
    horses
    lions
    orcas
    snakes

astral world
beaten, woman
beautiful
beer, drinking
birth, of giving, without pain
    babies born
blood, pools of
body; body parts
    disfigured
        feet, web toes, extra digits
        hair
            cut
            hair ornaments
    legs paralyzed
bored, disinterested
breathing through face, chest, entire body area
Buddha, reclining like a
business, of, difficulties in
calculating
camping, campgrounds, of
car, driving a, dangerously, intoxicated, stoned
cars, automobiles, buses
    automobiles, motorcycle
car, sabotaged
child, children, about
    danger, in
    dead from drugs or poison
    must leave her
clothes, cape, sequined, soft, bright, glowing
college, football weekend
colored
communal living, of
confused
    incomprehension when spoken to
country, foreign
crimes
cruelty
Dalai Lama, gentle and sweet, being blessed and accepted, by
danger
    brother, impending
    but calm
    fear, without
    must hide
dead; infant, fetus
    people, of
        friends, long deceased
        relatives, long deceased
distorting everything
dreaming, of
drugs, illegal, must conceal
earthquake, impending
epidural, all must have
escape, of
excrement, without disgust

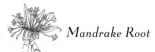

Mandragora Officinarum   Mandrake Root

exiled
falling, into abyss
family, own
    sister who is manic depressive, of
fear felt in heart
fearless
feats, capable of challenging mental and physical
fights, martial arts, use others' strength against them
floating, looking down on self from above
food
friends
    meeting, of, at theater
    recognize, does not
    will not help
frightful
guest, unwanted
guns
    shots
haircut, of bright red hair
home, of
hospital
hotels
house, houses
hurried
husband chased, grabbed, kissed wife
insulted, by husband
intoxicated, stoned
island, on
journey
joyous
kindness and love of spiritual teacher
kleptomania, must conceal
knives
knowledge, knows where everything is
ladders, chutes, hidden
legal forms, regarding inheritance for a baby
lesbian, she is a
lewd, lascivious, voluptuous
lost in train station
love alone heals, hatred never ceases with hatred
manipulated
marijuana, smoking
masks
    of wolf
meditation retreat, Vedanta, in a cave
metaphysical
mice
mistakes, writing
moral issues and acceptance of others
mountains, of
murder
mutilation
nakedness
paralyzed legs, pushing chair to walk

parties, of pleasure
    drinking beer and smoking
        wearing pink dress and a wig, looks weird but does not matter, just aspect of body
passing through a building (wall), body is
peaceful
peacemaker
people, of
    living in her home, no privacy
plans
police
prostitute
purchase, making
pursued, of being
    must hide
    police, by
racism
religious
restaurant
running
    rushing about, not enough time
sailboat
scientific
scolding (fighting)
seduction, brothers, seducing me
sharks
ships
singing
skating, ice
slaves, packed into boats, journeying home
snow
    snow storms, of being out in
stabbed, woman was
strange
threatened, neck, felt was
toilet
torture, training for it
train
trapped
travel (cured symptom)
trespass, someone is, bad intentions, with
unsuccessful efforts to, talk
vehicles
helicopters, rafts
violence
volcano, inside dormant
watched
walking, of
    expressway, on, going wrong way
water
    pond, dark, foreboding
        men thrown into, drowning
    swimming in Mediterranean, without fear
    waves, high
waterfall

   wax man
woman
   big hair, tiny, dwarf-like
   comforted her
   naked
   tall, then short
women
   female energy
work
world, end of the
youth, time of
DWELLS ON PAST DISAGREEABLE OCCURRENCES
EMOTIONS; opening deeply and profoundly
ENVY
ESTRANGED
   family, from her
   society, from
EXERCISE; anger increases energy for
FAMILY members, wants to be with
FASTIDIOUS
FEAR
   animals who are outside her door
   danger, of impending
   happen, something will
   insanity, of losing his reason
FORGETFULNESS
FORSAKEN feeling; isolation, sensation of
HOME; desires to, go
HOMESICKNESS
HURRY, haste, tendency; occupation, in
IMPATIENCE
INDIFFERENCE
   apathy, children, to her
   towards others
INDIGNATION
INDUSTRIOUS; mania for work
   efficient
INSANITY; madness
INTOXICATED; as if
IRRITABILITY
   anxiety, with
   bite, with impulse to
   casual conversation, with
   causeless
   easily
   general
      heat
      hurriedness, with
      sleepiness, with
      takes everything in bad part
      trifles, from
      waking, on, agg.
      working, when
   hurriedness, with

ISOLATION; sensation of
JEALOUSY
LATE; rushed
LAUGHING; serious matters, over
LOSING, things
MANIA
MEMORY; weakness, loss of
  names, for proper
  time, for
MEDITATION; deep well-being
MISANTHROPY
MISTAKES; makes
  names; in, calls things by wrong
  time; in
MOOD; alternating
  changeable; variable
MORAL, affections; want of moral feeling
MUSIC; amel.
NO, cannot say (cured symptom)
OBSTINATE; headstrong
PHILOSOPHY; ability for
PLAY; desire to, playful
QUIET disposition
REFLECTING
RELIGIOUS AFFECTIONS
RESTLESSNESS; nervousness, general
  nervousness, general, pressured
RUNS; rushing
SADNESS; despondency, depression, melancholy
  thinking; ephemeral nature of life, about
SCHIZOPHRENIA
SELF-DEPRECATION
SINGING; morning
  humming to herself
SPACED-OUT feeling
SUICIDAL; disposition
SYMPATHETIC; compassionate
  animals, only for
SYMPATHY; desire for
TALK, talking, talks; indisposed to, desire to be silent
  indisposed to, philosophy, about
  agg. all complaints; boredom with others, yet animated and interested with her own
THOUGHTS; clearness of
  collect, cannot
TIME; loss of conception of
  passes too slowly, appearing longer
  passes too quickly, appears shorter
TRANQUILITY; serenity, calmness
TRAVEL; desire to
UNFEELING; hard-hearted
UNSYMPATHETIC
WEEPING; tearful mood
  tearful mood, amel. symptoms
  asthma, during spell of

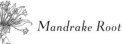

Mandragora Officinarum   Mandrake Root

	respiration, with difficulty
	general, sad, thoughts, at
	music, from
	sympathy with others, from
	sad thoughts, ephemeral nature of life
	WELL; feels very, deep well-being
	WHISTLING
	WORK; all day without stopping
	satisfying
HEAD	HAIR; affections of, baldness
	ITCHING; scalp
	scalp, spots, in
HEAD PAIN	GENERAL
	morning
	morning agg.
	morning agg., waking, and on
	one-sided
	sides, left above temple, behind left eye
	talking, agg.
	walking agg., while
	alcoholic drinks, from
	daytime
	eating amel., after
	extending to face
	jar, from any
	LOCALIZATION, forehead
	forehead, sleep, before
	left side
	sides, morning, waking, on
	right
	DULL
	PINCHING
	POUNDING
VERTIGO	INTOXICATED; as if
EYE	DRYNESS
	DUST; as if in
	LACHRYMATION; left
	during coryza
	PAIN; pressing, left, behind, worse exertion
VISION	CLARITY; of
	PIERCING; seeing with extra clarity
NOSE	CATARRH
	general, extending to, sinuses
	CORYZA
	lying, amel.
	DISCHARGE; general, posterior nares, choanae, change of weather agg.
	mucous
	thin

	watery
	ERUPTIONS; inside
	inside, left
	ITCHING
	OBSTRUCTION
	cold air, agg.
	cough, during
	weather, wet, damp, during
	PAIN; rawness
	rawness, coryza, during
	posterior nares
	SNEEZING
	eyes watery, with and perspiration
	paroxysmal
	tingling, from inside nose
SMELL	ODORS; imaginary and real
	cigarette smoke
	jasmine
	rose
	sandalwood
	SENSITIVE; to odor of, flowers
EAR	NOISES; in
	PAIN; cutting, left
	general, pressure, on, amel.
	warmth, wrapping up amel.
HEARING	ACUTE; circulation all over the body, seems to hear
FACE	CRACKS; corners of mouth
	corners of mouth, right
	ERUPTIONS; general, nose, tip
	painful, nose, tip
	throbbing, nose, tip
	vesicles, mouth, corners of
	HEAT; flushes
	PEELING; lips
	lips, lower
	lower, right
	TENSION; of jaws
MOUTH	APHTHAE; tongue, top of
	DRY; with thirst
TASTE	DIMINISHED
	INSIPID; watery, flat, food tastes
THROAT	CATARRH
	HAIR; sensation of
	MUCOUS; night
	PAIN; burning
	rawness

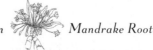

Mandragora Officinarum   *Mandrake Root*

EXTERNAL THROAT
    CLOTHING, agg.
    CONSTRICTION; neck band feels too tight
    SWELLING; cervical glands

INTERNAL THROAT
    DRY; with thirst

STOMACH
    APPETITE; capricious, hunger, but knows not for what
      diminished
        morning
          business, with
      increased
        hunger in general
        ravenous, canine, excessive
      wanting
    EMPTINESS; weak feeling, faintness, hungry feeling
    ERUCTATION; bitter
    HEARTBURN
    HICCOUGH
      morning thirst
    NAUSEA
      eating; agg., after
      waking, on
    PAIN; burning, eating, agg., after
      cramping, griping, constricting
      griping, constricting
        drinking, amel. water
        eating, agg. after
        eating, agg. during
    SATIETY; sensation of

THIRST
    THIRST
      unquenchable, constant, sipping of cold water
      night

ABDOMEN
    DISTENSION
    FLATULENCE
    FULLNESS; sensation of
      sensation of; nausea, with
    PAIN; cramping, wandering
      general; urinate, with urging to
        stool, agg.; during, diarrhea
      stitching, sticking, stool; before

RECTUM
    CONSTIPATION
    DIARRHEA; general, forenoon

STOOL
    DRY
    HARD
    SOFT

BLADDER	*PAIN*; general, urinate, during urging to
	    cramping
	    pressing, pressure in

URINE	BURNING, hot

FEMALE	DRYNESS
	ITCHING
	  burning
	MENSES; bright, red
	  gushes, in
	  late
	  painful, dysmenorrhea (cured symptom)
	  thin
	PAIN; general, wound, healing
	  lancinating
	    uterus, extending to back
	SEXUAL; desire
	  diminished
	  increased

RESPIRATION	ASTHMATIC
	  cold weather, agg.
	  light, amel.
	  lying, back agg.
	    stomach, propped on elbows, amel.
	  night, midnight, agg.
	  wet weather, agg.
	YAWNING; general, evening

COUGH	AIR; damp, agg. ASTHMATIC COLD; on becoming DEEP

CHEST	APPREHENSION; heart, region of
	CONSTRICTION; tension, tightness, heart, grasping sensation
	EXPANSION; sensation of, rib cage
	OPPRESSION; lying, back, agg.
	  touch, agg.
	PAIN; cutting, heart, region of
	  Cutting; mammae, under, right
	    respiration, during
	  general, heart, region of
	  pulling, after meal
	PRESSED IN; as if

BACK	PAIN; aching, lumbar region
	  aching, lumbar region, evening
	  drawing, dorsal, scapulae, below, left

EXTREMITIES	COLDNESS; general, lower limbs, legs DIRTY; hands, sensation of hands, sensation of, washing no help

Mandragora Officinarum   *Mandrake Root*

DROOPING; of upper limbs
ERUPTIONS; desquamating, fingers, nails, about
  eczema; upper limbs, hands
  elbow; itchy
  hip; itchy
HEAT; general, upper limbs, hands
HEAVINESS; tired limbs, lower limbs, legs
ITCHING; hand, palm
  hand, palm, scratching, amel.
  fingers
NUMBNESS; insensibility, lower limbs
PULLING; sensation, upper limbs, thumb
  sensation, upper limbs, thumb, on waking
SWELLING; leg, dropsical
  ankle, dropsical
TENSION; shoulder
TWITCHING; upper limbs, fingers, first, thumb
UNCOVER; inclination to
WEAKNESS; upper limbs, upper arms, lying in bed

EXTREMITY PAIN

ACHING; upper limbs, fingers, first, thumb
  right
    waking her after midnight
  wrists, left
CRAMPING; lower limbs, foot, right
  drawing inward
CUTTING; hip, left
GENERAL; lower limbs, knees, ascending stairs
  lower limbs, toes, right
SORE; bruised, fingers

SLEEP

ANIMALS; with
FALLING ASLEEP; early
HEAVY
NAP; with animals
NEED OF SLEEP; great
  little
POSITION; back on, knees drawn up, left, on, and hands on chest
PROLONGED
REFRESHING
  as though meditating all night
SLEEPINESS; afternoon, agg.
SLEEPLESSNESS; desires, but fruitless
  general, activity from too much
    dreams, from
    night, latter part of night, in
UNREFRESHING
  rise; indisposed to
WAKING; difficult, morning
  four p.m.–five p.m.
  three a.m.
  dreams, from
YAWNING

PERSPIRATION	EATING; agg., after ODOR; offensive SNEEZING; from

GENERALITIES	AFTERNOON; one p.m.–six p.m., agg.
	AIR; seashore, amel.
	COLD
	  air, agg.
	  becoming, agg.
	  from damp places
	EFFICIENCY; increased
	ENERGY
	  abundant
	  lack of
	EVENING; six p.m.–nine p.m., agg.
	EXERTION; physical, amel.
	FOOD, and drinks; alcohol, alcoholic drinks; agg.
	  alcoholic drinks; agg., intoxicated easily
	  chocolate; desires
	  coffee; aversion
	  farinaceous; desires
	  frozen; desires
	  meat, desires
	  milk; desires
	  peanut butter; desires
	  protein; desires
	  salt or salty food; desires
	  spices, condiments, piquant, highly seasoned, agg. (cured symptom)
	  sweets, desires
	HEAT; sensation of
	  vital; lack of
	LASSITUDE; tendency, alternating with, activity
	SENSITIVENESS; alcohol, to
	SLUGGISHNESS; of the body
	  of the body, morning
	WEAKNESS; enervation, exhaustion, prostration, infirmity, alternating with, activity
	  left
	WEARINESS; general, patients, from seeing
	  general

JOURNALS..*Mandragora*

EDITOR'S NOTE: *Punctuation, abbreviations, and individual stylistic nuances of the original journal entries have been preserved wherever possible.*

> Prover #1 • Male • 41 years old

Day 1
♦ Perhaps more emotionally distant. I felt less connected, empathic, than is my norm while speaking with brother on telephone.
♦ Dream: A reptile—perhaps a crocodile? I am the crocodile? A man has had his arm eaten by the crocodile, yet I am not horrified. Somehow he deserved it. I felt an emotional distance. Not really caring. Later I thought that was strange that I felt that he deserved it. An aggressive feeling.

Day 2
♦ Emotional flattening. Shallow feeling. I usually love riding my bicycle. I didn't have my usual joy. Felt "I've got to get there." Functional.
♦ Energy dropped off at 4:00 p.m. or 5:00 p.m.
♦ Some itching of scalp.

Day 3
♦ Dream: I'm in an apartment on the top floor of a building. I hear a gunshot, maybe a cry. As I open the door into the hallway a woman scolds me, says I shouldn't concern myself, that I will just bring suspicion onto myself. I feel trapped, isolated. I notice that people are taking my *Science News* (a subscription magazine), using them for a project I'm not invited to participate in. I grab them (like a child who takes back his toys) and bring them back to my room. I open a door to the apartment where someone died and people immediately come out and scold me. They tell me to run to escape. I go down a fire escape but it becomes clear I'm seen. So I head back up to search for another way out. I see Uncle N., tell him about my studies. But he, too, suddenly has to disappear because of danger (guns?), and I can't follow. The feeling was intrigue, danger, scolded, suspicion. Exclusion from the group, falsely accused.

Day 4
♦ Dream: Went to look at a room/apartment for rent. It was located in the house adjacent to one I had grown up in, and in the dream the landlord actually lived in my childhood home. The landlord had complete say over how this apartment was to be furnished. He ordered spraying of insecticide, and was demanding the removal of certain ornamental furnishings, and offering simple but unattractive replacements. The

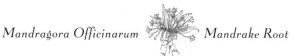

Mandragora Officinarum   *Mandrake Root*

neighbors, other tenants, are all aloof, unfriendly, uninviting. I'm asked to participate in a coin toss to help decide what could go on the wall. I tell the landlord, "You're the owner, but he's the decorator." The landlord is angry at me.

♦ At the Health Center where I work, I was asked to re-do a form explaining need for granting medical leave for a student with chronic fatigue. On the form I had written "see attached progress note." I was told that this was insufficient and that the student had not signed a release. I asked for the chart and easily found the medical release note (and plenty of documentation). I felt harrassed.

Day 5

♦ Thoughts are scattered. Difficulty focusing, worse in the evening.

♦ In a group check-in found myself taking a long time to get the words out. A feeling of great emotional distance between myself and group.

♦ I put an ad in a local paper as a homeopath. I got a call from someone who accused me of advertising that I was selling health insurance. I couldn't believe it. I was feeling scolded. She promised to send me the ad. I was so shaken I went and looked in a newspaper at my ad. Fortunately it still said homeopathy!

♦ Driving home at night through the fog, reminded me of the "cobweb" of fogginess of my mind.

♦ General: Energy good until 9:30–10:30 p.m., in spite of early waking; then energy crashes. High energy but ungathered. Going from one task to the next with a sense of urgency to complete them.

♦ Head itching in spots, better by scratching, but almost instantly emerging in other points.

♦ Increased hunger, for warm/hot food, for fruit. It wasn't cravings for particular foods but I would forget to eat and then when I thought about it I was ravenously hungry. I would grab whatever and it didn't matter what.

♦ Increased thirst.

♦ Fullness in lower abdomen, with mild nausea. Feel I would be relieved by a bowel movement, but none comes.

Day 7

♦ Again woke up early, about 5:45 a.m. Was lying in bed when telephone rang at 6:15 a.m. It was my youngest brother, who recently had sent me an angry letter falsely accusing me of intentionally breaking his sofa (when I visited him) and of arrogantly lecturing to him. I have had trouble relating with my youngest brother and don't understand our conflict. I had traveled cross-country to try to mend our relationship and thought the counseling we had done had gone well. But afterwards he didn't call or write for months and then he called at 6:00 a.m. He seemed manic. That was very upsetting. He said, "Let's call a truce." He went on with pressured speech, was hyper-verbal. Was talking inappropriately about his patients. About sexually coming on to them but afraid he would be sued. I had to be careful what to say because he would feel attacked. He said I should have been a stock broker. And I said yeah it would be nice to have money. Then he said, "You need money?" Like I was trying to get money from him. I listened to him with sadness and trepidation, but also with less emotion than I might have normally. Like he was in a fog, I am in a fog. But brooded about his condition, about how I might help, yet probably couldn't do much, for most of the day.

◆ Brought my new used car to mechanic to fix horn. He had said beforehand that he could work with the extended warranty. But when I came to pick up the car they said they hadn't received pre-authorization, implied that I may have to pay. Wouldn't let me drive away until they were sure they were going to receive payment from the insurance. I became angry and said, "I feel like you're holding me hostage." They relented and gave me the key.

◆ Continue to feel very task-oriented, busy. Can't just "be," so I "do." Very productive of things that had been waiting to get done, but not feeling centered or joyful. More frenetic.

◆ Still disconnected from people. Don't feel my usual empathy.

◆ Will eat anything to satisfy increased hunger; not so important what it is. Less mindful of meals, mealtimes.

◆ Clutching feeling in my heart or behind my heart at 9:00 p.m. Something clutching at it. A hand clutching at it. Sensation of my heartbeat later than the clutching pain. Fear of death or heart attack.

Day 8

◆ Sadness, but feel more connected to self. Reflective.

◆ Desire company. Company ameliorates.

◆ My dog and cat and I seem more connected. I'm more empathic with them (served them dinner before I scavenged food for myself).

◆ Not attentive to meals. Just scavenge food from the fridge and eat unceremoniously.

◆ General: Very tired, low energy. After some work, lay in easy chair. Difficult keeping energy up playing games with my son, wanted to go to sleep.

◆ Post-nasal drip.

◆ Sore throat from post-nasal drip, onset late afternoon as I bicycled through cold drizzle. It went down into my larynx and had hair in the throat sensation. No relief, no matter how much I coughed.

Day 9

◆ Dream: Genital mutilation. Not much feeling about it.

◆ Dream: Anxious about picking up six-year-old son from Sunday school class after church. I'm stuck on an elevator that goes up and down and spins on its axis. The elevator is as large as a room, which keeps going up and down without stopping or opening its doors. In desperation I push open a door and leap out. I'm not hurt, but I think I may have injured someone else in the elevator by that maneuver. My focus is on my son. I was desperate, anxious and guilty. Guilt over hurting someone to get out of the trap. Very isolated. No resolution of dream. Mental state on waking: sad, feel disconnected from people. Later that day I was reading the church newsletter and there is a piece that says, be sure that you walk your child to the class because last month a child ended up in the wrong classroom.

♦ Dream: I am a student in a French class. I had been comfortable with the usual (female) teacher, but a male substitute teacher, visiting, takes over the class. At first he is pleasant and respectful, but then he asks increasingly challenging and impossible questions. Then he scolds us for not knowing the answers, for our alleged inattention, and I wonder, "Why am I taking French anyway?"

♦ Desire company, but don't have energy to seek it out. Even if others were present I wouldn't be able to connect because they couldn't understand my state of mind. I wouldn't be able to relate to theirs. A lack of focus, scatteredness. Wasted time on the internet, looking for some sense of community.

♦ Energy level very low, especially in the afternoon. Napped from 2:00–3:00 p.m. Asked twelve-year-old daughter to entertain six-year-old son.

♦ Nose had raw feeling at root, posterior nares. Obstructed. Thin coryza.

♦ Throat raw, burning. Worse swallowing.

♦ External throat: swollen tonsillar nodes.

Day 10

♦ Concentration difficult; want to do something different, but don't know what.

♦ Distant from people. Pause before speaking with thought. How am I ever going to make myself understood?

♦ Locked myself out of car. Felt better when locksmith told me he had a 24-day-old baby. Seemed to give perspective. What's an inconvenience like this compared to miracle of life and inevitability of death?

♦ More empathy for pet dog and cat. Taking better care of them.

♦ Mood is dark, low. Feel lonely but being with people doesn't help.

♦ Missed choir practice because of this feeling and sore throat, low energy.

♦ Napped after dinner.

♦ Scalp itching

♦ Flushes of heat on face, while feeling generally cold.

♦ Swollen tonsillar nodes. Hurts to talk loudly. Sore, raw.

♦ Sillier with the kids in a way they like. Caricature more than usual and jesting.

♦ Fogginess about my connection to God and myself.

♦ Scavenge for food. Animal thing. No ritual, just feed the belly.

♦ Constipation. Wanting to have a bowel movement but not able to.

Day 11

♦ Dream: I signed up for a class on flying an airplane. I was at a rural community college-type campus with some old military cargo-type planes lying around. There were just a few "good old guys' and myself in the plane. It didn't seem very organized. I was very apprehensive, feared we would crash, that I would die, that I would never see my kids again. It took off unexpectedly while I was in the airplane lavatory. I ran back to where the seats were, holding onto the seat backs to keep myself from falling. The other guys laughed in a friendly but mocking/jesting way, but I was really scared. The plane seemed to be flying very unevenly, accelerating then decelerating, leaving puffs of black smoke behind it, and flying too close to ground. It seemed we would get entangled in the branches of the trees. I became increasingly

frantic while the other guys became increasingly critical of me. I became isolated from the group, scolded for my fear and immaturity and lack of confidence in them.
- I'm usually so in tune with my kids even when we're not in the same room. Son went upstairs to get dressed. He started to cry out. Normally I would have been there right away but I felt detached. Daughter got there first. Normally I would have felt the pain and been upset by it.

Day 12
- Very chilly in evening. Shivering.
- Irritation in larynx causing cough, which does not relieve. Like a hair in throat. Worse in the evening, and worse from speaking.
- Transient aching pain in bones of fingers in evening.

Day 14
- Throbbing headache after disappointment in business (new patient canceled appointment).
- Backache in lower back in evening.

Prover #2 • Female • 51 years old

Day 0
- When I first got the remedy I held the closed bottle close to my face with my eyes closed shut. Beneath my eyelids my eyes were sensitive and able to see long distances. Felt awareness of heartbeat and nasal area. Super sensitive clarity of senses. Awareness of abdominal region. Temples, nasal cavities, the spaces seemed very clear. Space on each side of spine, wherever there wasn't organ or bone. Like a sense of hollowness, a clarity like menthol. Then I took the remedy. It tasted very sweet.
- Dreams: Large public lavatory with six toilets of stainless steel, all were blocked with tampons, and there was blood all over the floor. Robin Williams was there pretending to be a woman. I kept flushing and was embarrassed trying to get the blockage down. Dreamt I must write that this was about female energy. In the dream I get a card and write this down. The dream continues in the house with other women, my sister and niece. She is anorexic and manic depressive. The house is huge. When I wake up I am relieved that I wrote it down and then I realize that I didn't write it. I'm anxious to go back to sleep but can't.
- Can't go back to sleep—wide awake—but anxious to not go back to sleep. Sort of doze until 7:00 a.m.
- Rib cage feels expanded, as though increased capacity. (Like a four-legged animal, round into cage.)
- Slight headache above left temple, behind left eye. Lachrymation of left eye.
- Slight stiffness on left side of neck.
- Left arm feels weak, even though I'm lying in bed.
- Whole left side feels weak.

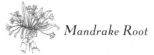

Mandragora Officinarum   Mandrake Root

Day 2

- More assertive in circumstances with a particular person I can be wimpy with. I said, "No, this is what I want." Then I noticed that usually I am self-apologetic. A voice says, "You don't have to be like that." My voice dropped and I felt I was stopping a habitual attitude. I was more assertive with patients, reassuring them that they would be better.
- Dream: I am in some sort of retreat situation, and there is a progression of places we are suggested to go to—certain rocks and caves. I keep being told by the staff of the retreat it is Vedanta—this word again and again. I follow the route, sit on the bare rocks, go in the caves. One is a long horizontal split on the top portion on the rock. I lie in it, aware of my breathing, lying like the reclining Buddha. There is a party planned—I don't much want to go, but it is part of the retreat. I wear a bright pink long dress, and a wig all different shades of pink. My own hair is tumbled in a high ponytail of dark chestnut ringlets around the top of the wig. I think it looks weird but am aware it's just my vanity and it doesn't matter. The same situation recurs with the variation that my hair is short (and no wig). I remember getting it cut but am surprised he cut it so short. Again I am a bit upset but feel, "never mind, it's just an aspect of my body." All night I am aware of being at a spiritual retreat, and with people who are aware and guiding. When I get to the party building—I can just pass through it and into another space where there is no party happening—but rather a talk going on about "Vedic Breathing." A woman instructs us to breathe in through our whole nasal frontal face area for the first day. On the second day to breathe through our entire chest area and the third day through our entire body area. All through the dream, I am repeating, "Veda, Vedanta, Vedic."
- Wake 6:00 a.m. (early for me) refreshed—as though I had been meditating all night.
- I work all day very well without stopping.
- I felt again as though I had been meditating with awareness and deep well-being.
- Feel dizzy, almost intoxicated. My eyes see very clearly.
- No appetite until 4:30 p.m. and just eat a little. Feel sweaty and nauseous after lunch that I had to have with friend. At dinner slightly nauseated. Eat little.
- Wake at 6:00 a.m. and work without stopping until 3:30 p.m. Very efficient, good concentration, etc. (better than usual).
- Feeling of deep well-being.
- Notice my eyes feel very "piercing." I'm seeing well—not just physically—but with extra clarity.

Day 4

- Woke early again (4:30 a.m. and couldn't get back to sleep).
- Felt really tired and rather impatient with patients. This morning I couldn't wait for the day to be finished. Very unstable, hot with instability. Would almost feel steam rising from my sweater. Hot and irritable. Have to control myself not to be snappy and irritable with everyone.
- Went home at 4:00 p.m. and took a nap—feel better after.
- Dinner with friends and feel really tired—yawning all evening.
- Dream: I am on Thai Air going to Thailand. We fly really low—through city streets—and then along the canals of Venice. It's a huge jet, but it lands halfway though the

journey on a little bamboo platform. I am not at all scared, and in the dream I keep wondering why I'm not scared. In real life I hate flying. In the dream I think I'm not frightened because it is Thai and the Buddhists make it safe. It takes off again—along a little street—and I see it heading toward a building, then the sails of a galleon (ship). I shut my eyes tight and think, "This is it!" But it's ok. We come out far under a canopy of a sports pavilion with crowds cheering as we take off to the skies. I definitely feel a bit shaky.

♦ Dream: My sister and others belonging to a spiritual community that I used to belong to (in real life). They are to go to a meeting/training with the main teacher. The training has some title like "Aggression, Force, and Violence Necessary in the Future." She attends this and comes back and tells me that they were all trained to give torture and if necessary kill people—as the future was likely to become so dangerous and we would all be threatened. They were shown how to fix electrodes in people and give shocks—and other really horrible things. It was a secret training and she wasn't meant to tell me. I felt glad I had left the teaching—and also frightened they thought this kind of thing necessary. I also remember Buddha's words—"Hatred never ceases with hatred—by love alone is healed"—I thought I would stick to that if the worst came to the worst!

♦ Dreams of scary situations, but I am not really scared. A kind of lack of emotion in a way. Maybe it is more low-key. I felt a balanced state. Funny spiritual thing with fear and danger but being ok.

Day 5

♦ Singing all morning. Made up songs. Singing, whistling, and humming. Very unusual. Normally I don't like playing music.

♦ I feel well and happy it is the weekend and Halloween. I am touched by the holiday. Windows were beautiful. A time of remembering people that have passed on. Little pumpkins and little children in costumes. I felt a depth to it.

♦ I feel in the evening my energy plummets quite suddenly. This is the second night I've noticed it.

Day 6

♦ Irritable with other people's slowness (in shops and with a patient who speaks vaguely and too lengthily). I also feel I don't want to just talk for "no purpose." This can make me sound irritable I think—I notice it when my sister calls, and two other friends, that usually I will chat for ages. Things need to be "to the point."

♦ I'm liking smells—of the air and also of essential oils—sandalwood—rose—jasmine—delicious.

♦ Otherwise I'm feeling rather "stuck" mentally in that I want practical efficiency. In my dress I notice the last two days I've worn sweat pants and a sweater, not caring much what it looks like. Just feeling good to be cozy and comfortable.

♦ My legs have felt cold night and day.

♦ Dream: Driving in a car with my kids. I don't know if I'm driving or someone else, but it's really dangerous driving. Squeezing between two trucks going really fast, and fast around corners. I'm more disturbed than scared. We go to a seaside holiday place on the

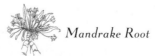

Mandragora Officinarum   *Mandrake Root*

Mediterranean. We all go straight into the sea. It's night and the sea is very dark and quite warm. We all get pulled out quite far by a current. I shout to the children, "Be careful, it's a strong current," but with none of the fear that I would expect to have. We go in there safely and I remark that it's probably really polluted as it's the Mediterranean. There are people cooking hamburgers on the beach. We get one. I realize we have no coffee so there is a trip to shops to get coffee and a percolator or drip system. It's 8:00 p.m. and I realize that we've missed a meditation session at my old center (the spiritual teaching I used to be involved with). I'm not very sorry.
- Dream: A patient says that on the questionnaire of her former homeopath she was asked, "Did she ever take a shower with a homeopath?!" I said that was totally weird, and she said that she had seen a strange homeopath. She had given her loads of antibodies in potency as well.
- Dream: Of a train journey. In the dream I think, "This proving has a lot of travel images."

Day 7
- I am definitely appreciating and wanting music, which is unusual.
- I am definitely not wanting to just "chat" with friends as I normally do. Talking but only insofar as it's practical. I feel perfectly friendly—it's not anti-social—but rather, it only seems necessary to say what is necessary, no extra. Not wanting to talk philosophy.
- Not very dreamy. I'm not verbally or emotionally creative. Notice I'm also being quite focused and efficient, and probably because of this.
- Not feeling fear in the dreams where normally I would do so.
- I like making things with my hands (have been painting and sewing). Happy making things with my hands.
- Pain in the knees going up steps. I think this is new.
- Dream: Hair cut.

Day 8
- Dream: Having to get my hair cut (second time that dream).
- Dream: Living in a house that is being shared with another family. I feel really sad in the dream that I gave up my previous house that was all my own. In this one there is no privacy; there are other people all over the place.
- I wake feeling grumpy and a bit down.

Day 9
- I feel it's very hard to listen to people. My irritation is more about them talking. This makes it hard with patients. I feel very impatient and bored, yet I notice I am quite animated and interested if I am talking!!
- I'm also tired. Not much sleep last night due to my two new kittens jumping on me. It's not another feline remedy??
- I feel very hot, especially my hands. They feel hot and sort of grimy. I wash them several times. It doesn't help.

- Dream: Meeting the Dalai Lama with D. He (D.) does all the speaking and I feel sad that I haven't thought of anything worthwhile to say. When the visit ends I am crying, and the Dalai Lama says, "Oh! I am so sorry. Instead of making you happy, I have made you sad." He takes my face in his hands as he talks, very gently, very sweet. My feeling was very blessed and accepted. Warm that he would do that.

Day 10
- Relieved not to see any patients today. Don't feel like calling the patients I have to, but I do. I get it over with quicker than usual; I'm more decisive about what they should do, etc.
- Eating meat; have had it three nights in a row. Unusual.
- Body temperature not so hot today. Times of feeling cold.

Day 11
- Definitely feel cold.
- Can't wait for the end of the week. Definitely tired of speaking to patients.

Day 12
- Relieved to be home—no phone calls to make! I enjoy being with the kids and painting, making things. Family and home = Good!
- Dream: Someone asks me about Jack Kornfield. It's a woman who sells kittens. Although it sounds corny, I tell her that he is an embodiment of love. Very connected to the practice of love and kindness as I tell her.
- Dream: My two new kittens fall into a river. I scoop them out.
- Wakened at 3:00 a.m. by one of the kittens. He wants to play, and we stay up for two hours. I feel really hot when I wake, and nauseous, but wide awake.
- I had real difficulties with my supervisor. I didn't feel irritable but I had a lot of patients and we kept missing each other.
- Summary: The spiritual theme struck me. I don't usually dream about the Dalai Lama. The irritability was, "This is what needs to be done." Other people said I was irritable. I was efficient. Emotions: Not being scared in scary situations. I felt well and clear.

Prover #3 • Female • 36 years old

Day 1
- At 12:00 midnight I took the remedy. Thirty minutes after taking the remedy, I felt a little dizziness for ten minutes while lying. Moderate intensity. Lasted five–ten minutes.
- Feeling of more blood circulation in head. Could hear the blood going through my head. More awake for fifteen minutes, then fell asleep.
- Stomach mildly upset. Digestion slow. Had eaten raw red pepper.

Day 2
- On waking, tinnitus was there and louder than normal.
- Little headache over left eye—above it. Pinching pain. Intermittent for about five minutes and then gone.
- Image of a white bird. Like a parrot or cocatoo. On a branch. Suddenly it was there. Eyes still closed, image suddenly came. Something light, not heavy. Felt peaceful.
- Two hours after being up, I was standing and felt my head and body were going around to the right. I was going to lose my balance and I needed to sit down. Lasted three to four minutes and then let up. I never sat down.
- 11:30 sleepy—tired—sleep for one hour.
- 2:00 p.m. very energetic, playful, alive.
- Went to a presentation about Yogananda and the Self-Realization Fellowship. Inspiring.

Day 3
- Energetic, good mood. "High" feeling to it. Was very active—more so than usual. Physically more active. Mentally better concentration, more awake, more alive.
- Tinnitus on awaking.
- Jehovah people ring on my door. I can tell them very clearly and at the beginning that I respect them and I am not interested. Incredible, normally I would need a lot more time to tell them diplomatically that I am not interested (difficult to say no). Telling my feelings, normally I would let them in. Felt good. Normally I have trouble setting boundaries. Came out spontaneously—surprised me.
- With a friend—I don't usually share what I'm feeling (only when really comfortable). This time—I don't want to keep it for me; I want to share it. It was the first time I didn't keep it in. Was able to share and let go. Felt positively afterwards. My friend was surprised—he misunderstood. This happened by mail. I wrote a letter.

Day 4
- Little headache—went to bed at 2:00 a.m., physically tired, heart pounding.
- Energetic, empowered, open minded—more spiritual, meditation.
- Doing things that are waiting for months to be done—impatient but peaceful—don't waste my time—more compassion for others—better listener—very quick, clear thinking.
- Last two days a number of friends calling me in crisis and telling me the crisis and getting support. I could be more concentrated with them and more compassionate. Three friends in two days.
- Little headache on the front side before sleeping

Day 5

- Headache at night was worse. Right-sided. Like a band from the shoulder to the eye, pain constant, crampy, worse lying down, better standing, worse hot temperature, hot room, better rubbing point on shoulder, better not concentrating on the pain. I did have this headache for years regularly one or two times a month, but not in the last year. Headaches were changing and more irregular now.
- More aware now that headaches have to do with suppressed emotion (anger, sadness, disappointment). This time, anger was a reaction to my friend. I received her fax on Monday and I was very disappointed. I feel now more sensitive, more assertive. Instead of letting it go, I try to deal with it. I answer her letter with kindness but I am clear with my feelings. Normally I would have said, "Let's forget it." I would have let it go. This time I reacted more sharply and wanted to deal with it.
- Very tired but energetic!!
- Evening very tired, headache comes back, right side. Left upper side of right shoulder blade, point very painful, inflamed, better to not move, relax.
- Menses without pain or PMS. I normally have cramps, sore lower back and abdominal pain. I would be very tired and dull. Also very sensitive emotionally—weepy and irritable. Generally, three days of being "ill" and very tired. Like beginning a cold. This time: NO PAIN AT ALL!!!

Day 6

- This morning headache over eyes, then right-sided, from shoulder to right eye.
- Mind very awake, sharp.
- Good energy level even with headache.

Day 7

- More impatient, more assertive.
- Energy good.
- Headache finished yesterday at 5:00 p.m.
- Menses with no pain at all.
- I drank a cup of coffee at 2:00 p.m., didn't realize it until later, felt guilty, nothing seemed to happen.
- Overall, like "bubbling life."

Day 8

- No problem with spicy Indian food I had yesterday (normally stomach hot with poor digestion, and waking up during the night).
- Before I took the remedy, I bruised the back of the right hand, between the second and third fingers. One day before the remedy I felt numbness between the two fingers and 50% of the back of the hand; the numbness has persisted.

Day 9

- Very energetic but going down a little (90%).
- Dream: Feeling of fear in the heart.

♦ 5:00 p.m. great disappointment with myself (I didn't say no when I wanted to, doing a favor for a friend!). I feel how the anger about myself eats up energy. Later I feel better.

Day 10
♦ Energy 60%.
♦ 3:00 p.m. headache began with chills, dull pain on nose root and eyes. Then left side, started slowly, pain from left shoulder to left eye, better fresh air, being active, worse lying down, lying on painful side.
♦ Old symptom, tinnitus louder since then.
♦ Dizziness for ten minutes.
♦ 12 p.m. headache over occiput, left eye.

Day 11
♦ Energy 60%.
♦ Feel tired because of headache, disappointment with headache, discouragement.
♦ Sleep well. Once awake because headache, blood pulsating in whole head, tinnitus louder—headache left side, left shoulder to left eye.
♦ 4:00 to 5:00 p.m. very tired, could sleep.
♦ 8:00 p.m. tired, headache comes back a little, perhaps because phone call of friend, disappointed with myself.

Day 12
♦ Tired. Sense of struggle. Discouraged because energy from first week of proving, 100%, went away, this morning somewhat 20%.
♦ Feeling of struggle and discouragement in the heart, in the chest.
♦ I want to cope and try to put my mind in the stage of what was 100% energy (power of thoughts).
♦ Today I feel especially like some years ago in my job—life is a struggle, I try hard, sometimes it seems to go and then it falls apart. First I feel optimistic and idealistic, I am trying hard, and then I get disappointed, discouraged, I don't get anywhere, the feeling of hurt, sadness, I am not good enough. While I am writing these I feel more this state and I want to get out of it. I get the sense I don't want to deal with this state, I try to suppress this turmoil that wants to get out, tears, suppressed feelings, suppressed anger, suppressed sadness, suppressed disappointments.
♦ After tears I feel somewhat better. I want to function today.
♦ Headache left side, extending from shoulder to forehead, especially inside, behind, between eye and ear. Dull, sometimes stitching pain.
♦ Mouth is dry.
♦ 1:00 p.m. dizziness for fifteen minutes.
♦ 3:00 p.m. pressure on head and eyes, feel tired.
♦ 5:00 p.m. dizziness for ten minutes—since then, stitching in one spot under the left jaw sometimes.
♦ 6:30 p.m. heart seems to pound faster for fifteen minutes.
♦ 7:00 p.m. right ear tinnitus worse for several minutes.

- 11:00 p.m. somewhat little headache from morning back, went away during the morning at 12:00 a.m.
- Lots of energy, 70% back.

Day 13
- Energy about 60%.
- No headaches.
- I saw R. yesterday evening in a presentation about homeopathy.
- Dream: In a nice Italian villa with different houses, a beautiful garden, swimming pool. I am a guest among others of R. there. My room is a mess, a lot of papers I have to put in order (a normal state in real life for me). My brother has a birthday and he is also there in another house. There are a lot of friends and acquaintances of his. It is late and we all go to bed. I am concerned about my brother that something will happen to him. He seems to be alone among his friends, and it seems very difficult for me to reach him. I am looking at someone, guards perhaps (?), close the gates to the villa.
- A little sadness in my heart, perhaps because of my brother in dream.
- 11:00 a.m. stitching in left upper back for half an hour.
- 6:00 p.m. very tired.

Day 14
- Wake up tired—energy 60%.
- Feeling some fear of danger in the heart, of being outside driving to a conference—went away during the day.
- Feel good, 70% energy.
- Tired after whole day conference. It was a very inspiring day, powerful women speaking about spirituality, femininity, psychology, astrology, religion, vision of the future of our world and the energy of femininity. Visions for the next millennium.

Day 15
- Tired—energy 70%.
- I spoke with my supervisor, he has written ten pages. He is a very sensitive listener and very thorough, he gave me good insights and thoughts. I feel much better after speaking with him about my fragility points (difficult to say no, feeling of being taken advantage of).
- A lot of awareness about myself and others, digesting thoughts and the conference of yesterday, "Women Visionaries."
- There was a situation where I promised a friend I would buy them a camera. I went to Fisherman's Wharf—an earlier time there I was cheated. This time I was determined not to do it again. This guy gave me a hard sell. At the moment of paying, he tried to raise the price! Same thing happened—I paid the higher price. I had anger about myself because I allowed this to happen. I was also upset that it was unfair. I got in the same situation and fell for the same thing despite my best efforts.
- I had another experience of not saying NO. A woman friend was going through a crisis with her husband. She's crazy. She had fallen in love with a man on the Internet. She told me the whole story. She was very alive in the crisis. The marriage was more a

friendship. She wanted to travel to meet this man. She asked me to take her to the airport. She was asking me what to do. I said, "Do it." The inner conflict came up around having taken a stand without knowing the whole situation. Also conflict around having been taken advantage of by my friend. This was the deeper conflict. I wanted to say I wouldn't take her to the airport, but I wasn't able to—I took her on Friday. This brought on a headache.

◆ My main issues are being taken advantage of and not being able to say no when the situation was not right for me.

Day 16
◆ Energy 70%, tired.
◆ I put my hands on my abdomen and repeated, "Healing my womb, my wounds" and I had to cry. There was a feeling of pain, hurt, wounded. I felt better after crying. A woman friend calls me, she is in a difficult love affair situation. I realize that my feeling she had taken advantage of me last week was my delusion. I am compassionate and let my ego go to listen to her.

Day 17
◆ Dream: I am in a house. I am with a woman friend. She is lesbian, she is very lovely and caring to me. Suddenly she is gone, feeling of loneliness. I look outside, the sea is surrounding the house and there is a little boat moving in the waves. I go outside and ride on the boat. It is my mother's house; it seems to be closed in the front. I look from the boat to see if she is there, or if a window, a door is open. Why is all closed? She told me she was there. The wind and the waves move the little boat from one side to the other of the house. Suddenly the sea is gone. I go out of the boat and go to the house. A group of girls appear; they are looking at some flowers outside of the house. Peaceful feeling. Now the house is open, my mother is there. I tell her I couldn't come in because the house was closed. Feeling that something was opening deeply and profoundly.
◆ Today I feel more centered—I am more aware about a lot of things: about the bigger picture of the world, the universe, how all is one, about life, about friends surrounding me, about their worries, about their friendships, my life, my inner voice, my ego which is in my way, my path, my mission, my fragility and vulnerability, my body.

Day 18
◆ Tired and ok.
◆ 2:00 p.m. and 3:00 p.m. very tired, little headache over left eye, pressure.

> **Prover #4 • Female • 43 years old**

Day 1
♦ Was trying to talk myself out of going to a meeting of alternative healers. Just wanted to sit and read, be absorbed by something instead. Went on to the meeting in the afternoon. Enjoyed the women at the meeting. The home where it was held was beautiful and decorated with my taste in art. I wanted to stroll around and take it all in. The view of the mountains with a nearby storm was inspiring. Several of the women present I was intrigued by and felt a connection with. The brochures were beautifully hand painted. I wanted to use them for my patients. I shared the communal feeling. Felt let down when I came home and found that the brochure offered vague and mystical descriptions of her healing work with spiritual, poetic quotes, not very appealing to me. Expansive feeling at the meeting with feeling of disappointment afterwards.

Day 2
♦ Awoke this morning with dramatic healing of my chronic lower right lip peeling and cold sore.
♦ Feel more energy. Good pace and better prioritizing than usual.
♦ This morning noticed new pulling type of pain in left back below scapula, and more tension both sided, mid-thorax in back. Occasional sharp pain in the region of my heart seems associated at times. Not very distracting, not persisting, just a fleeting awareness. Feel that my heart and emotions are involved. Not aware of sadness or other specific origin.

Day 3
♦ Repeated remedy.
♦ Good energy.
♦ Occasional reminder of back tension/discomfort, left side mainly, still fleeting. No heart or chest symptoms. No new symptoms, no details remembered.

Day 4
♦ Good energy.
♦ Some mid-back bilateral muscle tension only, again fleeting awareness only, no localization, nothing anterior.

Day 5
♦ Computer pointer failure, had to turn off computer to reboot without saving info, lost important letters and seven days of proving journal. Spent rest of day trying to reconstruct data, not especially upset, take things like this in stride usually, perhaps even better this time.
♦ I nearly torched my place this morning when the metal can candle on my night stand ignited the paint on the outside of the can. Lucky we were awake and the tissue box wasn't closer!

Mandragora Officinarum   Mandrake Root

- Long, busy day and still have good energy.
- Still have peeling lip and most of my fingernails.

Day 6
- Energy amazing.

Day 7
- Awoke with good energy. Aware of peoples' appreciation of nature.
- Persisting lip peeling.

Day 8
- Dream: I colored President Clinton's eyes with a felt tipped marker, green or blue, right over the pupil. Later wondered if the ink was toxic or not. Would I get into trouble since it probably was not non-toxic?
- Spent a good part of the morning at the nursery selecting trees for the now open yard, trees with colorful flowers, red bud and crepe myrtle, and a Japanese maple. Planted the trees then took a long bath.
- One very irate mom, not interested in my reassurance that her child had only a virus. Couple of callers angry at me this weekend, unwarranted, very unusual. I was very gentle with them and let it go.
- Felt dirt in my eye under my contacts most of day, too busy to flush them. Sometimes gone but would return until contacts removed before sleep.

Day 9
- Re-dosed remedy.
- Awoke today with good energy. Felt overwhelmed at times but plowed right along with amazing stamina.
- Difficulty connecting, coordinating with supervisor
- Occasional pulling back pain, left better than right-mid-back, no chest radiation or pain. Fleeting, not distracting or persisting ever.
- Lip is peeling.

Day 10
- Energy unusual, friend wondering if I may be bipolar. This remedy must be acting. I'll have to do a differential diagnosis, bipolar type II?
- Soft grit sensation under my contacts at times, allergies?
- Lip peeling not any different.

Day 11
- Awoke this morning very lost. Flitted around one thing to another in my office, no motivation, no direction.
- Awoke with menses. Very unusual. Usually I am very lackadaisical during the late day and evening before my flow. Premenstrual lack of energy and motivation arrived late for

me. Flow, fresher blood and thinner, heavier than usual. Typical oblivion to potential mess and kept forgetting liners.
- Couldn't get my act together.
- Lip still peeling.
- No muscle/back/chest symptoms.
- More nail-biting in morning when frustrated trying to plan a useful day.

Day 12
- Dream: Beautiful and inspiring. An unrecognized acquaintance man was showing me and another person his home with wonderful art pieces of sculpture and wall hangings. More impressive were the fountains, natural ponds with waterfalls, well-designed. There was his wife working on a new piece of an animated hologram of a rainbow, people walking within a landscape, all inside a large box, very non-television, can't say why, maybe three-dimensional, or iridescence? Husband very proud and loving. She had done all the creations in the home. Very friendly and down-to-earth.
- Dream: Small group, friends? Finishing a dinner in someone's home and being led downstairs to den where the couple had set up a little theatre where they showed slides of fetuses/babies who had been aborted and buried, founded by this group of Right-to-Lifers. Slides showed frontal views of bodies curled into balls with heads bowed into knees, arms folded at sides, fists. No open positions, no side views or extended limbs, no faces. Purpose was to show the tragedy of all these babies unearthed. I was noticing that this couple had lots of weapons showcased, collection of handguns and machine guns, antiques. Feeling was that I was trapped by conservatives, no debate or arguing of any points being made, just observing and making mental notes.

Day 13
- Unusually unaffected by stressors of work.
- Lip peeled and bled today, cold sore continues.

Day 14
- Dream: Interviewing old ladies each in her own home, all with Southern drawls, just matter-of-fact info about themselves. The feeling—I was minimally interested in topics discussed, bored.
- On impulse bought several books for Christmas gifts. Reading them on the drive found them not what I wanted after all. Another example of my feeling excited about materials that I later feel disappointed about.
- When I voided my bladder, it seemed to go on forever, no burning or spasm, normal urine.
- Fleeting, wandering abdominal cramps after breakfast, didn't last more than perhaps one-half hour. No diarrhea or constipation, no nausea.
- Lip peeling as usual, right side.

Day 15
- I seem to be more tolerant of the cold on this remedy.

- Pitting edema of my ankles and shins.
- Lip still peeling easily.

Day 16
- No edema, no back pain or tension, no cramping.

Day 17
- Typing my journal late, making whole lot of mistakes and corrections, which has been strange and peculiar about this whole journal.
- I've been more aware of my posture (not ever good) since starting the remedy, come to think of it. Not straightening up or stretching, just aware when I'm standing or walking that my vertebrae are lined up vertically with curvature and flexibility. I have had this awareness, but mostly trying to correct my posture, when I've been physically fit and active in the past and I'm more aware of my muscles at those times. This is different somehow.
- My penmanship has been very illegible and shortcut lately, more than before, possibly progressing since the remedy.
- Bit thumbnail short and notice the pain.
- Lip is also painful today, peeling not different.

Day 20
- Better cold tolerance.
- Dream: In a retreat. Looking for my purse. Banquet of food spread. We all slept in the same room. I was seeking privacy. It was taken for granted that there was no privacy. It was OK because the other people were interesting.
- Dream: About flowering trees.
- Lying down with my dog. Taking a nap with the animals.

Summary
- Was in a funk before the remedy. Took three doses. My funk was an energy problem. I was calling in sick. I felt suicidal and not wanting to go on. I felt overdue for a remedy. I had a dream the morning of the remedy. I was looking forward to it. I woke up with the dream of an oil lamp that was given to me and I was going to use it at a spiritual talk. It would be private at her table. I never got to see the speaker. Yesterday I opened a catalog and saw the lamp of my dream.
- Dreams of retreats.
- Typical dream is looking for my purse.
- Dream about flowering trees. Went to nursery and picked up pink flowering trees for my yard. Several references to birds. Humming bird in yard. Large lemon tree and that tree was pruned. It was getting into lemon flowers.
- Traveling. Seagull with one leg.
- References in my journal about bird feeders.
- Several patients got angry with me. Expressed anger. No real reason. I was very effective in an allopathic way on this remedy. I wasn't touched by homeopathic symptoms.

At other times frustrated by allopathic medicine. Problem in that I identified two women friends who I was disappointed with. The connectedness was lost because I could see there was a way that they would connect.
- No physical symptoms. Was energtic. Fleeting left flank pain.
- Sharp emotional pains in my heart day two or three of the remedy. Knew it was my heart, and emotional.
- Later realized I was more aware of my spine than usual. With remedy was aware that my vertebrae were lined up and flexible.
- Peeling of lip on left side.
- Had mistakes all thoughout my journal—many typos.
- Recording on phone was messed up. N. was unable to reach me during the first week. Erased seven days of journal on my computer. Lost really important letters too.
- Dream of waterfalls. Being shown home of acquaintance. Waterfalls all over the place. Animated hologram with a rainbow and landscape. Feeling of awe about the woman artist.
- Very bloody menses. Blood was thinner and brighter. Delay in PMS. Usually the day before menses. Happened the day of my period. Was quite lazy.
- Talked about lying down with my dog. Taking a nap with the animals.

Prover #5 • Female • 46 years old

Day 0
- General: Worked today and it was perfect. Went to a wiener roast at night and it was perfect weather. Energy level good. Walked after work. Took the remedy at 5:00 p.m.
- Head: Some sneezing and sinus drainage.

Day 1
- Slept really long and hard—eight hours. Felt sluggish and didn't want to get up. Yawned a lot. Napped 7:30 to 9:30 p.m.
- Did homework, but couldn't concentrate—weather is too nice.
- Felt an increase in appetite. Wanted meat.

Day 2
- Awakened at 3:00 a.m. with a dream.
- Dream: About going fast. I was driving with my sister in a car on this big bridge/hill. Went down really fast. She was scared and I was exhilarated. Missed the exit and ended up in a corn field. Then I was getting on a carnival ride. It was going fast too.
- I felt sleepy today. Took a nap between patients in the afternoon.
- Low energy but worked anyway, which helped. Went to bed at 9:00 p.m.
- A lot of flatus, even though I had my normal morning stool.

- Sneezing and mucous today. Slight head pain behind left eye when I worked out, which increased pressure to the area.
- Eczema worse on left hand today.

Day 3
- Another dream at 3:00 a.m.
- Dream: My husband and I were at a hotel and I wanted to walk home. I walked on an expressway and was going the "wrong way," but in the right direction. I stood in a line to buy a swimsuit for $100. A friend said I was supposed to stay out of the sun while doing a proving. I put on the swimsuit and the salesgirl told me it was $300. I felt they were ripping me off, so I punched her, gave $100 and wore the swimsuit as I left the store. When I left, I found the "right" street—Union Street—and went home.
- Slept well and actually felt like getting up in the morning.
- Felt angry today. Got mad at my trainer. So I upped the stairstepper and worked out harder. Did have more energy.

Day 4
- Awakened at 3:30 a.m. with a dream.
- Dream: I was at my office and two boys, engineering types, were looking at my implant case. I left them looking at it. When I came back they had melted wax all over the screws and crowns. I was angry and chewed them out.
- Dream: I was in the town where I went to college, living with some friends. It was a football weekend. I was sitting at a bar under an umbrella talking to my lab man for implants. Told him what had happened in my implant cases.
- Didn't sleep well after the dreams.
- Had a scissor-like headache behind the eyes. I took a Motrin.
- Diarrhea three times today before noon. Possibly from black beans?
- Worked out. Weather changed from sunny to cloudy. Possibly the headache was sinus which is related to the weather change and that is "normal" for me.

Day 5
- Took the remedy again.
- Hard to remember my dreams.
- Dream: Have a few images. My husband and I were chaperoning my son's class. I was wearing black and riding in an airplane. Had to take the train home. I played peacemaker for the girls in the office at a hotel room. They were arguing about the heat. I said, "Turn it off at the vent."
- I just realized in the past few days four major things that went wrong in the office after I took the remedy.

Day 6
- Dream: Of going to a friend's house to get my haircut. My hair is bright red. It's a big party and a lot of my friends are there. All are drinking beer and smoking. Everyone is getting their hair done. A new male hairdresser cuts mine. My husband came up to me

and said, "No sex." I said, "Ok," turned away, and left. He chased after me, grabbed me, and kissed me. We decide to have a "high school" relationship and just make out. That made me feel really good. That's all I wanted anyway—to be hugged and kissed. Then a friend and I were in an airplane in Washington, D.C. There was a glass top on it and we flew upside down so we could sight-see.
- There was a plumbing water leak today in the office. Soaked the carpet. Had to turn the water off for the whole building.
- Went to a Halloween party. Danced and had two drinks.

Day 7
- Felt like shit. Woke up 6:00 a.m. with a pounding headache, especially behind the left eye. Pulsated whenever I moved. I took a Motrin. At 7:00 a.m., I vomited everything in my stomach. Then I had three bowel movements by 9:00 a.m. Felt like the worst hangover I had ever had, as if I'd had a half a bottle of vodka. I had my usual red wine with dinner, and then had two gin and tonics over the next three hours at the party. I danced constantly and didn't finish my last drink. Much more sensitive to the alcohol than normal.
- Spent the morning in bed. No energy. Haze of a headache all day. Finally felt like myself around 7:00 p.m.

Day 8
- A good day. Started the day with yoga. Taught Sunday school class and got a lot of reinforcement from everyone. Then worked on a write-up. Took a case for homeopathy and feel like I did a good job. Don't know the remedy but I got the case. Talked to my preceptor. Made a really good dinner for the family, which I don't do very often.

Day 9
- Tough day at work. Five cancellations. I haven't had that many cancel in a day in years! Able to fill the canceled appointments.
- Worked out and that helped me immensely.
- Lots of mucous and sneezing, gloves burned my hands today.
- Slept quite well, but heavy. No dreams.
- Sinus is related to weather change. Northwest wind and rainy all day, 45 degree temperatures—yuk!

Day 10
- Good day at work. But exhausting.
- Eczema worse but sinuses better.
- Really felt sad this morning. Put on some music while working on a patient and started to weep. Felt better after that. Walked at lunch and the sun came out. Felt better after the walk.
- No bowel movement.

Day 11
- No dreams. Slept well. Awoke at 5:30 a.m. with a bowel movement.

Mandragora Officinarum   *Mandrake Root*

◆ Good concentration—finished a write-up. Worked on homeopathic case to send to my preceptor. Did yoga and worked out with R. Played ping-pong with him and won!! Very surprising because I haven't played in years. Told him it was because I wasn't attached to winning.

◆ Feel a lot of anxiety about my son's poor grades and attitude towards school.

Day 12
◆ Lots of normal physicals—ezcema, sinus with blowing nose, good bowel movement.
◆ Work was good today. But an air/water syringe leaked water—probably a washer.
◆ Good energy and worked out after work for one and a half hours.
◆ Wanted to eat all day but really didn't feel hunger. Ate a lot of spaghetti and meatballs for supper.
◆ Dream: Remembered a dream image. I was fighting—using some sort of martial arts. The key was to use the other person's strength against him.

Day 13
◆ No dreams but restless sleep. Awake from 1:30 a.m. until 3:00 a.m.
◆ Some sneezing and bowel movement at that time. Ate too much, too late.

Day 14
◆ Dream: I gave birth. I'd been in a social situation—at a party. Started to bleed and a man put his hand there and stopped it. Then I was happy because some friends were moving nearby. Now I had someone to refer to for cranial. I lay down on the floor and gave birth quickly to a boy. Got to cut the cord all by myself. No pain. I looked at husband and said, "Another baby."

Day 15
◆ Taught Sunday school today and was very emotional. I couldn't read because I kept crying. And the crying spread—D. and B. cried also. Really felt drained throughout the class. We were reading about love and sadness.

Day 16
◆ Quite an emotional day for the office. Unbelievably, my hygienist lost her kids in a custody battle. She was hysterical. I tried to calm her.
◆ Slept well but the high winds awakened me. Rainy and thunderstorms.

Day 17
◆ Hard to sleep last night because of my concern about my hygienist. Today she was quiet, didn't sleep at all last night.
◆ The weather was constant winds, often up to 60 mile per hour gusts. We had to eventually evacuate our building in the afternoon, due to an ammonia leak from a chemical tank. All weather-related (hopefully not the remedy).

Day 18
- Slept well and long.

Day 19
- Slept well. No dreams. Woke at 5:00 a.m. and finished typing journal.

Prover #6 • Female • 40 years old

Day 1
- Maybe slightly calmer. Slower. Normally I am more irritable and hurried. Both were better on the remedy.
- Menses started.
- Dream: I was at a spiritual gathering where each person was going to say something important. One friend was not allowed to speak. I insisted she be allowed to speak. She said something inappropriate. I went to the leader and asked why, and he said the friend had done something bad.

Day 2
- Maybe calmer, not sure.
- Good energy.
- Had hiccoughs in morning on way to school. They stopped, but up until 2:00 p.m. had occasional hiccough, involuntary.

Day 3
- Still calm.
- After dinner had bile come up in mouth—bitter—very flatulent too. Bloated, gassy all evening.
- Dream: About grandmother. House just painted. The color and feel of the house was peaceful, cheerful light and pastel colors. Beautiful. She is peaceful and I am. I never dreamed about her before. She has been dead for ten years. It was a calm and serene atmosphere. Pastels, pink and peach. I don't like pastels. I usually dream about my kids and anxiety. She was wonderful.
- Dream: Of S.
- Perspiration still odorous.

Day 4
- Great mood, happy carefree. More joyful than last few weeks.
- Thirst not as bad as before. Not waking up as thirsty.
- Typical period although slightly lighter flow.

Day 5
- Head a little fuzzy today and yesterday. Woke at 5:30 a.m. from a phone call. Slept well, can't remember dreams. Feel good, happy again.
- Headache at 10:30. Usually caffeine takes it away and it did, but it was stronger than before.
- Still not as thirsty.
- Vaginal itching, on labia. Better after shower. Showed up end of day Wednesday. Worse from scratching. Burning. This is the most marked symptom.
- Odorous perspiration still there.

Day 6
- Calm. Energetic even with lack of sleep.
- Itching on labia. Crusty feeling, dryness. Needing to itch but burns, worse from scratching. Very dry eyes.
- Dream: In a car with the H. family. It isn't the right car, but they won't listen. I know it is not right but am frustrated because I cannot get that across.

Day 7
- Slept late, feel groggy.
- Eyes burning all morning. Wanted eye drops. Dry feeling in eyes.
- Itching still there.
- Slept hard and well.

Day 8
- Rested. Calm.
- Eyes still dry.
- Not as thirsty.
- Still itching.
- Dream: Who should I take as a patient next?

Day 9
- Loss of sense of taste. Things are bland. Even candy isn't sweet. Corner of mouth has blister. Dry. Hurts to open mouth wide. Cracked, right side.
- Dream: Traveling with a large group to a campground. We have boats and kids, many people I do not know. Lots of confusion. My children are there and receive gifts from their dad. I have to hide them. Other children are winning contests. All are confused. Mixed in all this is meeting new people, all with children. I am just floating around in this chaos. Relaxed and happy.

Day 10
- Woke up tired even though slept well.
- Dream: I go to have a pedicure and they make me stand in a machine that takes a picture of your body. Then they scan it, three different outputs, and want me to pay $75 to read each evaluation. I am so mad, so indignant. I keep saying, "Just do the pedicure!" Finally I leave in disgust.

Day 11
- Dream: My youngest son is riding with me in a car. I keep having to ask him to step on the brake because my hands are full. Even though I knew it was dangerous. We are driving along, I am rinsing the soap out of my hair and see an old friend with her daughter, someone I am not friends with anymore. I see her child and feel very jealous.

Day 12
- Dream: I had to work in a tall building in Paris. I took the train in. I was alone in the building and very scared. Couldn't find may way back to station. Confused. Friend is there but won't help.
- Abdominal pain. When my bladder was full, instead of having the urge to urinate I had an incredible pain replacing the urge. Pressure and cramping low down.

Prover #7 • Male • 38 years old

Day 1
- Took dose today before bed.
- Was watching Discovery Channel—there was a show called *Snake Bite*. Researchers were collecting snake venoms. They were searching for a Black Mumba—this snake could kill a person in five minutes. They discussed how snake venom of the same snake may be different—when living in different locations (chemically different).
- My daughter began venting anger in the evening. She was feeling she is unloved, angry with her mother. She was cursing and demanding—wanting to be equal with us (she is eleven years old). Feeling persecuted, put down, not cared for. She wants sympathy, wants to be loved. She is weeping. We had a discussion about how we could get on better in the household. My daughter asked for more sympathy—she wished she could be treated like she was when she was a baby. We sang her lullabies and gave her affection at bedtime. She was happy.

Day 2
- Dream: I am out in front of the property I grew up on. It is night time. The property has three houses on it and ours is in the middle. I see suspicious headlights driving on the property. I feel someone is trespassing with bad intentions. I realize my mother is alone in the house and may be in danger. I go off to investigate the possible intruder. Feeling of possible threat.
- Dream: Someone is showing me a map of the U.S.A. that has earthquake activity. The person says there were earthquakes that day of large proportion. I look at this map and there is a horizontal quake line running from coast-to-coast, the highest Richter scale number along the line was 9.0. I think, "Wow, that must have been horrible where it got that bad."

Day 3

◆ Back to work with a busy schedule. Today was an unpleasant day. Things that have been frustrating in the past were heightened today. Two patients did not show up for their appointment. Two patients called at the last moment to re-schedule their appointments. This has happened off and on before the proving, but today, it was heightened. I was angry with my Maker—I was cursing God. I try to do the right thing always, I do my best work—why should I have to put up with this bullshit. I am trying to support my family, and it is very difficult. People don't care and are irresponsible. I schedule patients for an hour plus, so it is very upsetting when they just don't show up. The feeling is anger, frustration, and disappointment.

◆ I have had allergy symptoms in the past—sneezing and runny nose. Sensitivity to east winds and cats. They are usually mild, and sporadic. Today my sinuses felt as if I had a cat under my nose all day. My nose ran clear, thin, mucous discharge all day. I had to blow my nose every five minutes throughout the day. My nose had a tingling, unpleasant feeling most of the day. This also provoked some strong sneezing. These are old symptoms, except intensified and constant. When I went to bed this night, these symptoms got 90% better as soon as I laid down, which was very peculiar.

◆ My wife took my daughter to the orthopedic doctor today. She is fine, very little discomfort at this point. He literally spent two minutes with her, and decided to cast her arm without explaining anything to my wife. My wife said the doctor glanced at the x-ray, palpated her arm, and said he would cast her. He wasn't sure if the arm was broken, but this was the best procedure. The bill will probably be $300–$400. I feel resentful that being a practitioner of acupuncture and homeopathy, I have to work a full day to earn what this doctor makes in five minutes. Our insurance will reimburse most of his bill and we will pay the difference. Even though the state has put me through vigorous requirements to be licensed, calls me a primary health care provider, health insurance coverage for my services is extremely minimal. This makes it difficult to earn a decent living. The feeling is anger, resentment, ripped off.

Day 4

◆ The nasal irritation and discharge was about 75% better today. I still had some clear mucous from my nose. But it was much reduced. Now I am a bit stuffy. I had two patients forget their appointments today. I called them, but felt less angry today.

Day 5

◆ I developed a painful spot on the upper right side of my tongue. It seemed like a canker sore or apthae. It was a small painful point on the top of my tongue.

Day 6

◆ Traveled to San Diego for Oriental Medicine Symposium.

Day 7

◆ Busy all day in classes. Nothing peculiar overall. Canker sore on the top of my tongue began to disappear.

Day 8
- Busy all day in classes. Just before I arrived back home from traveling, late in the evening, I was listening to the radio in my car. An extremely beautiful rendition of the old Byrds' song (Turn! Turn! Turn!—There is a season, turn, turn, turn. . .) began to play. I had an overwhelming sense of grief and began to weep. I had to pull over for a few minutes to let the emotion out. I thought, "What a painful world we are passing through. Everything that we cling to, must leave us."
- That evening my wife had the flu and I was not sympathetic. I felt overwhelming grief and no joy in my life. Lasted five minutes and it passed.
- Watching another nature show and there was something on wolfmen. They were talking about the study of wolfpeople. Then PBS is showing a Stramonium plant. Thought this is synchronistic and weird.
- Dream: I caught an Orca (whale) and it was tied to a rope. The whale took off and was spinning, and one of my patients was telling me to be detached. Dreams dark and sinister.
- Dream: I was climbing up shrubs or trees. I was following two men, and I was looking down on them. They were smoking cigarettes or marijuana. One of the adults was carrying a child who had died by drugs or poison. I had a sick feeling.

Day 10
- Several nights later my daughter woke up afraid of the wolfman. The chair in the bedroom was turning into a wolf. Came into bed and was happy and comfortable.
- Dream: Being given guard duty. Climbing a ladder. Following someone up the platform. Losing my footing. I had a thought of catching pigs below. I spoke sarcastically that the job was menial.
- Dream: I was treating a patient and told him about the proving. He fell into a deep sleep. He had a dream that his sheep were in danger. He is a police officer. He felt like a shepherd that needed to protect his sheep.
- Dream: Frightening. My daughter ran out of her bedroom and said someone was trying to come in the window and get her. I went in and saw a shadow and the dream ended. The feeling was fear and having to meet the danger.
- A general theme was looking down on things and dangerous, dark situations.

Prover #8 • Female • 43 years old

Day 1
- I was sanding my bedroom floor. Instantly I glanced at my friend R. and he was covered with feathers and a beak and I was repulsed. I was thirsty and went for a glass of water and stopped myself because I had just taken the remedy.
- Felt chilly in an hour. There was sand dust everywhere. I was sleepy. Went into the next room and fell asleep. The noise of the sander didn't bother me. Fell asleep with the dogs and cat. I felt relaxed and light. My mood went way up. I felt going off somewhere. It was nice.

Day 2
- Dream: I was ice-skating in Holland. I enjoyed the gliding motion on the ice—felt free. Sky was very blue and I don't remember any sun, but it was light everywhere. I was wearing a burgundy coat with a brown fur collar and muff.
- My cat woke me up meowing and meowing like crazy. This was so unusual—as she is a very quiet kitty. She just wanted me to pet her and give her attention.
- Dream: I was at homeopathy class, but it was in a resort place. Actually we were in the Swiss Alps and skiing between classes. I loved the cool crisp air—very high altitude. The snow was clean and white.
- Cooler than usual.
- Decreased appetite.
- No interest in sweets, no chocolate.
- Could not finish dinner—easily filled. Homemade chicken noodle soup.
- Went out with my daughter. I was very impatient with traffic even though traffic was fairly light. Irritable, people in my way. Sitting in restaurant I was telling my daughter about a woman and I couldn't find the word for woman and called her a "thing." Lost my keys twice that day. My daughter commented that I was not able to focus well. Teased me, calling me a "bird-brain."
- Driving daughter to school and had sharp pain in abdomen. Went to bathroom and had diarrhea. Out of the blue. Unusual.
- I laughed a lot.

Day 3
- Energy high.
- Felt well but not really interested in anything; felt like doing nothing—just relaxing.
- Experienced a sudden sharp pain with diarrhea—watery. Lasted about 20–30 minutes and then completely gone.
- Sex drive low.
- Experienced difficulty with remembering people's names. Thought that was funny.
- Thoughts were fuzzy. Hard to concentrate at work. Had strong desire to go take my constitutional remedy to "feel normal."
- Dream: Talking with a doctor that I work with about business and I was feeling trapped and unhappy with him. I was unable to speak up and I wanted to run away.

- Dream: I bought a new van but felt financially trapped because the payments were so high.

Day 4
- Feel very slow and sluggish in the morning. Had to really mentally discipline myself to get up in morning. Just wanted to stay in bed with my two dogs and two cats. Had moved the birdcage with my two birds right by my bed. I wanted them to be close to me. Felt like I wanted all my animals around me. They seemed to like that. Animals were more affectionate and clinging to me. I liked it.
- Woke up feeling brain-dead.
- Emotionally felt flat in morning. Spacey—concentration poor. Started reading repertory on Psorinum and could follow that—felt my brain starting to function again.
- I noticed that my appetite was down. I wasn't thinking about food. Wanted something salty. Bought potato chips but they tasted like cardboard.
- No more diarrhea.
- Driving to work I wanted to take LSD to wake my brain up.
- When I got to work at 1:00 p.m., my mood suddenly shifted.

I felt alive. Energy increased. Lots of laughter. Felt a better clarity with listening to my patients. Mood remained cheerful.
- When going home it was dark and the mountain pass is very curvy. I was having a hard time gauging my speed and was a little afraid to drive—felt like I was going to go off the road. Felt like I was in a bardo state—a state of nothingness and luminosity. Got home. Listened to a tape of *Tibetan Book of the Dead*. Fell asleep as a lump quickly with my cat cradled in my arms—just like a baby. I felt completely relaxed.
- Urine was hot and a little scalding twice today. Never experienced that before.
- For about ten seconds, the skin on my fingers and palms itched and itched. Hives on my left hand—went away. Palms very red and itched so bad I scratched them on the sharp corner of the dresser.
- Craving peanut butter. Tasted wonderful. Some cheese—good. Drank seven glasses whole milk—very satisfying.

Day 5
- Dream: Friend was visiting, walking down trail to waterfall, and it was beautiful. Blue sky, fall leaves. Daughters were ahead and we caught up to them. At the top of the trail it changed and my mother was there with her friend J. (both dead). J. was an astrologer and my parents' mentor. During the dream I asked my mom why life was so hard. They told me not to worry. The feeling in the dream was freedom, peace and wonderful. Playful and relaxed. Beautiful afternoon. One of the nicest dreams I've had. I remember thinking we had crossed into the astral world and that was why the colors were so rich and temperature was perfect. Then we all continued on the trail—uphill climb. We then were driving through red rock, like in Sedona, Arizona. There was a brewery there, passing out free beer. Beer was very thirst-quenching—it tasted different than regular beer. This was a perfect tasting brew. It was made from this special water and it had plant juices mixed in. Then the trail ended at a beautiful lake. I remember asking if this was

the Amazon? No, it wasn't. I was really happy then because there was my sailboat that I have wanted. Woke up. Felt good. Felt peaceful.

Day 6
- Video machine broke—tape got stuck in it.
- My computer system went out—just left it alone. Did not want to deal with it.

Day 7
- Felt tired after work.
- Was supposed to go to a meeting and felt like I did not want to be around people. Wanted peace and quiet. Wanted no noise and no distractions.
- Needed more sanding paper for my Profiler sander. Called the hardware store in town and lady in the paint department said they had it in stock. Drove into town—it was snowing and cold. They did not have the sanding paper—the lady acted like she was too busy to help and went off with another customer. Then I asked a male salesperson—he just laughed and said I must have talked to the wrong person and walked away. I was feeling angry. I did not want to drive an hour to the Home Depot. Then I stomped up to cash register to buy a few other items. Two men asked, "Is something wrong?" They were the new managers and spent time checking where else I could get the sanding paper. I felt like they cared.

Day 8
- Dream: Living in an old Victorian-type house with my mom and sister. My sister brought home this "homeless" man who was very attractive. Looked like a healthy version of Jim Morrison. I did not like him and mom felt the same way. He was recently paroled from the federal penitentiary and had to wear an ankle alarm. After three days mom and I were frustrated as my sister and this guy just sat around the house watching TV and eating. Even though mom was upset, she kept making excuses for them. The man and I went out and bought a motorcycle—a red Honda Gold Wing.
- Craving for muffins and then could not finish even one.
- Went shopping at the mall with my fourteen-year-old daughter. She needed more clothes. Usually I hate the noise and crowds at the mall. Felt detached and was even patient with my daughter while she picked out clothes. Pleasant time.
- That evening got my period—very different as absolutely no PMS. No heaviness or discomfort, no bloating. Did not experience the usual "improved mood on first day of menses."
- Feeling disconnected.
- Did not go to Halloween Party. Felt like I did not want to socialize with people. Rather be home with my animals. Felt a distance with people.

Day 9
- Most unusual period of my life. Sudden gushing and heavier flow than after childbirth. Worst menstrual period, ever. Heavy. Bled on the floor and stained the wood. Never bled this heavy before. I usually have PMS. No PMS. Menses was thin and watery and lasted less than a day. Really odd.

♦ Experienced left hip joint pain for about one hour. Odd—no limitation of motion—just a sharp deep pain.

Day 10
♦ Menses stopped completely by afternoon.
♦ Work day went well. Frustrated—computer went out.
♦ Energy good.
♦ Finally resolved work negotiations—feeling more connected with friends. More sociable and friendly at work.

Day 11
♦ Busy morning—energy high.
♦ Continued to want to just be in bed reading and animals with me during evening.
♦ Totally frustrated about computer.

Day 12
♦ Invited my group of friends to go out and have margaritas this weekend. Felt more of a party mood.
♦ Appetite improving.
♦ Sex drive starting to pick up. More lively feeling overall.

Day 13
♦ Computer completely messed up. Frustrated as can't check and answer e-mails.
♦ Dream: I was eating with some friends and these sharks kept swimming around us—like dogs begging for food. Everything was blue. No fear of sharks, and I remember thinking one of them had lost a tooth. In reality I do not like sharks at all!

Day 14
♦ Went out with five friends and drank two margaritas—loved it. Liked the salt on the edge of the glass. Talked about my future plans and wanting to try a recreational vehicle (RV). Lively discussions, etc.
♦ Dream: I was in this large Victorian house. Boarding there. It was warm and "summery" outside. I went to check on my male friend who was dressed in an old-fashioned suit. He was lying down and I pulled his arm—it came off—it was made of wax. The whole body was wax. I was upset and started to cry. I went outside and this very nice older lady who was dressed in Victorian style (blue dress with lace collar) talked to me. Told me not to worry and that my friend will be back tonight. He had some things he wanted to do. His spirit had just left his body temporarily. I did not feel so alone then.

Day 15
♦ Snowed in. Really happy to stay home and read and talk on phone. Took an afternoon nap. Rearranged furniture and cleaned.
♦ Worked on remedy write-ups but NO computer. Frustrated with this computer.
♦ Appetite continues to increase—craving bread.

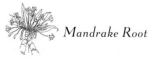

Mandragora Officinarum   *Mandrake Root*

◆ Left ear was hurting. I've never had ear problems. Pressure and pain. Popping, throbbing, sharp. Worse pressure, better from heat and warmth.

Day 16
◆ Left ear pain gone.
◆ Dream: Mice everywhere, cute little mice with big heads and little bodies. Mice had an awful lot of teeth. I did not want to kill the tiny mice—had to gently sweep them into newspaper in order to carry them out. It was spring outside. One mouse hid inside my bed and I could not get him.
◆ Dream: I was at a restaurant with this man; we were a couple. Another couple was with us and they were African American. The table next to us had four white people who were very rowdy and seemed drunk. This was a very pricey and stuffy restaurant. The four of us and the four rowdy people were "plants" to see if this restaurant discriminated against people of color. The four of us were sipping some wine—the restaurant manager was clearly perturbed by the rowdy ones and hovered around us. It felt like he was hurrying us to finish and then leave. He was overly attentive and did not give us time to enjoy the food.
◆ Spent afternoon looking through my father's pictures and mementos. Cried . . . ended when I found all these pictures of my brother (he committed suicide when he was 18 years old) that I had never seen. Later made the connection of the "wax-man" in my dream with my brother. The feeling was he is not coming back tonight but I will see him again. Theme of spirit world going back and forth.

Day 17
◆ Felt organized and clear-headed at work. Cheerful mood. Refused to deal with computer problems.

Day 18
◆ Resting quietly in bed about 9:30 p.m. while reading and all animals in bed with me (except birds)—heard garbage can fall over again! Went out and yelled at the dog in the garbage. "Dog" stood up and looked at me. It was a black bear with white spot on its chest! Then another larger black bear appeared. Then a third little bear came up to the bigger ones. I ran inside and felt totally "blown away." It felt totally surreal. Watched the three bears from my window with my cat. All the animals were completely quiet. I called the Sheriff's Department and wanted to know if someone could just drive by and scare the bears. No one could. The bears finally left.
◆ Slept poorly—woke up at any little noise.

Day 19
◆ Frustrated that computer won't be fixed for at least another week. Fantasized about new career as a computer technician, "Good pay, regular hours, no emergencies."
◆ Tired all day from poor sleep. Kept thinking about the bears.

Day 20
- On my way to homeopathy class.
- Felt very guilty leaving my animals. More than usual.

Summary:
- Overall I felt like I didn't want to be here. I'd rather be on the other side because it is prettier, nicer and more fun.
- At work I had to shut off the remedy and do my work. One of the people at work said I was different and more moody. I wanted to get the work done, go home and go to bed.
- Dreams of work, being busy.
- Singing more. Handel's Messiah, Creedence Clearwater Revival, McKenna, Gregorian Chant. Would calm me and put me in another world.
- Chilled, wanting extra clothes.
- Slept on my back, unusual for me.
- Had a hard time connecting for a few days.

Prover #9 • Female • 55 years old

Day 1
- Irritable, beyond anything I can remember feeling for years. Pressed for time. Someone else's schedule. I reluctantly agreed to meet my daughters' friends for an outing. We had to grab a quick breakfast rather than have a leisurely one. Had to give my order three times. Given the wrong change, moved three times to find comfortable place to sit. Just settled, busboy came by to sweep around us/under foot. I wanted to scream at him or push him away.
- Ate hurriedly. Feel fat, ugly, mean.
- Called N. to report in. Told her about my morning irritability. She thinks I shouldn't retake the remedy. I am away from my normal environment and want to check this out in usual setting. I feel irritated with her and stubborn. I plan to retake the remedy in my home.
- Stomach: craving something, hard to satisfy, protein, sweets.
- Constipated.
- Twitching right thumb, pulling inward on waking.

Day 2
- Feel more normal. Forgot remedy in Phoenix. Forgot to call N. Rested.

Day 3
- Back home. Irritable, restless, pressured. Called Phoenix for remedy to be sent fast mail. $27. Have to take a day late.
- Very tired.
- Heartburn, cramping, burning in epigastrium ten to fifteen minutes after eating lentil curry soup. Relieved fifteen to thirty minutes later after water, two chocolates. Lunch!

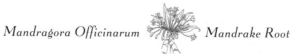

Mandragora Officinarum   *Mandrake Root*

◆ Aching pain, right thumb extending to wrist. Woke me up, after midnight and before morning.

Day 4
◆ Felt normal, calm, accomplished a lot. Re-took remedy.

Day 5
◆ Felt efficient, confident, not rushed. Very busy.
◆ Dream: A woman has a small restaurant and Bed & Breakfast in Point Richmond. I am in the restaurant. It's a cozy cafe, homey place. I find out there might be a vacancy and that she charges $30 a night for a room and meals. I am looking for a place to stay. She is behind a high half-door. I can only see her head and shoulders. She has big hair. Lots of blond curls piled up on her head. Very made up. Middle-aged. A rather stern woman. I am asking her about a room. I tell her I am a student of Hahnemann, I will be needing a room on the weekend once a month. I am trying to impress her with my reliability. She is considering my request. (I'm not sure if I imagined this or it is part of the dream—she comes from behind the counter/half-door and she is a tiny, dwarf-like person).
◆ Ate little, too busy.
◆ Bloating, gas.

Day 6
◆ Busy all day, felt low-level of pressure to accomplish more. Worked on write-ups after movie until 12:30 a.m.
◆ Slept in.
◆ Less hunger, still craving sweets.
◆ Dream: Communal living situation. I have a relationship with a man, and the freedom to live as a single woman. There is an older man. He lives here also, although not all the time. He is in his late sixties, an aristocratic patriarch. An artist. Picasso-like. A movie is being done of his life and of his ancestry. It is very important to him. He is learning things about his heritage he didn't know before. He has suggested to me that we will be lovers. It is a certainty in his mind. I am attracted to the idea and am considering it. There are also two younger men living in the house. They live as close roommates, sleeping in the same bed, yet act more like brothers. They are involved in some playful seduction with me. The older man knows about it. He is not threatened and comments that he knows what they have to offer, something rather mundane, while he has secrets of love-making I have not yet been introduced to. There is a scene where the older man goes off with some other young women to prepare for the movie shots. There has been a big meal and I am cleaning up after it. Two women are doing laundry. I move between both tasks. The younger men, boys, are asleep in one room. I discover that the older man could have great influence in my career. I am considering whether I want to have sex with him to get in his good graces or if I just want to have sex with him or not. He is back home, taking a nap somewhere. It is just the two women and myself around. I wake up.

Day 7
◆ Poor sense of time. Lost track of it. Late getting ready for evening out, really rushed.
◆ Difficulty remembering names of places, evening.
◆ Legs: Woke to feeling in legs like mild anesthesia. Very heavy feeling in both legs. Woke twice with muscle spasm of right foot drawing inward, especially small toe.
◆ Dream: Friend L. wrote a play (saw movie *Beloved* last night, the play is very much like the movie). It is her first play. Someone saw her script and wanted to produce it in a small theater. It is really more like a large parlor. I plan to attend and in order for me to do so I need to have an epidural (I don't know why). Then I have to get myself there with paralyzed legs. Because my legs are so numb I have difficulty, through traffic, etc. Finally manage by pushing a chair in front of me for support. The play is terrific. There are one or two important people there to see it. At intermission I find myself at another friend's house trying to leave her a message on her laptop about the play. She, M., and L. find me there so I can just tell them what I think of the play. I am crying. I urge them to see that it become produced nationwide. I then find myself back at the theater parlor. A wild mountain cat, the size of a small dog, is in the room with a couple of other pets and a few children and some adults. I am very distressed. I want someone to take the wild mountain cat out of the room before it hurts or attacks someone. It is menacing. Some woman walks by and casually pets it thinking it is domestic. I think the children are in danger. I want her help, but L. is busy with the production or talking to people who can promote her play. The cat either finds its way out or someone gets it outside. I am attempting to make my way to the chair to sit when I realize I am the only person who has had an epidural to come to the play. I am confused. I thought we would all have one.

Day 8
◆ Plan to push through at work until finished, get call from friend I haven't seen for awhile, change plans and take a break, go to dinner.
◆ Chest pain mid-sternum, like fracture with pulling, shortly after evening meal. Lasts 15–20 minutes.

Day 9
◆ Made up for lost time. Worked at computer early morning to late at night. Completed a good amount of work. Satisfied with result.
◆ Woke early morning with aching pain right thumb and general pain, aching left wrist, resolved spontaneously.
◆ Dream: A midwife's family home. She has a birthing room in her house. There is an odd assortment of people making up the family. I am visiting. A meal is being prepared. A young girl is cutting an orange on the floor. I note the poor practice of that in my mind. I look around. There doesn't seem to be much food. It's sparse. A patient and her family are somewhere in the house, she has delivered. I am talking to the midwife about her practice. The scene shifts and the midwife exposes the fact that she has eleven toes on one foot and something like eight on the other. They are web toes and small extra digits. The meaning of this has to do with something about babies being born with anomalies and how they can be accepted. Her family did not know until this time that

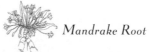

Mandragora Officinarum *Mandrake Root*

she had abnormal toes. The overall theme has to do with moral issues and differences and acceptance.

Day 10
- Some difficulty thinking.
- Threw diaphragm and cervical cap models into trash after wrapping in paper towel.
- Feeling a bit insecure.
- Stool loose, brown, soft, with gas.

Day 11
- Smelled the strong scent of cigarette smoke briefly while driving home from work at 6:30 p.m.

Day 12
- Had a patient hang up on me at 3:00 a.m. when trying to evaluate her labor status over the phone. What she was saying and what she sounded like were incongruous. I was monitoring my irritation and probably sounded distant. When her husband called back an hour later we made a plan to meet at the birth center. I went to the birth center to prepare for her. Instead she went to the hospital and told them I wouldn't admit her to the birth center. She was complete, willing to push for one half-hour, then wanted an epidural. Glad for it. Slowed her progress so that midwife following could take over. I didn't want to be around this woman for her sake as well as mine. Not good energy to welcome a baby.

Day 13
- Determined to finish write-ups, worked well. Still feel a little outraged at treatment from patient. Wondered what remedy she might be.
- Evening out for 50th birthday. Colleagues believe I am seen in a different light; dance, was social. Seldom seen as light-hearted or playful. Felt a bit off-center by end of evening; probably drank too much wine.
- Very rushed, accomplished all tasks in time allotted, just barely.
- Tired but could not sleep, had too much to do.
- Stools more regular; soft, no constipation consistently.
- Dream: Getting ready for an evening out. Rushed. Not enough time to really get ready, take a shower, press whatever I am going to wear. Another woman is getting ready also, we are going out together with a couple of men. She is ready. I am throwing things together trying to find something I can wear that is suitable. The men arrive and I am caught not dressed, the bed unmade, the room strewn with clothes.

Day 14
- Enjoyed time with my daughters, granddaughter. Declined invitation to baby-sit. Contented.
- Forgot to pack overnight clothes, general personal care items. Not even a book. Follow up on several small details.

- Tired. Forced myself to go to an open house in hopes of networking with homeopaths. Rested late afternoon and had a resurgence of energy until 10:00 p.m.
- Ate fish tacos and beer.
- Joint of right big toe painful, probably from dancing.

Day 15
- Contented. Drifted through the day. Nice.
- Crave sweets, had popcorn, more thirst.

Day 16
- Felt like I needed to beat the clock. Several personal things I needed to finish up.
- Discovered that my downplaying most everything in the hospital gives the impression I don't know what I'm doing and am caught by surprise. Too late smart they say.
- Dream: Someone from an old and wealthy family gave me a very old piece of cloth and a sequined garment. I am to keep it until a baby who is being brought to me from some other state grows into adulthood. There is some problem legally for her to be in my care or my state. She is being sent by an obstetric doctor I know who also sent duplicate papers for me to fill out so that we have covered the legal problem. I open the package to see what this sequined garment looks like. It is beautiful and has an elegant cape which comes to the floor with a small rolled collar and buttons down the front. The colors are soft and bright. It glows. It is beautiful. While I am distracted I lose track of the baby but know she will come back to me when the time is right. I talk with a local doctor about the problems of the papers and the inheritance of the old garments. They are precious. I find the baby in the care of a group of people. She is fine. The papers are with her. I am confused about whether I sign the birth certificate as if I had delivered or if I make other alterations in the papers that will allow her to stay and then clear any problems with her gaining access to her inheritance when she becomes an adult.

Day 17
- Joy. Time with good old friend. Philosophical insightful discussions over breakfast.
- Very forgetful.
- Time passes slowly, or seems altered, loss of sense of time. Impatience, mild, for responses to e-mail, phone calls, etc. Feels as if more time has gone by.
- Had hunger, craving that was insatiable and couldn't figure out what it was.
- Woke up with pain in right thumb and spasms in right small toe.
- Chronic constipation went away.

Mandragora Officinarum   *Mandrake Root*

| Prover #10 • Female • 48 years old |

Opening Summary
- I did crazy things to get here. I missed my plane by five minutes. I missed the second plane also by five minutes.
- My mind is really unfocused and it has been like this for weeks. Whenever I talk about this I totally lose it. I feel like I'm having a nervous breakdown. I can't think clearly. I can't focus. I really haven't attributed this to the remedy. My life for the last year has been really stressful. The main thing is I haven't been able to think clearly or transfer my thoughts to paper. I haven't been able to write in my journal. My daughter helped me transcribe the bits of paper that I wrote on.
- I took the remedy. Woke up with a right-sided headache in the morning. This has been predominant throughout the proving.
- Yesterday I woke up with the headache. I had planned not to come to class, because I had so may other commitments. It was the last day of a class with thirteen-year-olds. That was the priority. I happened to pull out the schedule and saw the proving meeting. All of a sudden it hit me that I have to be here. All rational thought disappeared. I had to be here for the proving meeting. I made numerous phone calls and rearranged my course and I had to get here. I wanted to get this over with. There was no way I was going to make the plane but I had to drive to the airport anyway. I parked the car and put my suitcase in the shuttle van. Then I realized I wasn't going anywhere. I had a terrible headache still. I called my daughter and she calmed me down. I called everyone again. I went to lunch and got a cup of coffee and it tasted terrible to me. I had two dreams about drinking coffee two nights. I never actually drank it. One in a village scene with a beggar making coffee and I sipped it. I felt if I drank it I would antidote the proving. But there was no memory after that.
- I've been forgetful. I can't remember names of people, things people told me. My scenario is my house: getting up and getting ready doesn't take a rocket scientist to get going in the morning. If I didn't get the umbrella immediately I would forget. All of a sudden I would be in the bedroom unable to remember what I was doing.
- One day I was home alone all day. That afternoon I had a dark heavy feeling. Depressed and dark and heavy. I thought to myself, "This is why people commit suicide." I wasn't hopeless, the feeling was just there. That was the only day I felt that feeling I had when my husband died. I had a depression on top of everything. It has been hard for my family. I have always had it together and don't get upset easily. I am always the strong person. My daughter has had a hard time seeing me like this. There aren't many other people I've told about it. I've been isolating a lot. I called someone else who was proving to ask if she was having a similar experience and the phone was disconnected and I couldn't deal with it. Forgetful, isolated.
- Things that I don't normally do. When I've been home I've had to be really organized and am easily disorganized. I've had to take care of the piles. I spent an afternoon cleaning out my closet. I don't do that sort of thing. All the blouses on one side, all the dresses on the other. I had many pressing things to do. I did the same thing with my pantry, and that was so unlike me.

◆ My perception of time has been altered. Time has never been an issue but this thing has been knowing that forty minutes wasn't enough time. I'd have time but something happened and there wasn't enough time. I've been constantly late to things. Another issue has been with the group of twelve- and thirteen-year-olds I've been working with for five weeks. I love teenagers, and it has been a strength in my work. I have been so intolerant of these kids trying to make them pay attention. They haven't been abnormal, but I was unusual. On Thursday I tried to pay attention to the dynamics, and I think whenever there is chaos or disorganization I get really anxious. I think that is what I responded to in these kids. It drives me crazy to be with them.

◆ I am a person who walks every day. Better taking a walk. I have no desire to walk. I found a dog and he is a purebred springer spaniel, well taken care of. I was certain his owners would call me. No one has called me. I haven't taken him for a walk. That is unusual for me. Weird things that happened. I have spent endless hours trying to get my laptop computer to work. I've been on the line with my computer company, and really impatient with them.

◆ I bought batteries for my smoke alarm and for my remote control for my car. None of the batteries have lasted more than a day.

Physicals

◆ I don't get headaches. Thursday I had a headache all day and went to bed with it. My computer won't even turn on. I've had increased craving for water, especially at night before I go to bed. Craving for sweets has skyrocketed. I bought a bag of Hershey Kisses and put them in the freezer. I got up in the middle of the night and ate them until they were gone. Craving frozen chocolate. I've never done it before.

◆ Mood swings. I'm ready to see a psychiatrist. It is getting worse. I felt relieved getting here. I felt the importance of telling you all. This morning when I drove here it was foggy. I looked at my watch and the next thing I knew I was at the toll booth. I turned around. The next thing I knew I saw the Albany exit. I said, "Enough is enough" and I turned around and paid attention. I still almost missed the turnoff. The main thing is the inability to think and focus clearly. Everything else is a result of that. Forgetful, not being able to remember things. I've gotten to the point of having a breakdown, a major depressive episode.

Day 2

◆ Right-sided headache, woke up with it. Off and on for next three to four days. Felt lighter in spirit today, not distracted or feeling stressed. Could it be that I am going to Yuba City today—(emergency room work for weekend). Though I have dreaded "Hell Week" I feel excited today.

◆ Had a flat tire. <u>Extremely</u> long time getting it fixed, did not bother me even though I had a long drive ahead of me. Headache still there at midnight.

◆ Dream: I am with my family at a gathering—my mom was worried about cooking a roast.

◆ Dream: I lived in small village setting with outdoor tables and verandas.

Day 3
◆ Dream: Woke at 1:30 a.m. with vivid picture of an altar-like setting with candles burning. The thought was, "Oh, this is what this remedy is about—Spirituality??"
◆ Dream: Shopping with my daughter someplace like Mexico. Looking for clothes. She bought a yellow hair ornament that looked Cuban. She said it only weighed thirteen pounds and we could share it.
◆ Dream: I had to helicopter into someplace to go for a hike. I saw this "vehicle" that we were going to use for a river trip. It looked like a giant suitcase. I thought to myself, "How cool—that the rafts can fit in here."

Day 4
◆ Took remedy again.

Day 5
◆ Feeling like I am a pendulum—big mood swings—feeling "discombobulated."
◆ Dream: Young girl with me at a house I did not recognize. Not sure if I was a man or a woman, or who this girl was. I made love to her, kissing and fondling her. I was experiencing both sides. Wondering whether to use a condom, but then it was over and I was holding a capillary tube that said the test was negative—I wasn't pregnant. I wondered if she was a prostitute.
◆ Dream: Cast-iron pan melted that I was washing while doing the dishes—before the taxi came?
◆ Dream: With best friend at Dr. H.'s house. She was copying a cookie recipe on a photocopy machine. Her sister E. (who is schizophrenic) was there. E. had been painting ALL weekend on small enamel items.

Day 6
◆ Dream: Went to a party with friends. I went up tram with friend, D., to talk. Felt attracted to him, or vice-versa. I came down in morning to find that people had overdone it. C., my ex, was very hung over and had been throwing up. I helped to clean him up. Then I am with same friends driving—the police are chasing us. All of a sudden E. took off, so the cops chased him. I took his stash (of what?) and stuffed it in a cupboard.
◆ Dream: Shopping with mom—she was almost bald.

Day 7
◆ Afternoon—home by myself—<u>very dark heavy</u> feeling, not sure if I could handle it—never felt that before—thought this is what people who commit suicide must feel. Did not feel suicidal, but afraid of feeling that way.
◆ Dream: Awoke with a feeling about a place?? Chasing a band of Indians, never overtook them... Saw ten "somethings" that signified their defeat... traveling with friends and a trailer to a place to camp. Driving up a mountain, came to the first site which was literally an acre of concrete. I could not believe that someone would think this was how it was supposed to be... what was this place for??? I tried to picture us in our lawn chairs and tents. I could see myself sitting at a small table studying.

Day 8
- Dream: I was working at a teaching hospital with my old medical staff. I got a page from Dr. B. asking if I was still going to come talk to them—the surgeons. I felt anxious that I hadn't remembered and was not prepared. I couldn't find his pager number and no one seemed to have it. I asked many, many people. I finally found a woman who had the number, and she had done some kind of a security check on me to work at the facility.
- Dream: About houses being authentic and not remodeled.
- Woke up remembering that I had forgotten to call my dad.
- Dream: I was at some kind of gathering outside—a wedding?? I had a small plastic bag with something alive in it. It turned out to be a kitten. I thought it was dead, but it started running around. A woman was selling hot drinks. I sipped one and realized it was a coffee drink. I paid for it, knowing that if I drank it, it would antidote the proving remedy. There was a deep cylindrical hole where I was standing with the kitten. A little girl fell into it. I laughed and helped her out.

Day 9
- Dream: Scene from an old house we used to live in... I was out in the wooden addition, pulled up planks on the floor and saw a huge snake. I tried to reach for his tail and he snapped at me. Then I realized that he was in water. A much larger snake with orange and red on its neck appeared, and it changed into a large shaggy cat or pig or sheep-like creature—not sure which. I was not afraid. It climbed out of the water and went to the back of the room. We opened the back door and let it out—then shooed it away. It seemed like a cat then. Another one climbed out, my younger brother put it out the same way. I ran outside and looked across the property as these creatures moved slowly eastward.
- Dream: I was in a kitchen with two women—one was my proving supervisor. She was making coffee. All I was wearing was a pair of red short-shorts that were too tight. I was cleaning, wiping off the counters, my hair was wrapped in a towel like I had just gotten out of the shower. I kept thinking that I should go get dressed, etc., instead of feeling that I had to clean the kitchen.

Day 10
- Dream: Vague dreams of animals—that had escaped from zoo??? Flash of a tiger jumping through cleft in adobe wall... something about grasshoppers—seems I was eating them??

Day 11
- Dream: With W. (best friend)—plans to go to Hawaii. She had carved army scenes from a green rock of marble.
- Dream: There was gravel in the hallway. I asked the janitor if I could have his broom and dustpan. He said it was against the rules. I grabbed it from him saying, "Don't be ridiculous, someone is going to slip and get hurt." I left, telling my work that I needed to go research the rules. Justice.

◆ Dream: Scene in laundromat. I was doing laundry and drying clothes in small drying compartments (not real dryers). I heard what sounded like a gunshot in another aisle. Three men were nudging each other like boxers in a ring. Feeling: not upset, just wondering what to do. I sensed that one of them had been shot by the other two. I could not run and was trying to figure out what to do. Climb in a washer and hide? Were they going to kill everyone there?

◆ Dream: Scene in a boxing ring. One fighter received a heavy blow and was stunned, wobbly; tried to fight it, his body could not—his brain? He went down on one knee and fell on to the mat. I was thinking what a brutal sport it is that we take so much pleasure in, watching such insult to someone.

Day 12

◆ Dream: I am medical personnel waiting for a patient. There are three to four people assisting a young man. Everyone seems to be having great difficulty. I approach and grabbed his right arm. I pulled off his prosthesis and saw a stump. He had a motorcycle accident some years earlier. I was living in a small town. A call came for all medical personnel to report for emergency. I was with EMS.

◆ Dream: I was driving late at night, tired, started to exit the freeway, next thing I remember, I am walking and have no idea where my car is. Did I wreck? Or is it parked on an exit ramp? It is the middle of the night. I call someone to see if he will drive me to find my car. We meet at a casino, he took me to a suite with lots of people staying in it. There was a woman (a mom) making prom dresses.

Day 13

◆ Dream: Me standing with back to mirror. I get a glimpse of my face. Am I wearing a mask of a wolf?

◆ Dream: The earth was covered white, snow and ice. I was driving large four-wheel drive vehicle and maneuvered the bad roads. I am not sure who was with me. Ahead I could see a huge mountain with the road clearly in view up its face. Later I am driving by myself, lots of traffic, going to some event. I pulled onto the median, men were working on the road... drilling something. They were all Asian men. It was difficult to get traction. The more gas I gave the more I was sliding around these men. I was worried about hitting their equipment—which out of the corner of my eye looked like a net or a web. I finally got going.

◆ Dream: I am driving down a windy road with a huge patch of ice coming up. At the bottom is the driveway of a family I grew up with. There is a little girl on a bike; I tell her to get out of the way because I was afraid I was going to slide into her.

Day 14

◆ Dream: Working at hospital, patient angry with me. Followed me to the basement... don't know what happened. I shot him and thought he was dead. There was a lot of bleeding from the head wound. I was calm, started to call security and realized he was still alive. He asked why I had shot him.

Day 15

♦ Dream: Small village somewhere with a lake. We were at the beach. At first just the three of us, my daughter as a little girl, her dad, T., and my brother K. I walked out into the water, which was very shallow. I was quite far out but still able to walk. It was almost as if I had taken a nap, woke up and looked back toward the beach. There were hundreds of African men all sitting together. I could hear them singing and playing musical instruments. Beautiful music. I also saw my old mare playing in the water by herself. She was making huge splashes as she pawed the water. I decided to go to shore to take a picture from the water, never before had I seen it like this. By the time I got there the Africans were getting on their boat. We realized that they had taken our ice chest by mistake, so I yelled at the boat to stop. I realized that the men were packed into the boat, like slaves, all lying down to fit in the hull. Yet they all seemed happy and said they were going home. I wished them a happy voyage. After that I walked down the beach to a village setting. There were tents set up like a crafts fair. Each stall was a different scene. One was an old saloon, and at the end of the bar sat an old friend, T. As my daughter and I walked in we were suddenly dressed in long 1800s style dresses. I told him that T. had been with us but that I had taken him back—to the hospital, to jail, to heaven? I said that he had a great time and had gotten to sail his boat. T. asked if T.'s skin had been ok in the sun? Because of his cancer?

♦ Dream: Next scene we are in my old playhouse as a child, talking about the beach. Y.'s cat started attacking the house. He was rowdy and scrambled up a large tree, then we heard a large thump as he fell out of it.

♦ Dream: I was in a bathroom and had two babies' heads, only the heads, and sensed that I had done something wrong by not creating whole babies, so I stuck the heads in my bag.

Day 16

♦ Dream: Scene—beautiful red, roan-colored horses in a valley, running, then swimming. My horse was white with a black trimmed mane... swam up to where I was sitting... was very loving, nudging me. I was tempted to jump on its back, but instead I dove deep into the water to see if it would dive also. We played for a while. It was a powerful swimmer and would retrieve objects that I threw. I was diving deep into the water, taking my granddaughter down with me to touch the bottom of the lake. She had learned to hold her breath. I remembered that we would both swim around and quickly burst up out of the water.

♦ Dream: Visiting old friend that had hiked the Pacific Crest Trail, many years ago. I was happy to see him. He and his family were caretaking a lodge somewhere up in the Sierras, and I was planning a visit. A friend of his entered the room, very scruffy, had been hiking all summer. We were tying his shoes for him. They were falling apart with big knots in the laces. D. was teasing him to buy some new ones. I offered him my new belt and I bound together all his hiking books, probably fifteen or twenty of them. I regretted giving him my new belt, said that he could give it to D. the next time I saw him. Inwardly I chastised myself for always getting myself into situations like that.

◆ Dream: Traveling in huge snowstorm. Two cars with friends and family into the mountains somewhere.

Day 17
◆ Dream: This dream seemed to last a long time, mountain trek. I was in the mountains with W., going to hike into a camp, lots of snow. Going to take a long time. Many people in town to hike and ski, scene like a gold rush camp. No accommodations, so people sleeping everywhere, buying tarps and blankets to sleep in. I have flip-flops on, I am very disorganized but not worried about it. Not even after a train ran over one of my flip-flops.
◆ Dream: We went into a store to buy tequila—there were about 50 brands.

Day 18
◆ Dream: Vivid dream of flooding city—colonial city? I was navigating my way through—some streets not deep water. Went into a shop with small toys or objects with sandpaintings on them. I took one of them.

Day 19
◆ Dream: I was cross-country skiing up to top of mountain. It felt good to be exerting myself so effortlessly. I came up behind someone ahead of me in the tracks... I was going to pass him, and was just about to say something when he became startled and tumbled off into the snow. I kept going—did not stop to help, mouthed that I was sorry. I came to a place where everything in the trail became slushy and turned to water. I had to maneuver myself up and over boulders and trees. I took off skis and was climbing a big tree. Then I was surrounded by lions. I had to lie motionless to hide—very afraid and worried about people behind me on the trail. I woke up feeling that I was traveling within my own body???

Day 20
◆ Dream: Traveling in Mexico. Eating in restaurant that ran out of papelles (whatever that is—I thought of potatoes.) D., my realtor, lived there. I thought, "Is this my second dream about this colonial city?" I purchased small stone figurines that represented spiritual worship. As I prepared to cross the border I am uncomfortable as if I don't have the proper papers. An Anglo woman is going through my things and I tell her that I would be happy to tell her what I bought. Later we stop at a small store to use the bathroom... very dirty inside. Someone has stuffed toilet paper into the vent on the floor. There is also a wad of paper on the wall that has feces on it. I am not grossed out, have seen it before.
◆ Dream: Camped at beautiful spot at water's edge. Have pulled rafts up on shore. I wonder in my dream why I keep dreaming of rafting.

Day 21
◆ Dream: A., my granddaughter... grasshoppers... dinosaurs...

♦ Dream: Something about CPR, a woman who came to my house in the middle of the night.
♦ Dream: Pyramid Lake scene... sitting at a small bar with my dad, my dad is a young man. He is talking about going to work at Pyramid Lake, I am going to drive him.

Day 22
♦ Woke early with bad headache.
♦ Last day of five week course with twelve- and thirteen-year-olds. Found course difficult and seems chaotic in our classes. I have usually loved working with teens—never so frustrating.
♦ 10:30 p.m.—Planned to fly to Oakland early tomorrow morning, looking forward to Hahnemann proving meeting. Pulled out my schedule suddenly, wondered if "Provings" scheduled for afternoon was a lecture or could possibly be the proving meeting? After several calls to Hahnemann with no contact, I reached classmate who confirmed that proving meeting time had been changed. Felt that I <u>HAD</u> to be there. Made numerous calls to change my flight—would arrive at Hahnemann at 4:00 a.m. Made other calls regarding: my class, dog sitter, etc. Missed plane by five minutes. No other flights would get me there.
♦ Dream: Image is of my mom being ill, not sure what is wrong, but I am rubbing her back. She can feel something inside not normal. Suddenly there is a thick, brownish liquid coming from her pores. I ask someone to get some gloves. I keep massaging her gently to get the stuff out of her. (My mother is still alive and well.)
♦ Dream: I stop at a shop late at night. A woman is putting on makeup. I look in the mirror and I have face powder, red lipstick and black eye makeup. It is very unnatural. The blush-on is not spread out evenly so I take one of her brushes and decide to steal it, except it is very long, a couple of feet. I stick it down the front of my dress, but it sticks out so I try to conceal it with my coat. At some point I decide this is silly to be doing this and I put the brush back down on the counter.

Summary
♦ Inability to focus/organize thoughts, very difficult/impossible to put thoughts on paper.
♦ Forgetful—very difficult remembering details, people's names, etc.
♦ Isolated/?disconnected—could not call anyone to express my needs—tried classmate one night—her phone disconnected.
♦ Need for extreme order at home: Even though I had so much work to do I spent afternoon organizing my closet—cleaned out pantry and sorted everything.
♦ Time issue: My perception seemed to be distorted—have totally misjudged time needed to do things.
♦ Difficulty in telling anyone how bad I am feeling.
♦ Very difficult working with group of teens (adolescent social action program)—usually I am patient, find them humorous—have felt irritable—wanting them to be more attentive, etc.
♦ Batteries lasted only a few days.
♦ Endless computer problems—spent hours on phone with computer technical service.

◆ No desire to go out walking, usually daily walks.
◆ <u>Huge mood swings.</u>
◆ Felt lack of excitement at news of my daughter being pregnant again—<u>NOT</u> natural response for me.
◆ Important dream I forgot to share: I had lots of dreams of animals, lots of distortion in my dreams, detached feelings in dreams prominent. My daughter also said she felt I had been very detached in recent weeks. It seems that I did not care about her. I was not aware of this. She also shared how out of character it was for me to bring a stray dog home, but I acted like it was not unusual. My voice sounded so sweet when I'd talk about Dog. I am now struck by how Dog has followed me everywhere in house—constantly nudging my hand.

Summary of Important Physicals
◆ Nauseated frequently.
◆ Recurrent right-sided headache.
◆ Warmer than usual—conscious of sticking feet out of covers a lot (not usual for me).
◆ Increased thirst, especially in evenings and bedtime.
◆ Increased sweet craving: bought bag of Hershey's Kisses.
◆ Definitely noticed stools—harder or drier, sometimes skipped bowel movement.

Prover #11 • Female • 38 years old

Day 1
◆ Dream: Woke with a start. Was going to be framed or manipulated to lie about my whereabouts regarding the disappearing death of J. (J. is a good friend of my husband's. I was closer to her myself at one time. At the time of the proving I was still feeling a bit wounded from an experience with her. I felt let down by the way she handled a situation in which we were all involved.) Someone was in another car watching me. Felt my neck was threatened.
◆ Dream: An older black woman and her companion were walking down the hall in an institution—she was sweet and kind. Then these two people who were wanting to escape encountered them. They had knives and were going to kill her. So she said, "Ok, stab me." One of the people threw a knife in her chest which hit but didn't really penetrate and then she knew she had a chance and started running. She had been so brave even though she was so frightened.
◆ Woke up tired. I think being super aware of writing down my dreams kept me up some. I'm sure it will calm down.
◆ S. and I went for a bike ride only to be one-half hour into it and realize the tire was about to blow. Not a big deal, but we had to turn around early.
◆ My bowel movement was delayed till evening and very hard. It was a relief to pass it.

♦ Had been wanting to get out and work in the garden for weeks and hadn't made it happen, but today I got out there and really cleaned out the beds and cut back plants. Getting ready for winter—collected walnuts. I've been feeling like a squirrel—storing up and preparing for the winter. Nice feeling.

Day 2

♦ Woke up at 3:00 a.m. with right-sided chest pain just under breast. Worse from aspiration. Sharp!

♦ Dream: I was on an island. It was geologically made up of a volcano maybe or some raised land. The inside was hollow. There were a couple of secret ladder/shutes that can get you down quickly. This is where the Hahnemann class met. Nancy and Roger were there. Lots of other students too. It was a good feeling of camaraderie between people. I was in charge of some aspect there. There were a couple of small children too. I remember holding one little boy. I think it was Nancy's or someone she knew well. There were a lot of complexities to being there. I had to get $30.00 to Roger for some reason.

♦ My brother called to offer us a round-trip ticket to anywhere British Airways flies, which is almost anywhere. That was pretty exciting! We're thinking of Bali.

♦ Had big cravings for greens today.

Day 3

♦ Dream: I was walking on a city street in Berkeley. It was a residential street. I was passing a house and I saw J., the gardener for Hahnemann. She had two dogs in her yard. There was a man or maybe two who were going to hurt her. She looked at her dogs and told them to attack. They just sat there, not understanding. I didn't actually see the men, but I could sense they were there. I just kept walking and didn't think until later that I could have/should have helped. She was beaten. But the next day she looked fine. Then I was to meet my friend K. We were going to go for a run and then to my women's group. She couldn't find the right clothes to buy. I just kept running around the block, waiting for her to finish. I tried to explain that it was no big deal. I felt patient with her and good that my running stamina was good.

♦ Dream: I was totally stoned (which I don't do). I was with my mom and sister outside of a building. A man approached us and started a conversation with me. I couldn't follow a thing he was saying. I couldn't focus. Just wanted to get away from them. In my haste I mumbled some excuse about needing water. As I was walking away, I realized I was holding a bottle in my hand. I felt foolish. I headed to my car and drove away. Being stoned, I felt unsure about my ability to drive well. Got to an intersection and wanted to turn left, but I wasn't sure how or when. Suddenly, I was looking down on my car from above (and the whole intersection) and I knew when and how to proceed. It was as though I was a bird looking down.

Day 4

♦ Before bed I took another dose.

♦ Dream: There was a knowingness that the world as we know it was coming to an end. We knew we had to stock up on water and essentials. I was at my friend M.'s house. It seemed as though I lived there. We got along well. The house had a bunch of rooms. Each was different with a bunch of irregular angles. I remember seeing the bathtub and noticing that it was oddly shaped: very long and slightly bent. I thought, "Now that is made for a very tall person!" Then I was sitting down on a couch. There was a television maybe five feet from it that was very unusual. It was a long rectangle. The screen was about eight feet long by three feet high. I thought the couch was awfully close to watch such a big television. My kids came home from school and my good friend came in the room. I looked up at him and he seemed so tall. He was maybe fifteen feet tall. Very strange. Such distortions.

◆ I've been on my own for the last two days and doing fine. But when my poor husband came home, I became snappy and irritable. I felt as though I could bite him. He actually put out his arm in jest (as we were both acknowledging my odd mood) and I really had a strong impulse to bite him hard! He says I'm unusually edgy, sharp, brisk. He says my movements are more jarring and hard.

◆ My usual allergy/snuffles have been really intense lately. I can hardly go a minute without blowing my nose. Irritating!

Day 5
◆ Restless night.
◆ Dream: Husband and I were at a Goodwill store. It looked like a good one with lots of great stuff. There were two or three black women in the front asking for handouts because they had been flooded out of their home. I didn't have what they were asking for. I would have liked to help them. Then we were in the back of the building; there was this dark foreboding pond. These black men were being thrown into it in these sacks. If they could work themselves loose and swim out then they were free; otherwise they were dead. We saw one die and one live. Awful.
◆ I went running and noticed how tight my shirt felt around my neck. I had the same experience two days ago. Can't stand pressure against the front of my neck.
◆ Dream: The principal of my daughter's high school called to tell me she had been noticed being "under the influence" (of drugs) at school, and she was failing classes. I called her father to tell him. He didn't believe it. I realized he was right, that S. deserved the benefit of the doubt, as she has always been an A+ student.

Day 6
◆ I've been so thirsty the last two days. My mouth and throat feel dry. I just want to sit over steam (thirsty for sips).
◆ Husband and I are on the coast in our trusty camper. We got here when it was dark and cold. I got so cold. We couldn't get a fire to stay lit. Everything is too damp. Got into bed to get warm. Soon I felt I couldn't breathe. Lying on my back was worse. Sitting up or on my belly raised on my elbows relieved. Soon I was feeling that I was having an asthma attack (which I don't typically get). I really couldn't get a breath and both my nostrils were clogged. Couldn't breathe through my nose at all. My husband fell asleep. I got almost hysterical. Started crying. Couldn't breathe, couldn't sit up because the head room doesn't allow. Couldn't go anywhere because we're in the woods and it's cold. I felt

afraid that I wouldn't be able to breathe. I started having deep coughs that felt like they came from the deepest cavern of my lungs. When my husband was doing some Reiki on me and put his hand on my chest, it felt like an iron weight. My lungs feel like they are being pressed in with pressure. Almost like being under water. With the light on I feel better. Heat helps. I long for the sun tomorrow.

♦ Dream: I was capable of extremely challenging mental feats. Intense mathematical equations. Then I was capable of great physical feats. But after running this great distance over rocks and difficult terrain, I was crossing a bridge. This woman was there with a board over a gorge and she tipped the board so that I fell into the gorge. Awareness of falling, knowing that I was going to die. No fear, but wishing that I wasn't going to die. Empathy with the woman who had killed me.

♦ Dream: A mysterious woman, beautiful, tall, very unusual looking, was having an affair. Later I saw her with few clothes on and she was short. Maybe four feet tall. Her body was odd, almost non-human. I couldn't believe my eyes. It was as though something was off but I couldn't place it.

♦ Dream: Some people put together a Christmas scene in their backyard using two very tiny deer. They were alive, real and eight inches tall. They just sat there and watched us as we walked by. I was charmed and amazed.

Day 7

♦ Was finally able to sleep with pillows propping my chest and head up. Still feel kind of shaky from last night.

♦ Have noticed some itchy skin eruptions on my left hip and left elbow. Reminds me of latent poison oak.

♦ Near the ocean, I can breathe well. It is nice to be here. Slept well.

♦ Dream: Buses everywhere. I was trying to find my daughter on one of them, feeling a little panicky. Then I heard/saw her in my mind's eye as though we were psychically linked (which we are often).

♦ Dream: I was with our friend J. He was part of an art class. Everyone was putting their artwork on the ground. Husband was using his Chinese chop/seals, with that bright red paint. It's almost an orange/red. People weren't paying attention to what they were doing and walking on his paintings. J. called everyone's attention to husband's work, as his was so exquisite. It was nice to hear an objective compliment.

Day 8

♦ The ocean air is so nice. No problem breathing.

♦ My left nostril has two very red and shiny sores just at the inner tip. They throb sometimes and are painfully sharp if touched.

♦ Dream: I had done something wrong and I was being asked to leave the country. At first I thought about how exciting that would be to start a whole new life. New surroundings, friends, lovers, jobs. I was quickly being driven in a car by a short Mexican man, his wife and a friend of mine. They were all engaged in a conversation. The driver was controlling the car from the back seat. He was so short I wondered how he could see. His wife was in the front seat. I guess she didn't know how to drive. He was driving

so fast through all this busy crazy traffic. I kept watching these almost fatal accidents. I searched in my purse and was glad to see that I had my passport. Then I remembered that I wouldn't see my kids again. Felt really sad.
◆ Woke up 2:30 a.m.
◆ Dream: A friend was showing me an abcess she had on her heel. When I saw it I couldn't believe how big and hard it was. She had worn high heels so much that her foot looked like a Barbie doll's, with the permanent arch to it. I told her she needs to stop wearing those shoes right away.

Day 9

◆ Still noticing a peculiar aversion to anything tight around my throat.
◆ My appetite is hardy. I'm eating things I usually don't. I ate sausage with breakfast this morning!
◆ Husband commented that I seem to be more psychic than usual. I've been reading his mind a lot lately. I'll just know what he's thinking.
◆ Dream: Nixon and Clinton smoking cigars together in the White House.
◆ Dream: Went to the grocery store with my dad. As we drove in we met up with Shirley Maclaine. She greeted my dad with familiarity. I joked that I can't go anywhere with him without running into someone he knows. She and I got to talking about how to prepare for when our society crashes. Where to be, what to have on hand. I enjoyed the interaction.
◆ Dream: Husband and I went to a movie. There were a bunch of his friends sitting together with one seat left. He sat down and refused to move. I looked around and saw the theater had many empty seats. But he refused to go and sit with me. I was so mad! I went to sit by myself.
◆ Dream: Motorbikes and wine.

Day 10

◆ Wake up tired. Couldn't sleep between 2:30 and 4:00 a.m. Got up to read.
◆ Started my period. It is on time. Got my usual cramps but they didn't last all day like they have.
◆ Got home from the coast to find our fish bowl half empty, with the two fish gone. I presume eaten by either a cat or raccoon. Very upsetting.
◆ I'm feeling very overwhelmed by everything I have to do before I leave for school and then Italy. It's hard to let it go and relax.
◆ Dream: Husband and I were on the coast of Italy. We had arranged to see some friends of his. They had come to our wedding and I knew them a little. I had been hesitant to meet with them since it was our honeymoon and I wanted it to be our trip. So I agreed anyway. We got to the arranged place and there they were. I went up to J. and gave her a hug. She seemed surprised, like she didn't know me. She asked me who I was. I was taken aback but didn't let on. Later husband said he wanted to spend the day with them. I was appalled. I felt personally insulted by her behavior as I was sure she had recognized me. I felt snubbed and hurt. Husband and I argued. I felt shitty. Then we were walking away from a high seacoast and realized we were going to get hit by a huge wave. I was

terrified we were going to get dragged in. We ran. It hit but we were ok. Another one was coming. I was afraid it would take husband. Woke up scared.

Day 11
◆ Started feeling really tired and foggy. I almost feel drugged. I've had two cups of black tea but it doesn't seem to help. I've been trying to work on homework but I just can't seem to focus my energy.
◆ We have raccoon problems like crazy. Just had a fish-and-game trapper here. Gonna trap 'dem coons! Set the trap, and in fifteen minutes we caught our first raccoon. I can hear all the other raccoons sounding with each other. Poor things.
◆ Allergies are getting worse. My eyes hurt, are dry and tired. I feel like lying down with a cold compress. My eyes have been so itchy all day. It's on the inside along the upper bridge.
◆ Last night I had severe cramps (menstrual). They were unusually sharp and felt like a dagger going through my pelvis into my back. Still have cramps today.

Day 12
◆ I feel like shit! I haven't been able to breathe all day. I'm actually starting to feel shaky again. Afraid I might go into another asthma attack.
◆ After walking around in a fog all day I almost broke down into tears. (Probably would have helped.) I can't concentrate, can't breathe, can't think! And I have so much to do. I need my mind and nose back!
◆ Stuffy nose, head. Nose dripping like faucet, clear discharge salty to taste. Constantly blowing nose, sneezing up to three times in a row—hard sneezes. Nose itches inside. The itch tingles like effervescence, goes up into my eyes which water. Eyes itchy. Want to rub them till they are puffy. Ameliorated bathing in hot water. Nose is sore and red. Hurts from blowing so much. Left nostril opening is red and ulcerated or somehow raw.
◆ Finally talked with Nancy. She told me to stop the proving. Suggested I take Sabadilla. I went in search. Turned my house upside down. (Felt like a drug addict looking for a fix.)
◆ Have been reading Ann Rice's book, *Armand the Vampire*.

Prover #12 • Male • 53 years old

Day 1
◆ Dream: Lots of traveling around, returning home or to a family reunion. Best part was returning home and seeing my daughter. I had such a peaceful feeling. I sang her a song of realization, that sort of turned into Bob Dylan's song, "My love speaks softly." Before that, I had been to a family reunion where they started talking about a matriarch of the family, named Mary, saying she had been "flexible," implying she may have had one or more affairs. Switch to a scene where older woman goes out to watch some salvage work, takes a bad fall and lays on the cold ground for a long time while people try to help her. This gave her a chill that presumably led to her death. Then I was in a kind of field hospital with lots

of little white tents. A nurse was putting camphor around my mouth and nose, and helping me breathe oxygen or something. After a while I noticed her hand was on my genitals. As attention shifted there, she started literally beating me off. Each time she would whip it, a little bit of semen would leak out, spraying over my face and everything. We were interrupted by a man, who said we'd better pack up and head out. I saw all the people in the encampment were doing that. The man said something about Wyoming. As I drove out of town, I passed the road where I could have doubled back to the reunion site, and kept going. Pretty soon I saw a sign that said "Entering Wyoming." I didn't really want to go there—I was afraid they had different laws. But I crossed the depression that marked the state line. I was looking for a place to turn around, then some young punks were following me, beating sticks together. I was afraid they would see my indecision. But finally they sort of passed so I could turn around. Then I turned around and was headed home to see my daughter. I was leaping across terraced gardens and feeling very joyful and peaceful.

Day 3
◆ Dreams confused, changing. One vignette was of my dad showing me some Japanese greeting cards he had bought, which expressed incredibly detailed matches to situations. They meant something meaningful to me. There was a wedding. I was trying to convey a message to the groom to look down at his tie or something, without really coming out and saying it (while he was getting his picture taken.) He wasn't really getting it, which was a cause of mirth.

Day 4
◆ Dream: Lots of driving. I traded cars with my ex, or somehow got her old car. My ex-stepson went with me to pick it up. I was driving it next to the curb, and my passenger told me I almost ran over a baby that was lying on the curb. I said, "That's the way it goes in this city."

Day 5
◆ No symptoms. Went to bed at 2 a.m. Woke at 3:30 a.m. with mucous in my throat. Went back to sleep right away. Woke at 6:00 a.m. and had a hard time getting back to a deep sleep. Got up about 8:00 a.m.
◆ Cramping stomach pain while eating in Chinese restaurant. Unable to finish meal. Goes away after about twenty minutes.

Day 6
◆ Went to bed about 11:45 p.m. Waking dream—I was with a person who knew where everything was—even underground things.
◆ Dream: Running wires in a strange building with my kids.

Day 7
◆ Took third dose of remedy around 12:20 a.m.
◆ Waking dream: Someone was asserting the tire shop had or hadn't done something to the tires with a block of iron containing chlorine. We were supposed to have a group protest.

Day 8
◆ Dream: I was getting ready to publish a scientific work. It was based on a classic text. I was updating, republishing, or somehow mirroring it. I had a kind of mentor, who was encouraging me. He was a sax player and he was there with another sax player who was also encouraging.

◆ Dream: We were on a ship or plane with some Tibetans. My partner asked if there was a bathroom. We were directed to the front, to the left. We went up to the cockpit and out the door. We found two large round pools of cold water. I hesitated before jumping in, thinking I should take my clothes off.

Day 9
◆ Dream: Met my ex-wife—she comes to work and I introduce her to my boss. She's telling me about a website, we're going over her list, she's very warm and friendly. She has trouble using the boss's phone; there seems to be a key missing.

◆ Headache about 5 p.m. after a fairly energetic discussion with a colleague. Craving for peanuts. Could not find peanuts, but ate some trail mix, which made the headache better.

Day 10
◆ 10:30 a.m. headache has been with me most of the morning. It is a dull ache, behind my forehead, in a band across the forehead. My shoulders feel tight, and I have this general oppressive feeling, I feel kind of hunched over. I want my shoulders to droop. The headache extends down into my face and I notice my jaw and face muscles are very tight. The headache is worse from the jar of every step as I walk through the parking lot. I have an "all gone" feeling in my stomach.

◆ Got very tired about 3:00 p.m. About 4:30 p.m. I decided to go home early. The headache was with me, on and off, mostly in the background all evening.

Day 13
◆ Dream: Planning a remodeling with a contractor. Cement extending, etc., to make a platform to sit. I think the idea is a shrine room on the front of my house. Other fragments—taking a stroll around a small college campus with a young person complaining about "money." Designing a ship. These all seem to be regurgitations of yesterday's experiences.

◆ Sleep position: On back, left leg drawn up, hands on chest.

◆ Driving home from work, about 8:00 p.m., tremendous tickling sensation in the middle of my nose. I start sneezing, which lasts for a minute or two, which gets me hot and sweaty.

Day 14
◆ Dream: I come into this narrow area near the ocean—on the beach, an embankment. A sheep crosses the road, just narrowly missing getting hit by a car. There are three or four dead sheep lying next to the embankment. A woman is there, says something, and we ride our bicycles up the road together. It's a rather narrow road. I'm next to the edge, which is uneven, and I end up pushing her pretty much out into the middle of the road.

She says that as a farm/ranch housewife, she has to have a lot of herbal medicines around. I start to tell her about homeopathy, but keep getting interrupted. We reach our destination at the top of the hill, and I lock up my bike. I'm concentrating very one-pointedly on the lock, rotating it to the number 100, three times. Then I'm done, and I turn back to her and start talking to her more seductively about homeopathy, then finally I see a look of interest in her eyes. She says, "Does this have something to do with the retreat you're in?" I say, "No." Another woman says, "One woman died of cancer in the last retreat," and explains more about the cancer. I wake up.

Day 15
◆ Took another dose at bedtime.

Day 16
◆ Waking dream: Seem to be having trouble logging in to a website.

Day 18
◆ Sometime between 7:00–8:00 p.m. I had a sneezing attack—couldn't stop. My eyes were watering and I got really hot and sweaty. It felt like I was coming down with a cold, and I reflected on the previous night's restless feeling, and thought for sure this was the case. But after the attack subsided I was ok.

Day 19
◆ Dream: I went to a fancy hotel and there was a place for me to eat at a big table in a private room. There was another couple there—I didn't know them but I guess I was going to be sharing the room with them. I thought I would go to another hotel to eat. I went to this very busy trendy hotel and couldn't find a place, and I wanted to go back to the original hotel but I couldn't. I ended up sort of rolling out a bedroll with a bunch of other people on the street outside (the second hotel). It seems they were all employees of the hotel that had been staying there but had been pushed out. One man took all his clothes off and was standing there. Long, full, blond hair. I noticed another man eyeing his butt. Then I saw the police captain down the street checking out the situation. I went into the hotel to warn the management their scene was about to be busted, and when I came out, the police had moved everyone and my stuff was gone. I sort of followed the group and eventually picked out another place to camp. I remember a part of the dream where I was plotting my income growth, trying to see how I could have enough for retirement. In another part, I had my car repaired at a gas station on a street that was under construction. When I picked it up, I got in, and when I looked at the dashboard it wasn't my car, but the keys worked. Someone else was with me. We were worried. My car was next to us but the garage had somehow cloned my car's identity and put it in this one. That was probably illegal. Should we call the police?
◆ My nose is a little stuffy this morning.

ROSA GALLICA

Ancient Yellow Rose

ROSA GALLICA [ROSA G.]
Ancient Yellow Rose

Rosa gallica
Family: *Rosaceae*
Miasm: Cancer

To many, the Rose is the loveliest flower in existence. Growing on the earth over 32 million years before the evolution of *Homo sapiens*, the Rose is deeply imprinted on our psyches, aesthetics, and imaginations. Few plants receive as much human attention or play such a significant role in art, medicine, folklore, trade, and religion.

Rosaceae, as a plant family, is enormous, having over ninety genera and 2,000 species of small shrubs, bushes, trees, and herbs. The two striking characteristics common to the entire family are five petals to the flower and an edible or beautiful fruit. Delicious and well-known family members include peaches, blackberries, apples, cherries, pears, and strawberries.

The original roses, *Rosa alba* and *Rosa gallica*, being hardy plants, have been willing members of cultivated gardens for over 5,000 years. (**GARDENS**) The first records of horticulturalists provide instructions on how to "force" the plant's growth during winter months hinting at the importance this flower held in the ancient world (*Grieve*). Sheila Pickles in *The Language of Flowers* writes:

> Nebuchadnezzar used them to adorn his palace and in Persia, where they were grown for their perfume oil, the petals were used to fill the Sultan's mattress. In Kashmir, the Moghul emperors cultivated beautiful rose gardens and roses were strewn in the river to welcome them on their return home.

The Rose markets in Egypt developed a tremendous business sending the most beautiful roses to the Romans who lavishly made use of the blossoms. (**MONEY**) Although rosewater was used to adorn the body, it wasn't until the early 1600s at a Persian wedding feast that attar was discovered. There a royal couple rowing through garden canals filled with rosewater noticed that the heat of the sun separated out an intoxicatingly fragrant oil (*Grieve*). Soon Attar of Rose became a lucrative export. Requiring sixty thousand roses to produce a single ounce and using ten thousand pounds of Rose petals to produce a pound of oil, it is one of the world's costliest essential oils (*Durrani*).

Rome's indulgent ruling class saw the Rose as "a sign of pleasure, [and] the companion of mirth and wine" (*Grieve*). Strewn on paths, floating in wine, roses gilded their halls for special banquets where sexual liaisons were a public activity. (**SEXUALITY**) Debauchery became part of the Rose's history and the "flower of the gods" became:

> . . . synonymous with the worst excesses of the Roman Empire—the peasants were reduced to growing roses instead of food crops in order to satisfy the demands of their rulers. The emperors filled their swimming baths and fountains with rosewater and sat on carpets of rose petals for their feasts and orgies. Heliogabalus used to enjoy showering his guests with rose petals which tumbled down from the ceiling during the festivities. (*Pickles*)

Rumor has it that, during one of these revelries, the volume of petals was so great as to smother some of the "less conscious" guests.

In spite of these baser excesses, the mythology surrounding the Rose and most of its history are bound together with love, beauty, and passion. In Greek lore, the Rose is the sacred flower of Aphrodite, the goddess of love; where her tears dropped to the earth, mixing with the blood of her wounded lover Adonis, roses grew. (**RELATIONSHIPS**)

The power of the Rose to captivate another's heart pervades our myths, folklore, and history.

> It is said that the striking Egyptian beauty Cleopatra won over the affections of Marc Anthony because of her alluring perfume, the scent of which was made of pure essences extracted from rose petals. Cleopatra's love for roses even extended farther than just wearing the scent. She once filled the floor of a room with rose petals when receiving Marc Anthony. (*Durrani*)

The poetry that is etched into our contemporary psyche from childhood verse: "Roses are red, violets are blue . . . " to Shakespeare's, "A rose by any other name . . ." to song, "My love is like a red, red rose" places the Rose as *the* symbol of romance. (**LOVERS**)

But passion exacts a price. Browning warns: "Roses are for fearless hearts, the ones that bleed and bloom again." More chillingly, Blake pens in "The Sick Rose":

> O Rose, thou art sick!
> The invisible worm.
> That flies in the night
> In the howling storm:
>
> Has found out thy bed
> Of crimson joy:
> And his dark secret love
> Does thy life destroy.

Considering that eighteenth-century physicians believed an "invisible worm" caused syphilis, Blake's poem is a reminder that sexual passion can take life as well as give it (*Essick, 58*). (**MORTAL DANGER**)

Danger and overindulgence appear to be woven into the Rose's history. During the fifth century B.C. the Emperor of China, obsessed with roses, had, according to Confucius, six hundred books in his library concerning their culture. "The Chinese extracted oil of roses from the plants grown in the Emperor's garden. The oil was only used by nobles and dignitaries of the court; if a commoner were found in possession of even the smallest amount, he was condemned to death" (*Flower History*).

Early Christians seeing the Rose as the symbol of paganism and immorality were forbidden to have any association with the flower, but these edicts were largely ignored and in time the church claimed the Rose as originating from the five sacrificial wounds of Christ, eventually becoming the flower most often referred to in the legends of the saints. Marilyn Cameron writes:

> A maiden, unjustly accused of wrongdoing was condemned to be burned to death. As the flames were about to be lit, she called to God to deliver her and make her innocence clear to all men. As soon as the flames leapt around her, they were suddenly extinguished, the wood turning into freshly sprouting Rose bushes. . . . Since then the Rose has been the emblem of Christian martyrdom.

But it is Mary, constantly surrounded by them in apparitions, paths strewn with them by devotees, legends of Rose petals descending from heaven to bless her, who becomes the *Rosa mystica*, the personification of the Rose in Western spirituality. St. Alphonsus de Liguori in *The Glories of Mary* explains: "Therefore on account of the ardent love with which her heart was always inflamed towards God and us, she is called a rose" (*630*). (**LOVING FEELINGS/COMPASSION**)

Throughout history, the heart and the Rose have been at the center of spiritual imagery. For the Sufi's, the ancient mystics of Islam, the Rose is the symbol of the opening heart, it embodies the enduring capacity to love and absorb oneself in mystical union with God. (**HEART**) The heart, like the Rose, starts as a tightly closed bud which, when exposed to the bright light of sun, truth, or love, gradually opens wider and wider until it bursts itself, disperses, and merges with the beloved.

Martin Luther, the sixteenth century priest who defied the Catholic Church, chose the heart and Rose as symbols of the Reformation. A red heart "full of faith" in God's free gift of love, set in a white rose "of unearthly joy and peace" became part of the seal of his church and a direct protest against a corrupt papacy. (**REBELLION/INDEPENDENCE**) Another independent spirit, Florence Nightingale, committed her life to nursing, unheard of for a woman of means in her day. Lewis Carroll immortalizes her life in "The Path of Roses," as he describes a woman's longing to help those ravaged by war but constrained by social norms. (**DESIRE TO HELP OTHERS**) The "path of roses" is revealed to her as a sacred call to shake off those constraints and bring healing to man's darkest despair "where war and terror shake the earth" (*953*).

The Rose as a symbol of independence and strength has its counterpart in meekness. How many times have we seen roses used to pave the way for a timid admirer or a repentant lover? In *Through the Looking Glass*, Carroll portrays the Rose's more passive side when Alice asks in a garden of live flowers, "'Can all the flowers talk?' 'As well as you can,' said the Tiger-lily. 'It isn't manners for us to begin, you know, said the Rose, and I was wondering when you'd speak'"(*158*). (**PASSIVITY**)

One person writes of a curative experience with the remedy, *Rosa gallica* (200c and 1M):

> The Yellow Rose [*R. gallica*] . . . has allowed my soul to receive, to open up and not fight for what I need. I would always aggressively go out and get others to come to me, to love me and to want me. In the past, I was hyper-vigilant in getting things working in my relationships. I was always going out to connect, being the "Glue" in my relationships. I felt if I was passive I'd get screwed. I'd die because nothing would show up. No one would want me or be able to take care of the relationship. The Yellow Rose has

allowed a deeper passivity, a receptivity, and in so doing has allowed me to attract a beautiful, loving, equal relationship. I've seen my own energy opening up, allowing my partner into my heart and receiving that energy into my life and being able to appreciate that way of loving. The Yellow Rose was like a bud that has kept blossoming in my heart and soul. It was something I could feel and still do. I experienced old lovers contacting me . . . I also noticed after taking the remedy I'd become aggressive and angry/agitated for a couple of days but then it would pass. . . .

Alongside this "rosy" picture of the Rose, we have thorns. According to Ambrose in *The Dictionary of Christian Art*: "The thorns of the rose were a reminder of human finitude and guilt as the roses in the Paradise Garden had not thorns" (*Dodd, 296*). (**GUILT**) Nineteenth century Sufi philosopher Khan describes the thorns as that part of the self that is crude and must be ground down in order to "bloom" into a more refined self. The poet Rumi writes:

> If your thought is a rose,
> You are the rose garden.
> If your thought is a thorn,
> You are kindling for the bath stove.

Reportedly, St. Francis threw himself onto rosebushes outside his cell in order to turn away from sin. Legend has it that the roses thereafter altered their basic form becoming a Rose without thorns and having tiny brown spots on its leaves resembling drops of blood. Today, outside Francis' cathedral in Assisi, these roses still bloom.

Poets through the ages have used the brief span of time it takes for a rosebud to appear and then disperse as single petals as an allegory for the brevity of a human life. The Yellow Rose in particular is connected to death, and is sent in great huge garlands and wreaths at the time of a funeral or mourning. (**GRIEF/DEATH IN THE FAMILY**) One of the most poignant legends of our nation's history tells of the sorrow expressed by the Cherokees when one-fourth of them died on the forced march from Georgia to Oklahoma. As the legend goes, "The mothers of the Cherokee grieved because they were unable to help their children survive the journey. The elders prayed for a sign to lift the mother's spirits and give them strength" (*Sullivan*). The next day, beautiful white roses with golden-yellow centers began to grow where each of the mother's tears fell.

During the Middle Ages healing powers were attributed to the Rose as well. "Ring-a-ring o' roses, A pocket full of posies, Ashes! Ashes! We all fall down." was a children's song during the time of the European Black Death, referring to the attempts people made to stave off the deadly disease and purify their blood by carrying roses in their clothing. This is not surprising since the blood red Rose was associated with curative powers from the time of the early Greeks and Egyptians, and honored with legendary medicinal properties. By the Middle Ages the red *R. gallica* painted on a shingle and hung outside a doctor's door had become *the* symbol for the healing arts and pharmacology, now known as the Apothecary Rose (*Kavanaugh*). This was not without reason. "We are told that Pliney, the famous medical writer of the Roman period, listed some thirty medicines made from roses . . . " and monks cultivated it for its medicinal qualities in spite of its pagan roots (*Krussmann 12*). Old herbalists used the Rose to strengthen the heart, stomach, liver, and bladder, treating respiratory infections, colds, fluxes, coughs, joint pain, hemorrhages, and nausea (*Grieve*). Even today, we know the "miraculous" effect of rose hips (vitamin C) for strengthening the immune system and fighting off viruses.

Nicolas Culpepper (1616-1654) suggests that among its many medicinal uses, rose sugar be made into a "cordial" to "quicken weak and faint spirits" and rosewater be used "either in meats or broths to smell at the nose" (*Grieve*). Five centuries later, with the resurgence of the use of edible flowers in cooking, we find the Rose with its young tips and sweet nutty flavor in salads, desserts, wine, and flavorings at the finest restaurants. (**FOOD/HUNGER**)

Roses come in all sizes, colors, and shapes. New roses are constantly being developed for their extraordinary beauty and longevity. From time immemorial, the Rose has drawn us to it, perhaps because its fragility, beauty, thorniness, and transitory nature mirrors the experience of life itself. In the Rose proving, all the movements of the heart: loss, grief, rebelliousness, independence, compassion, danger, passivity, and love come to the fore. Yet, the depth of this single flower's influence upon our world remains a mystery as deep as the human heart itself.

Rosa Gallica Themes

Ancient Yellow Rose

- *Old Friends/Lovers*
- *Relationships*
- *Heart*
- *Grief/Death in the Family*
- *Loving Feelings/Compassion*
- *Sexuality*
- *Lack of Responsibility*
- *Desire to Help Others*
- *Passivity*
- *Rebellion/Independence*
- *Guilt*
- *Mortal Danger*
- *Food/Hunger*
- *Money*
- *Gardens*

Old Friends/Lovers

#16 Situation: My first lover calls me after a fifteen year period of time. Bizarre. As I spoke to her, old feelings dredged up. She always withheld herself from me and I was never able to see her as her whole self. It would drive me crazy, she always had secrets from me. I longed to totally connect with her and be in her secret world. I loved her and wanted her so much, but I never fully connected. We broke and my heart ached for years.

#3 Phone calls from people I had not heard from for 10–15 years, just found my phone number. Old friends calling.

#2 Dream: . . . I talked to an old friend by phone, someone I am no longer friends with.

#16 Dream: Old friend, broken relationship (male) comes back. He brings me many sheep and many wrapped gifts.

#1 . . . Two years ago I was given a research fellowship to a foreign country, and this fellow there developed an obsessive stalking thing, a terrifying, horrible event in my life. I had to leave a year early. Out of the blue he called me (during this proving). He is a very charismatic person—he acted as if nothing had happened.

#2 Dream: Of an old lover whom I have dreamed of before, had very amorous feelings.

#5 Overwhelmed with thoughts of my ex-husband today. Obsession. I had to talk with him. Have not spoken in over a year. Nothing new between us, same old same old in talking with him. Just overwhelming urge to talk with him. Wishing I could have been more emotionally there for him in our relationship when we were together.

#4 Disturbing and vivid dreams of father and ex-sweeties, the male element.

Relationships

#13 Dream: Fragments. In an apartment, not mine, some family presence, sister? A middle-aged man, tall, lanky, longish dark hair with dandruff, in some relationship. We are getting together again. He lies beside me and I embrace him, signaling to sister we are indeed together. The feeling is that I am accepting him even though he is seedy and conceited. Though I like to clean people's scalps, I know it is not good to do his—that would bind us together—so I maintain an inner independence, though I let others see we are together.

#16 Dream: . . . I walk farther into church and find a woman in there. I ask her for pamphlets about relationships and she gives them to me. I have no shirt on and I am just aware of it. (It is unusual I would be in a church and asking for advice and especially entering with being only half dressed.) I then go home. I hold my son, although he is not my real life son, and I realize that I am for the first time angry and indignant that she, without any permission or request, was inseminated by another man in order to have this child. I yell at her and ask her why. She is very aloof and casual, and said something about how a friend thought it would be charitable.

#1 Dream: I was the wife of an aristocrat but didn't want to be anymore. He had a mistress and had no interest in me on any level. I felt sad and helpless. . . . I discovered him with a cache of erotic material in the closet. He was very upset and ashamed, but I thought if I was accepting, perhaps it would rekindle his feelings. It was calculating on my part. I did not really think it was all right even though I told him so. Somehow it worked and he fell in love with me. The feeling was happy, creative, effective.

#1 Feeling melancholy after watching movie, *An Awfully Big Adventure,* about a girl who is searching for love and is not loved in return. The whole movie is filled with people who love others who do not love them.

#2 Dream: . . . I was being pursued by two men flattering me, asking me for a date, etc.

#5 Dream: Advising a young girl to leave abusive relationship.

#10 Went to a workshop and did a conflict resolution exercise. I had great trouble coming up with an example of real life conflict with my partner.

Heart

#4 Expansion in the area of the heart chakra—a sense of expectation or excitement, like a feeling of being just so excited about something, like children get, about to burst.

#4 A sense of this being a sweet remedy—it has to do with the sensation in my heart area. It reminds me of a time I was wearing this necklace of rose quartz for several weeks and was incredibly emotional about everything, with bursting into tears for no reason. Same feeling of very strong emotion here. But it is not a feeling of grief, more a feeling of sweet emotion. The "vibration" is like when one is excited as a child before their birthday, or a treat that is about to happen

#5 Awareness of my heart, the vibration now felt there.

#5 . . . What made an impression on me was the image of opening to new opportunities, good fortune; heart energy in abundance, with a petty line that puts the brakes on things. Afterwards I thought, it takes great discipline to have an open and compassionate heart. If the mind is not aligned to the heart's generosity, much could be wasted in the distraction of mind's judgments and/or conditioned—learned habits, draining the heart without replenishing.

#5 In meditation, focus of the mind narrows, the heart opens generously to cries from a goshawk, the body relaxes into stillness.

#16 . . . We broke and my heart ached for years.

Grief/Death in the Family

#16 Dream: My sister dies in this dream and I am devastated. She is there present in the scene, although I know she is dead. I want to be away from relatives that want to console me. I pull away. Go on my own. They are dressed up, and I do not want to be and I do not dress up, but unsure, self-conscious. My sister warns me that my true inner state will begin to torment me if I do not change. She says that she is okay with death, looking out into blue sky and white clouds with a seascape. I am not sure what she means that I have to change about myself. Feeling: Grief, incomplete.

#10 Dream: I had done something that caused my ex-wife to not allow me to see my daughter anymore. She communicated this to me in letter. I read it in the dream and wept and wept. I woke up weeping, very unusual, never before.

#4 Dream: Being in boat on the sea. I get off to see a friend or lover. When I return there is smoke and the sky is red, I am told my sister has died, I feel the deepest and most real sensation of grief. I wrap my arms around myself and am rocking back and forth racked with sobbing. It is like the few times in real life where I experienced profound grief. Although it is my sister who died, people bring me things from an ex-boyfriend, as though he had died.

#4 Dream: Of my son dying, woke depressed, with anxiety and grief. He is away working in Reno, I was so anxious to phone him, I was very disturbed and it haunted me all the day.

#5 Dream: . . . We come to the end, the scene of a cataclysm. Blood-dimmed water is everywhere. A woman, still alive and wailing with grief, is sitting on the carcass of my grandmother. She is holding two twin dead babies. I feel her pain; it is excruciating, but I have no feeling for my own loss, the loss of my grandmother.

#12 Sadness about my mother growing old and still working hard. What is it going to be like when they die?

Loving Feelings/Compassion

#13 Went to counseling. First experienced a sadness that was not mine. I could actually feel myself feel my grandmother's sadness, knowing it was hers. Very odd, but unmistakable. This is the first emotional connection I have felt to her since I can remember. I remember her, but have not been able to feel anything.

#13 Husband and I disagree on so many little things. Sometimes it bothers me, mostly because I genuinely like him, as well as all the deep loving feelings. . . . I have been thinking, since doing this journal, of how much love I actually do express. I am not sure that it is a lot, especially to my husband, funnily enough. . . . A lot of love for my daughters.

#12 Feeling—putting myself in other people's shoes.

#2 Dream: I had newspapers on my living room floor and my friend peed all over the newspaper on the floor. . . . He got his jacket and said he had to leave. I thought to myself, nothing is more important than loving him and maintaining our relationship.

#2 Dream: . . . we talked about changing the diets and lives of children that I knew—African American inner city kids. I felt compassion

#1 Dream: Oprah Winfrey had developed a program to help save the children in the inner city involving carbonated water. I was really excited about this.

#2 Dream: A friend came naked to my house. . . . She had a huge number of moles and freckles on her back, all over, confluent, which made her appearance very unpleasant, almost freak-like . . . and I had great appreciation for her, and compassion. . . . A friend having an attack of some kind, seizure, mania, I felt compassion.

#1 Dream: . . . A gray colt came crashing in through the window and is biting people, savaging people. I am afraid of the colt and he approaches me. Then I think perhaps he is teething, in pain, damaged in some way. I have to go and intervene and help this animal. I put my fingers in his mouth and was massaging his gums, knowing he could bite me and crush my hand. His teeth are brown, wood-like and sharp, but I feel sorry for him. He is obviously content with the massaging, then I realize he is very sad and that he was abandoned by his mother and damaged. As I leave the restaurant he crouches at my feet and I cuddle him. I want to mother him. Was very frightened but he did not hurt me. Felt compassion and impulse to help even at the risk of my own health.

#1 Dream: A woman with a baby in a car accident in Russia. I was a doctor trying to save them in the street. A crowd gathered around her and did not want me to save the woman, said she was wicked, a slut. I had to make many efforts to persuade them that I should save her.

#15 Feeling sentimental, nostalgic. I am looking at, seeing people, places and realizing it may be for the last time, or not again for a long time. A bittersweet feeling.

Sexuality

#16 Dream: Hiding away in a little room with a woman friend and making love to her. I kiss her lips and they distinctly taste like salt (Natrum muriaticum). I am passionately connected with her. . . . In real life this woman used to dance in a topless bar or something. She had an interesting bent on sex, like men want it more if they have to pay.

#2 Dream: . . . A woman walked up to a person in the audience and made gestures of love and the person responded with facial expressions like, "Oh, tempt me, tempt me," in an amorous way.

#13 Dream: "Bill Moyers"—I was driving to some border or crossing. On the way, road was torn up on right side. There was some delay. As I was coming back to the car Bill Moyers came up to me—very friendly, affectionate, wanted sex. He accused me of being dishonest about it, i.e. I should. I did not have an affair, but enjoyed the feeling.

#5 Sexual energy went up. Playful and satisfying, open and genuine. It's great.

#6 Increased sexual interest. "Horny."

#6 Dream: At end of dream with my wife I see a girl in a short plaid green jumper-type skirt and open-necked white blouse. I say to my wife, "Why don't you buy that outfit and put it on," and I'm thinking she will look very sexy and my thoughts turn amorous.

#6 Dream: At a party . . . I treat one woman and we start to make love. I realize I need condoms.

Lack of Responsibility

#10 . . . I totally "forgot" about being on call for work this day, until 6:00 p.m. when I was called in! I have not forgotten on call in eleven years of doing it.

#14 [*Turned in journal, didn't come to meeting, despite prior agreement!!*]

#10 Dream: I went to pick up my daughter at school and there was snow on the ground. I threw a snowball at a group and hit one of the children. I just walked away, left him crying there, pretending I did not throw it.

#13 Feel sad and disappointed that one student is not passing the course. I resist making it my responsibility.

#7 Had a difficult time talking to son about responsibility—his coming home late and getting a "D" grade in biology because he is behind, etc. I have felt like I am having a hard time letting this "be," and unlike most heart-to-hearts, I only felt frustrated. I sense that he will not accept any responsibility and I want his motivation to change to be internal rather than external.

#13 It is unlike me to be so unreliable. This is five days later that I am filling this in. I always keep a commitment like this, and now I do not even seem to be bothered by the fact that I will have to fess up in front of everyone that I did not bother to do this regularly every night.

#7 Dream: Go to hotel looking for a place to put up German exchange students. Large blonde woman is there with a small new baby. Then a man I know appears and shows us around this huge multiple room complex that they are sharing, basement suites, very plush. When we return upstairs, a small, petite woman with long, curly fiery-red hair comes to take the baby from her adoptive parents because they're Jewish and the woman says Jews can't raise his girl. I'm upset, screaming, horrified, and especially because the Jewish parents just seem to accept and even seem relieved about this, because she has been such a wild little girl.

Desire to Help Others

#16 Dream: At social functions where two women asked me to attend a ball or something. I say yes to both, and then feel conflicted as to who I should go with, and that I may hurt one's feelings. Could not understand why I said yes to both.

#1 Dream: . . . A gray colt came crashing in through the window and is biting people, savaging people. I am afraid of the colt and he approaches me. Then I think perhaps he is teething, in pain, damaged in some way. I have to go and intervene and help this animal. I put my fingers in his mouth and was massaging his gums, knowing he could bite me and crush my hand. His teeth are brown, wood-like and sharp, but I feel sorry for him. He is obviously content with the massaging, then I realize he is very sad and that he was abandoned by his mother and damaged. As I leave the restaurant he crouches at my feet and I cuddle him. I want to mother him. Was very frightened but he did not hurt me. Felt compassion and impulse to help even at the risk of my own health.

#4 I went to stay at a friend's house and had to be careful to leave it fanatically clean. Need to be responsible, not put anybody out, completely abandoning my own needs, everyone else was going first, I had no idea of my own emotional needs.

#3 I got a phone call from someone who thought I was able to fix a computer program. I asked how she knew me. I have a MAC and she had an IBM—we were virtual strangers. The computer business is like a foreign field. I felt why me? Then perplexed and then a desire to help, intense desire to help. A feeling of no idea of what to do. Not typical. I try to help but this is not in a field I know. I have no idea of what I am doing.

#1 Dream: I was wishing I could bring an old abandoned garden to life. All that remained were the foundations of the bed outlines. Then an elderly man was sitting next to me and said he would love to finance the bringing to life of the garden. I was so happy. Then I noticed that there were many roses starting to leaf out, and there was a woman who was mulching the beds. I felt so happy and excited. I was also relieved there would not be so much work to do, as these two rose beds were very large. Feeling of responsibility and impulse to heal and help.

#4 I have an exaggerated sense of having to please other people more than myself. Duty and responsibility, to people, to animals. Lose sight of my own needs. Boundaries blurry.

#1 Curative report six years after the proving: This remedy helped my tendency to want to do for others at my own expense. This is a very heroic remedy—the feeling is so grand, as if you can save the world, a very noble feeling. Even as a kid I felt a calling from God to do for others. This remedy helped me get clarity on this state and put it back into balance. My tendency is to take on an enormous amount of responsibility. It helped me to pursue the tasks that come to me but have a detachment, to do the best work and leave the rest in the hands of God.

Passivity

#4 Dream: Of my head being half a walnut shell as a skull and a cigarette butt in it, being squished into it by someone with their thumb. Woke with a terrible headache.

#7 Dream: I'm on a bus after a very long trip, we pull into the station and I can see my husband sitting on the grass waiting for me. As we get off some of the people pass through a room and then the rest of us are stopped, we have to wait. Because the others have already gone through, I object and finally defy the person in charge in order to get to my husband.

#7 Thinking of all this, I am beginning to think that what I am dealing with now is different than I thought. I was seeing youth, versus older. Now, I think it is about active versus passive. The source of my irritation for days has been passivity, on husband's and son's parts especially.

#1 Dream: I was at my daughter's school to meet with her teachers about her proposed schedule for the autumn term. I am not happy they made her sign an agreement to work hard and obey school rules, a loyalty oath, like I had to sign at university. Normally I would have gone in and made a fuss about it, but very uncharacteristically, in dream or in waking life, I just accepted it because that is the school's policy, even though it was against my wishes. I do not agree and I do not make an effort to voice my opinion, nor do I feel upset. Very strange. My father is in the dream and he wanders into an ongoing class to speak to one of the teachers about the situation, and I know he will disrupt everyone, but I am passive and do not try to stop him. I know I disagree with his action, but I do not stop him. . . . I felt it was wrong to make a child sign a loyalty oath—like moral outrage, this is not right, but I was passive.

#1 Dream: I was living abroad, in a foreign house, went into the kitchen and saw a large man yelling and slapping my son in back of the head. Then I realized he was not my son and that he belonged to this man. I tried to tell him that there were better ways to motivate children than slapping them, but he just slapped him again. He was bleeding. I felt very sad and helpless. My son did not cry, just threw himself on the floor with his face screwed up in a stoic mask of anger, as if he were used to this and would not show weakness. Feeling helpless, frustrated and sad.

#4 I have an exaggerated sense of having to please other people more than myself. Duty and responsibility, to people, to animals. Lose sight of my own needs. Boundaries blurry.

Rebellion/Independence

#16 Dream: . . . With a group of students with Nancy and Roger. We are trying to push a tree down. I say, "Why do we have to do work for you when we should be studying homeopathy." I rebel and leave the group, and go on my own.

#13 Another day not recorded—what is this, a latent teen rebellion?

#7 . . . I cried and had memories of how I was at that age, a rebellious teenager/young adult—angry, life was hard. I identified strongly with the kids in the writer's group and even felt some kind of attraction to the wildness and intensity of feeling in one of the young men who was smart, but rebellious.

#2 I am content, joyful, full of grace and expanding in the knowing of who I am. I am a child of God. Freedom is detaching from the opinions of others, the prejudices of others, the fear of others.

#7 As a theme I think of independence, struggle for independence.

#13 Dream: . . . Though I like to clean people's scalps, I know it is not good to do his—that would bind us together—so I maintain an inner independence, though I let others see we are together.

Guilt

#16 Dream: Hiding away in a little room with a woman friend and making love to her. I kiss her lips and they distinctly taste like salt. . . . I am passionately connected with her. I notice my two children are in the room saying, "Dad, when are we going home?" I think, "My god, they are going to tell their mother," then I feel guilt. No guilt up to that point.

#3 I did notice stress at work. I deal with low income women—we are short midwives and do not have enough to cover the hours, 100 hours for the week. I said, "No!" and was very adamant, I didn't care. I felt very guilty after this. A couple of people came up to me afterwards and praised me for being clear, but I still felt guilty, influencing them to stand up for themselves. I usually stick up for rights, so it was a reversal to feel guilty about this.

#16 Dream: . . . I notice a beautiful shedded skin of a snake. When I lifted it, there was a large snake which looked venomous. I grabbed it by the throat as did my father. I want to kill it as I was afraid of being bitten. I choked it, my father let go. I stared into its eyes as its life went out. After it died I felt great guilt that I had to kill it. It lay limp on a table.

#1 Dream: I was a clerk in a store and I had murdered someone and varnished them to make them look like merchandise. I thought it was the perfect crime since the victim had disappeared from the store and was never seen again and I had an alibi all day at work. I felt guilty that I had done this but I had a strong sense that this had had to be done.

#1 Dream: My sister died of cancer, then my elder son killed himself. Feeling was terrible guilt and grief that I could not prevent his death and that he had wanted to kill himself. Very guilty, sad. I felt I would go mad with these feelings.

#4 Wake up every morning—very disturbed. Feeling of being guilty and grief, not pleasant.

#10 I even played hooky from work. Felt guilty about that. I have not done that for years.

Mortal Danger

#1 . . . [Real Event] Something sort of horrible happened today—I received a very frightening phone call in the morning from Washington, trembling afterwards. Feeling outraged, pacing in the house. He had stalked me ten years ago, and I had not heard from him in ten years.

#14 Dream: In a house out in the country, wanted to walk in woods, afraid something would happen to me. A little ways out a man appeared with intention to do me harm. I looked in his eye and became fierce like a wild animal, he backed away. I ran back home. When I returned home, later in the week, he was there with a family member, as her lover. I was freaked, awoke feeling frightened and vulnerable.

#7 Dream: . . . I leave a friend's house on my bike and get lost, and end up in a back dirt road at a house. I am attacked by an older man, no one I know or can connect with anyone. He is skinny, balding, mean and creepy. He is trying to rape me and I am throwing food at him. I get away and try to tell someone about him.

#1 Dream: On a bus, and two men say they are assigned as my immortal protectors. They are both "number 12" on a long list of people who are competing to win by killing all of the others, until they are "number one." But they tell me being number one means all the others try to kill you so they can get your spot. I somehow understood that even though they say I am "it," meaning the one they protect, I also know that "it" means number one and that I am in mortal danger from them and other unseen enemies. . . . We go to an alley, into a bar and we have very little money. They want to eat well and richly, and say if the waiters give us trouble we'll just kill them. Somehow I have authority and I insist we can only eat what we can pay for, so we get sandwiches. I forced them to bend to my will. They are very unhappy, but it is very important to me to do the correct thing and act ethically. I was also aware of being in dangerous place, and know it is a matter of time until I face mortal danger.

#14 I notice the prevalence of disturbing dreams related to survival. Something keeps happening that is related to a death-life situation.

#16 Dream: At a pit—told it is 1,400 feet deep—with two men and it felt as though it was a punishment. One man says, "To hell with fear," and jumps in the pit. Then we are all falling in space bounding off the walls. Fear.

Food/Hunger

#16 Appetite increased last two weeks. I am hungry a lot and will eat and want more. Gained two to three pounds last few weeks.

#13 Uninterested in food, buying, cooking food. So many meals. I thought we should all go on a fast.

#16 Dream: . . . being brought lavish food and pleasures.

#13 Noticed had gained a lot of weight over the last three years, 12–15 pounds. Suddenly it does not feel good. I decide to cut out sweets, but at the open house, I eat some goodies.

#2 I awoke very hungry, extremely hungry. I eat well but this was different.

#2 Dream: An old lover who was cooking eggs at his house, then in another house with eggs on the floor.

#3 Wasn't hungry, knew I should eat, but I did not feel hungry.

#9 Traveling home from conference, I decided to start a new "diet"—a completely different way of eating for myself. (I am <u>not</u> one to "do diets.")

#5 . . . Stomach: no appetite at breakfast, finally ate just to eat at 10:30, and now I feel sick from it.

#12 Dream: Old man fixing a vacuum cleaner. I was upset because I could fix it, but I was eating cheese on bread, so I decided to keep eating and not help.

#7 Continue to have little interest in food, no real cravings or hunger driving me. I had been getting hunger crazed like when I was pregnant, but that feeling is gone. Wandered around supermarket looking for something appetizing without much luck.

#7 Dream: . . . He is trying to rape me and I am throwing food at him.

#13 . . . Reach for carbohydrates when I feel my body needing raw veggies. Habit? Weird.

#8 A continued obsessiveness with smoothies . . . strawberries, bananas.

Money

#5 ... "I am so fed up with the world of buying and selling!!!" When will we wake up, and move beyond the lower aspects of materialism!! What is beyond?!!

#16 Dream: Walk into a church office. No one is there in front. Lots of money for charity on desk, no one watching it. It could easily be stolen, I think. Not that I would steal it.

#13 Main concern is finances. Not fear so much, as aware that things need to change if we are to keep daughter at a certain school.

#5 Inclined to play Lotto (numbers lottery), never thought of it before. . . . Bought a Lotto ticket! Thoughts enmeshed with brooding feelings about money, status, power, respect—not my everyday sort of musings.

#12 Opened up a pair of jeans and found $20 in jeans at Salvation Army. Had needed $20 earlier and then what I bought cost exactly $20.

#5 ... Conversation with a friend yesterday turned to the San Francisco scene of big money with its huge emphasis on style with incredible restrictions on what is and is not acceptable. I don't quite understand it. What has felt different with the proving is "get it for myself!"—about material things—rather than the "let it come, let it go" I am familiar with, with regard to material things, money, assets, resources.

#2 Dream: A fat woman asked how much the toast was. I said, "Fifteen cents."

Gardens

#1 During the day, calm and peaceful, worked in the garden.

#1 Dream: I was wishing I could bring an old abandoned garden to life. All that remained were the foundations of the bed outlines. Then an elderly man was sitting next to me and said he would love to finance the bringing to life of the garden. I was so happy. Then I noticed that there were many roses starting to leaf out, and there was a woman who was mulching the beds. I felt so happy and excited. I was also relieved there would not be so much work to do, as these two rose beds were very large.

#4 Very connected to a kind of elemental or nature world (not totally unusual, but more so than usual). Feel connected to the plants and trees and flowers. Again, the sense this is a sweet, almost angelic remedy.

#4 Dream: Garden—walking in it—of the house I used to live in while I was in London. The neighbor next door allows me to buy her house and now I connect the two. My ex-husband is there and is happy as he can grow more flowers. A rose tree is broken and he mends it together again.

#5 Sumptuous, sensual images, desirous of beauty, beautiful things—melons, gentle flowers.

#12 I feel like being outdoors, getting hands dirty. I force myself to garden, weed, etc. but once I am doing it, it is fine.

#13 First roses blooming, I felt such joy.

ROSA GALLICA RUBRICS .... *Ancient Yellow Rose*

MIND   ABSORBED, buried in thought
ACTIVITY; morning; exhausted in the afternoon
ANGER, irascibility; breaking things
  teenagers, in
  tendency; accused when
  violent
ANXIETY; exams, before
  conscience, of
    on waking
  vertigo, during
AVARICE; desires more than she needs
AVERSION; work, avoids going to
BENEVOLENCE
BITING; fingers
BROODING
  money and status, power, over
  unpleasant things
CAPRICIOUSNESS
CARES, worries; full of
CENSORIOUS, critical
  husband accuses her of being
CLAIRVOYANCE
COMMUNICATIVE, expansive
COMPANY; aversion to, agg.
  desire for, amel.
  to contact and hear people
COMPASSION
  with son
CONCENTRATION; active
CONFUSION; night
  disoriented like, "where am I?"
CONTENTED; himself, with
CONTRADICT, disposition to
CONTRARY
COURAGEOUS; heroic, noble
DEFIANT
DELUSIONS
  animals
    elephants, of
  connected; to nature and elemental world
    to plants, trees and flowers
  dirt, dirty; he is
  drugged, he has been
  fleas crashing, hopping, biting her
  gold, precious metals, gems
  heart opening to cries of goshawk
  must please others
  neglected; duty

persecuted
protection by guardian angels
  by spirit guides
pushed against a wall, she is
sensual images, melons, gentle flowers
sink, heavy, is as though through the bed
sweet, angelic
violated, she is
visions, bones dancing
DESIRES; get it for myself
  help others, to
  open and compassionate heart
  outdoors, getting hands dirty
  talk to ex-husband
  useful, desires to be
  youth, to be young
DISGUST; money and materialism
DREAMS
  active
  advising girl to leave abusive relationship
  amorous
    old lover, tempted by
  animals,
    crayfish
    ducks, caged baby; saving them
    horses; rambunctious
    horse; sad, abandoned, damaged
    lizards, poisonous
    snakes
    spiders, black widow
  body, body parts; head; is half a walnut shell with a cigarette butt in it
  child, children;
    age 14 committed suicide
    in bathtub submerged but well
    wanted to save, inner city
  city; inner
  compassion for African American city children
  condoms, needed; embarrassed by people laughing
  consolation, aversion to
  counselors giving advice
  danger
    acting ethically, during
    determined to do what is right
    impending
    two men immortal protectors
    unseen enemies
  dead; people, of;
    grandfather
    grandmother
    infants, twins
    sister
  death
    dear one, of
    family, in

  lasting after waking
  relatives, of
  sister, of
  son, of
   suicide, by
defying the person in charge
doctor saving mother and child
embrace, desire to
ethical behavior
fight
  martial arts, of practicing
flying
friends; appreciation and compassion for
  having a seizure
  naked with moles all over, freak-like
  old
frightful
  mob action from the crowd, of
futuristic transportation
gardens
  connected to the neighbor
  husband happy growing flowers in
  mending broken rose tree
  old abandoned, bringing to life
  walking in
gifts, given to me by friend
grief
  at death of sister
  elder son, suicide
  profound, like in real life
  son dying, anticipation of
  twin babies, dead
guilt
  due to death of son by suicide
  over kissing lover and concern wife will find out
happy, creative, effective
helpless
helplessness, feeling
hippie, with nothing to do
hurried driving
inadequate, not smart enough
injuries; my son to, by a man
invaded, feeling
jewelry, pin; old charm from 1881
long
love, fallen in
lover, old
  returns and brings her gifts
loving my friend and maintaining relationship
loyalty oath
males
man; attacked by; tried to rape me
many
memory lost for phone number

men
missing out on something
money, could easily be stolen
murdering
   the perfect crime; had alibi
number twelve
parents, of, deceased
party, in ballroom on New Year's Eve
   two women agree to go to ball with
people, of; crowd
powerlessness
professor, sociology, who I respected
pursued
   of being; by two men; asking me for a date
   woman; fat, by
quarrels
   slapped; my son is, by a man
rape; pursued for the purpose of
remorse
   anxiety; of conscience at killing snake
responsibility
   towards others, my safety at risk
roses
rose tree is broken and is mended again
   sad
      over death of son by suicide
      over husband's lack of interest in her
      tears, with
   save the world for others
   saving people, of
technology
unpleasant
unsuccessful efforts
   trying to find someone
urinating, of; desire for; but could not
urinating on the floor; of friend
vivid
water
weeping
   sad
   tears, with
wild
   girl child with red hair, parents give her up
wild animal, I became fierce like a
DUTY; a strong sense of
   to animals and people
EMOTIONS; sweet sensation in heart
   felt in chest and heart area like a strong vibration
EXCITEMENT, child, as a, before their birthday party
   excitable; in area of the heart chakra
   sweet emotion
FANCIES; absorbed in
FEAR
   company ameliorates

duty; being unable to do her
stalker, of, who found her after ten years
FREEDOM detaching from opinions and fears of others
FRIENDS, old, coming back into one's life
FRUSTRATION
   at son's lack of responsibility
GRIEF; waking, on
HOME; desires to; be at
IDEAS; fixed
IMPATIENCE
   driving, during
INDEPENDENT
INDOLENCE, aversion to work
INDUSTRIOUS
IRRITABILITY
   morning; waking, on
   night; waking, on
   noise, from
   passive people, with
   weather, in rainy or cloudy
   with lack of respect shown to me
JOY
   grace in the knowing who I am
   roses, at sight of first blooming
LOVE; family, for
   especially daughters
   sudden return of old lover into her life
   unexpressed, toward husband
MEDITATION; resistant to
MISUNDERSTOOD, feels
MONOMANIA
MOOD; alternating
   capricious
   changeable, variable
OBSTINATE
OFFENDED EASILY
PASSIVE
PERTINACITY
PHILOSOPHY; ability for
PLAY; gambling, passion for
POWERLESS feeling
RAGE, fury
   phone call from stalker who
   rediscovered her, at
RESPONSIBILITY
   lack of
   strong, making lists of lists
   strong; social
   to others, abandoning her own needs, everyone else goes first
RESTLESSNESS
   nervousness; daytime
   nervousness; night; bed, in
   nervousness; anger, from
SADNESS, despondency, depression, melancholy; waking; on

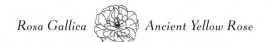

Rosa Gallica   Ancient Yellow Rose

SENSITIVE,
  external impressions, to all
    night
  noise, to
    night
  reprimands, to
SENTIMENTAL
  at seeing friends and places for the last time
SHRIEKING, screaming, shouting
  teenagers, in; at parents
SLOWNESS; motion, in
STALKED; she is
SYMPATHETIC, compassionate
  feels sadness of others
TALK, talking, talks;
  desire for chit-chat
  grunting like a pig
  sleep in
THEORIZING
THOUGHTS; sexual
  tormenting
TRANQUILITY, serenity, calmness
TRIFLES; important, seem
WEEPING, tearful mood
  tendency; sleep; in
  tendency over materialism
  over lost item
  trifles, over

HEAD   ITCHING; scalp

HEAD PAIN   GENERAL; morning
  morning; waking, and on
  evening; seven p.m.
  coughing, on
  exertion of; body
  heated, from becoming
  motion; agg.
  pressure, external; agg.
  stomach; disordered, with
  weeping, after
HAMMERING
LANCINATING; forehead; above eyes
LOCALIZATION; forehead; evening
  forehead; eyes, above
    extending; occiput, to
  occiput; pulsating
    morning, on waking
    lying, while
    pressure; amel.
    extending; temples, to
Temples; right

VERTIGO	ANXIETY, during
FEAR, during
HEADACHE; during
MENSES; during; agg.
TURNING
internally
EYE	AGGLUTINATED; morning
DUST in eyes, as if
IRRITATION
ITCHING
left
PAIN; general; right
waking, on
SWELLING; sensation of
VISION	BLURRED
NOSE	CORYZA; hay fever, annual
EPISTAXIS
left; during coition
ITCHING and crawling and tickling
SCAB; right nostril; with yellow green, bloody discharge on
blowing nose
SNEEZING
EAR	DISCOLORATION; redness
DRYNESS; behind
HEAT; left
INFLAMMATION; external; skin behind ear
NOISES in; general; left
cracking; right
PAIN; general; right
left
lancinating
STOPPED sensation
morning; waking, on
WAX; increased
HEARING	LOST; stopped sensation, with
FACE	ERUPTIONS; lips
SENSITIVE
ULCERS; lips; lower
MOUTH	ERUPTIONS; palate
INFLAMMATION; gums; right side
SWELLING
TEETH	PAIN; toothache in general; right
THROAT	ITCHING
PAIN; general; morning; waking, on
sore; pressure, on
TENSION; right side

Rosa Gallica   *Ancient Yellow Rose*

STOMACH	APPETITE; capricious, hunger, but knows not for what, or refuses things when offered
	   increased, hunger in general; waking, on
	      afternoon
	   wanting
	     morning
	DISORDERED
	ERUCTATIONS; general; amel.
	HICCOUGH
	NAUSEA; drinking; after
	   with stopped ear
	PAIN; general; drinking, after

THIRST	NIGHT

ABDOMEN	DISAGREEABLE sensation
	DISTENSION
	   morning; waking, on
	   menses; during
	FLABBINESS
	NUMBNESS
	PAIN; general
	   hypochondria; right
	   ower part; one spot over left ovary
	   liver
	   inguinal region; left

RECTUM	*CONSTIPATION* DIARRHEA; morning *FLATUS*
STOOL	FLOATING in water FREQUENT *ODOR; offensive* SOFT
BLADDER	FULLNESS; sensation of URINATION; dribbling by drops frequent; night
MALE	SEXUAL desire; increased

FEMALE	MENSES; clotted, coagulated
	   copious
	   late, too
	   protracted
	   short, too; one day only
	SEXUAL desire; increased
	SPEECH & VOICE
	VOICE; weak
	RESPIRATION
	SIGHING
	COUGH
	EATING, from

CHEST	AGITATION, heart
EXCITEMENT sensation, in heart area
excitable; in area of the heart chakra
PAIN; general; heart
PAIN; general; mammae; right; extending to heart
BACK	TIGHT feeling; cervical region
PAIN; general; crossing legs agg.
extending legs agg.
flatus amel.
cervical region; right side
cervical region; extending; shoulders
dorsal region; scapulae; left; under; agg. turning
head to right
lumbar region; left
STIFFNESS; lumbar region
TENSION
EXTREMITIES	ERUPTION; leg; rash
HEAVINESS, tired limbs
ITCHING; fingers; thumb
fingers; thumb; cold amel.
scratching agg.,
NUMBNESS; upper limbs; left
upper limbs; right
cold; becoming
fingers; left
extending; upwards
first finger
foot; sitting
STIFFNESS; lower limbs
morning
PAIN; general; numbness, with
upper limbs
fingers; first
extending to; upward
lower limbs; walking
knee; morning; rising
leg; left
SLEEP	*DEEP*
SLEEPINESS; noon
afternoon
one p.m.
two p.m.
POSITION; abdomen, on
side, on; left
RESTLESS
UNREFRESHING; morning
WAKING; midnight; after; two a.m.
midnight; after; three thirty a.m.
early, too
PERSPIRATION	ODOR; sour

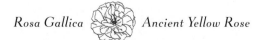

SKIN   DRY
ERUPTIONS; herpetic
  itching
  rhus poisoning
  vesicular; red

GENERALITIES   FORENOON, nine a.m. - noon; eleven a.m.; amel.
AIR; open; amel.
  desires
BITING sensation, bug like; fleas, as of
COLD; becoming
COLDNESS; morning
  night
FOOD and drinks; bacon; desires
  chocolate; desires
  drinks; desires smoothies
  farinaceous food; desires; which aggravate
  pizza; desires
  potatoes; desires
  salt; desires
  tea; desires; sweet
  wine; agg.
HEAVINESS
  internally; menses, during
    enlargement, and, sensation of like a sleeping elephant and couldn't move
PAIN; small spots
RESTLESSNESS, physical; fear, from
RISING up; amel.; bed, from
SIDE; left
  right
TOBACCO; desires; smoking
TREMBLING; fear, from
WAKING; on
WEAKNESS, enervation
  alternating with; activity
  working hard, as from
  menses; during
WEATHER; rain, agg. during
WOUNDS; bleeding; freely
  heal; slow
  old; pains, in

JOURNALS..*Rosa Gallica*

EDITOR'S NOTE: *Punctuation, abbreviations, and individual stylistic nuances of the original journal entries have been preserved wherever possible.*

> Prover #1 • Female • 41 years old

Day 1
- I took it at night right before bedtime. About 20 minutes after I took it, in bed (it usually takes half hour to fall asleep) I felt a heavy feeling like a narcotic. Great heaviness in body, I couldn't move. I felt like a very large animal, so massive, like a sleeping elephant, it would have a hard time moving.
- Then fear gripped me, with vertigo for one minute. I had a very powerful feeling of fear with a sense of internal spinning for one minute.
- I was anxious about doing this proving because I am a sensitive prover. I tried to be detached, tried hard to stay this way at that moment, the feeling of heaviness stayed with me.
- I awoke at 3:45 a.m. with a sense of having been active in my dreams. Many dreams all night long, of trying to help people, trying to act ethically in the face of danger, and difficulty with determination to do what is right. A series of dreams about being in the inner city. When I woke to write these, felt very heavy, like I had been drugged.
- Hard to get out of bed.
- Dream: Oprah Winfrey had developed a program to help save the children in the inner city involving carbonated water. I was really excited about this. I play an instrument—I was planning a fundraiser with her. Having trouble practicing and my husband made a comment, ridiculed me—I played it in an amateurish way. I was hurt, offended and picked up the instrument, told him how offended I was and walked away.
- Many "saving dreams": Dream themes: of saving people, my personal safety at stake.
- Dream: A woman with a baby in a car accident in Russia. I was a doctor trying to save them in the street. A crowd gathered around her and did not want me to save the woman, said she was wicked, a slut. I had to make many efforts to persuade them that I should save her. I felt personal danger, fearful of mob action from the crowd. It was my duty and personally I had to save her. I had this feeling of inadequacy. I thought I was not smart enough, had not gone to (good enough) medical school. With instrument dream I felt I was not a good enough musician.
- Dream: On a bus, and two men say they are assigned as my immortal protectors. They are both "number 12" on a long list of people who are competing to win by killing all of the others, until they are "number one." But they tell me being number one means all the others try to kill you so they can get your spot. I somehow understood that even though they say I am "it," meaning the one they protect, I also know that "it" means number one and that I am in mortal danger from them and other unseen enemies.

♦ Same dream: We go to an alley, into a bar and we have very little money. They want to eat well and richly, and say if the waiters give us trouble we'll just kill them. Somehow I have authority and I insist we can only eat what we can pay for, so we get sandwiches. I forced them to bend to my will. They are very unhappy, but it is very important to me to do the correct thing and act ethically. I was also aware of being in dangerous place, and know it is a matter of time until I face mortal danger. Again the theme of ethical behavior in the face of danger.

♦ Uncharacteristic dreams for me in the a.m.

♦ During the day, calm and peaceful, worked in the garden.

Day 2

♦ In the night I felt a strange passivity.

♦ Dream: I was at my daughter's school to meet with her teachers about her proposed schedule for the autumn term. I am not happy they made her sign an agreement to work hard and obey school rules, a loyalty oath, like I had to sign at university. Normally I would have gone in and made a fuss about it, but very uncharacteristically, in dream or in waking life, I just accepted it because that is the school's policy, even though it was against my wishes. I do not agree and I do not make an effort to voice my opinion, nor do I feel upset. Very strange. My father is in the dream and he wanders into an ongoing class to speak to one of the teachers about the situation, and I know he will disrupt everyone, but I am passive and do not try to stop him. I know I disagree with his action, but I do not stop him.

♦ I had other fragments of dreams like that, things happening around me and I could not intervene, disagreement yet acceptance. I felt it was wrong to make a child sign a loyalty oath—like moral outrage, this is not right, but I was passive.

♦ Dream: In a restaurant with my husband, looking out the window at the horses outside being rambunctious. A gray colt came crashing in through the window and is biting people, savaging people. I am afraid of the colt and he approaches me. Then I think perhaps he is teething, in pain, damaged in some way. I have to go and intervene and help this animal. I put my fingers in his mouth and was massaging his gums, knowing he could bite me and crush my hand. His teeth are brown, wood-like and sharp, but I feel sorry for him. He is obviously content with the massaging, then I realize he is very sad and that he was abandoned by his mother and damaged. As I leave the restaurant he crouches at my feet and I cuddle him. I want to mother him. Was very frightened but he did not hurt me. Felt compassion and impulse to help even at the risk of my own health.

♦ Restless sleep.

♦ Woke up groggy with an occipital, throbbing headache.

♦ Was very sensitive to noise and movement at night and woke frequently when my husband moved. I felt very irritable at him for waking me.

♦ Headache lasted all day—occipital—endured it all day (laughs). By 4:00 p.m. it spread to temples. Temporarily better with pressure, better only while pressing. Worse lying down.

Day 3
◆ The first few days were not so relevant. Something sort of horrible happened today—I received a very frightening phone call in the morning from Washington, trembling afterwards. Feeling outraged, pacing in the house. He had stalked me ten years ago, and I had not heard from him in ten years.

◆ Noon, friend came to stay with me. I felt fine with her, happy, not worried while she was here. Evening, felt fine, normal, put phone call into perspective, not worried nearly as much.

Day 5
◆ Dream: I was living abroad, in a foreign house, went into the kitchen and saw a large man yelling and slapping my son in back of the head. Then I realized he was not my son and that he belonged to this man. I tried to tell him that there were better ways to motivate children than slapping them, but he just slapped him again. He was bleeding. I felt very sad and helpless. My son did not cry, just threw himself on the floor with his face screwed up in a stoic mask of anger, as if he were used to this and would not show weakness. I was trying to make a plan to get custody away from him. Feeling helpless, frustrated, and sad.

◆ Several days after that terrifying phone call, horrible things going on. Still in this state I could not intervene, feeling powerless. The horrible thing: two years ago I was given a research fellowship to a foreign country, and this fellow there developed an obsessive stalking thing for me, a terrifying, horrible event in my life. I had to leave a year early. Out of the blue he called me. He is a very charismatic person—he acted as if nothing had happened. He called me unexpectedly. I called a lawyer—sought a restraining order. I felt violated and attacked.

◆ During day felt fine except for headache.

◆ Dreams with guilt and grief. I could not prevent things from happening and feeling personally responsible.

Day 6
◆ Woke at 3:30 a.m. till 4:00 a.m. or so, thinking.

◆ Dream: I was a clerk in a store and I had murdered someone and varnished them to make them look like merchandise. I thought it was the perfect crime since the victim had disappeared from the store and was never seen again and I had an alibi all day at work. I felt guilty that I had done this but I had a strong sense that this had had to be done.

◆ Dream: I was the wife of an aristocrat but didn't want to be anymore. He had a mistress and had no interest in me on any level. I felt sad and helpless. Then I decided I would open a healing center in the village, which gave me a sense of purpose. When I went to tell my husband of my action, I discovered him with a cache of erotic material in the closet. He was very upset and ashamed, but I thought if I was accepting, perhaps it would rekindle his feelings. It was calculating on my part. I did not really think it was all right even though I told him so. Somehow it worked and he fell in love with me. The feeling was happy, creative, effective.

◆ Dream: My sister died of cancer, then my elder son killed himself. Feeling was terrible guilt, and grief that I could not prevent his death and that he had wanted to kill himself. Very guilty, sad. I felt I would go mad with these feelings.

◆ 11:00 a.m. feeling sad when husband feels what I say is critical when it is not. Feeling misunderstood and bad. Want to be alone.

Day 7
◆ I was in the City at night and got chilled.

Day 8
◆ Woke with aching in the right eye.
◆ Facial skin is sensitive.
◆ Acute symptoms: sensitive and irritable. Took echinacea and vitamin C.
Developed a cold sore on lower right lip. (These symptoms are common when I get a cold.) Cold gone in a couple of days.

Day 10
◆ Cannot recall dream events specifically, but the feeling was similar to dreams of first few nights—feeling responsible and obligated to help others when my own safety was at risk.

Day 13
◆ Woke with headache, persisting after 11:00 a.m., worse pressure, motion.
◆ Feeling melancholy after watching movie, *An Awfully Big Adventure,* about a girl who is searching for love and is not loved in return. The whole movie is filled with people who love others who do not love them.

Day 17
◆ Dream: I was wishing I could bring an old abandoned garden to life. All that remained were the foundations of the bed outlines. Then an elderly man was sitting next to me and said he would love to finance the bringing to life of the garden. I was so happy. Then I noticed that there were many roses starting to leaf out, and there was a woman who was mulching the beds. I felt so happy and excited. I was also relieved there would not be so much work to do, as these two rose beds were very large. Feeling of responsibility and impulse to heal and help.
◆ Criticism—any perceived criticism, sensitive to criticism. Episodes with my husband. If I would say something, I felt really wronged if he took it the wrong way, how could he think I would do that.

Curative report six years after the proving:
This remedy helped my tendency to want to do for others at my own expense. This is a very heroic remedy—the feeling is so grand, as if you can save the world, a very noble feeling. Even as a kid I felt a calling from God to do for others. This remedy helped me get clarity on this state and put it back into balance. My tendency is to take on an enormous amount of responsibility. It helped me to pursue the tasks that come to me but have a detachment, to do the best work and leave the rest in the hands of God.

Prover #2 • Female • 38 years old

Day 1
- Took it at 11:10 p.m. Slept lightly, different for me, I usually sleep deeply and well.
- Dream: I was in California to take a peace awareness training. Going to the training, I decided to leave and go back to Washington, D.C. with a friend who was not there in California. I had to get there to D.C. by 10:00 p.m. and then back to California by 6:00 a.m. for the training. My friend decided to stay in D.C., because she had three babies to care for. I was being pursued by two men flattering me, asking me for a date, etc. One of them walked me to the bathroom before I took a shower to get ready to go. There was a little child fully clothed stretched out in the bathtub, submerged but alive and well.
- I awoke very hungry, extremely hungry. I eat well but this was different.
- Lots of gas and also some pain with flatulence. Back was more painful, though better after passing gas.

Day 2
- Slept hard and awakened at 5:50 a.m. to urinate, but I did not. Stayed in bed.
- Dream: Of an old lover whom I have dreamed of before, had very amorous feelings.
- Had to get up at 6:15 a.m. Sleepy by 1:00 p.m.
- Very hungry for anything at 1:30 p.m.
- Took a nap from 2:15 to 2:45 p.m. Unusual, but enjoyed it.

Day 3
- I am content, joyful, full of grace and expanding in the knowing of who I am. I am a child of God. Freedom is detaching from the opinions of others, the prejudices of others, the fear of others.
- Dream: Driving in a car with a female colleague down a very wide street to meet a group of people standing in the street. We were in a hurry.
- Six weeks earlier, Memorial Day, I had a back injury, and have been recovering. On the remedy I experienced back twinges, dull ache and pain worse crossing my legs at ankles or extending legs.
- 11:00 p.m. took second dose because I was not aware of any reaction with first dose.

Day 4
- Could not remember dreams.
- Only getting six hours sleep due to seminar, but considering that, my energy is good.
- Slight awareness of throat on the right side (typically left side sore throat when stressed or fatigued), but no real pain.

Day 5
- No change in mood, still calm, peaceful. Became upset, angry when I was accused of "separating" from my friend in the seminar. My upset was not as great as usual and I surrendered to the process (seminar). Peace quickly returned.

- Still aware of throat, not better or worse.
- Back pain occasional, dull.
- Dream: A friend came naked to my house which was a movie theater. She had a huge number of moles and freckles on her back, all over, confluent, which made her appearance very unpleasant, almost freak-like. She was going to work in the theater for me, I had great appreciation for her, and compassion.

Day 6
- Right throat, felt tight in the gland, tight and constricted.
- Right gland sore to touch, though throat not really sore.
- Woke up with awareness of having had an unpleasant dream.

Day 7
- Constipated—unusual for me.
- Throat right gland still tight.
- Dream: An old lover and being tempted—unusual.

Day 8
- Dream: Of parents, my dad is deceased, and some high school friends and a colleague. Talking to my dad about keeping the Infinity car and buying a Camry, neither of which I have. I was in a hotel room and left, my colleague came back and took the room. I went with him because I was afraid I left the gas stove on.
- Not aware of throat today.
- Stool strained again in afternoon, none in a.m.

Day 9
- Sharp shooting pain in right gland. Lasted seconds then gone.
- Stool better today—passed more and not as strained.
- Dream odd, but unremembered.

Day 10
- Skin behind ear lobes, just near mastoid, irritated and dry, very rough and red on both ears.
- Dream: I dreamed I was in New York City in the Village, sitting on the ground as if homeless or a hippie with nothing to do. I talked to an old friend by phone, someone I am no longer friends with.
- Dream: Then I was at a New Years Eve party in a huge ballroom.
- Dream: Then I was at a counseling service looking for a woman named McQueen, who was about to go play a game of cards. She said I could come with her to talk. Another woman said I should stay and talk to two women who were not going to play, they could help me. I went home to my house with McQueen and we talked about changing the diets and lives of children that I knew—African American inner city kids. I felt compassion. My house was different, yet my house. There were large areas of the floor where my couches are, that were dug down to the base of the hardwood floors.

Day 11
◆ Skin behind ears still rough, inflamed, worse.

Day 12
◆ Dream: Of former friend from Seattle, I was in Seattle and she was driving back to Washington, D.C. with me. I went to pick her up, she went to get changed and it took her a long time to come back. Said to another friend that if she does not meet me soon, I will have to leave. We bought a lot of khaki shorts, my friend putting papers in her pocket, creating holes in the back pocket of the khakis. Then I was thinking of moving back to Seattle, near the University or Capitol Hill.
◆ Dream: Then I was at Judge H.'s house, my professor of sociology (mentor) 1976. I have a lot of respect for him, he's a big guy. I heard a lot of noise. I got dressed, went down the hall and saw two Caucasian women getting dressed in another room, one named "Licorith" and the other "Amethod." Both corrected me because I didn't understand the pronunciation. I went down the stairs to see the Judge walking down the hall with some other man. Then I was picking very large blackheads out of my elbow.
◆ For the past three nights I have been waking disoriented, like "where am I?"

Day 13
◆ Dream: A friend having an attack of some kind, seizure, mania, I felt compassion.
◆ Dream: A fat woman asked how much the toast was. I said, "Fifteen cents." She said, "No it isn't. You trying to mess with me?" She came after me and I ignored her, then decided I did not want to ignore her, saying something like, "If you don't believe me, too bad, I told you what I thought." Then she swung at me. I caught her foot and asked her if she wanted it. I put her foot up close to her face. I grabbed a fork and put it up to her throat and told her to leave me alone motherf....r. I put her foot down and walked away and cursed her.

Day 14
◆ Dream: An old friend/lover.
◆ Dream: My mom and dad and I were staying at my brother's. Dad went out but came in at 2:30 a.m. with Judge H. and two college professors. I came out of my room to tell them about my book and the Judge got teary eyes. Then I left after making sure the locks were on the door. I was in a passageway where there were a lot of Caucasians selling meat and crabs. Mom found me and told me her friend—the only Afro-American woman selling anything—was selling something else that was good, too.
◆ One of my assistants drank my water and I just gave her an evil look.

Day 15
◆ Dream: Same former lover as night before. I was also with the founder of my spiritual group, in a large circle with two other African American women, one woman wearing green and one in beige. My most former lover was saying something to my teacher, and he said, "You are just not going deep enough." I had some sour milk in a glass. I was waiting for them to come back when a woman, my friend's sister—who was Caucasian in

the dream, but not in real life—started playing with a white man who was swinging on a rope. Then someone's fourteen-year-old son committed suicide. Then someone was singing a song, but wrong verse, as a picture of Johnny Mathis was on the screen. A woman walked up to a person in the audience and made gestures of love and the person responded with facial expressions like, "Oh, tempt me, tempt me," in an amorous way. I was watching the show with some high school friends, and then I was in the stairway looking at caged baby ducks and other birds that were rare. The moderator was trying to raise money for saving them and feeding them. The mistress of ceremonies asked all of us what we had learned, and at my turn, I did not want to speak.

♦ Dream: I had newspapers on my living room floor and my friend peed all over the newspaper on the floor. He would not go to the bathroom. I just watched him. Even his penis dribbling urine at the end of urination. He got his jacket and said he had to leave. I thought to myself, nothing is more important than loving him and maintaining our relationship. After gathering up all the newspaper off the living room floor I was in a lab of some kind. My receptionist was asking questions about herbs and plants. A woman there answered questions correctly, "The herb he needs is Nepthilis," the woman replied. I thought she knew that because she was an herbalist, not a physician.

Day 17

♦ Dream: An old lover who was cooking eggs at his house, then in another house with eggs on the floor.

♦ Dream: Went to Nordstroms (a store) on the bike, realized I could not park there, so I wanted to go home. I went to the counter and I had a pin on, and a woman to whom I was attracted came up and asked where I got it. It was an old charm/pin, and my friend asked if I had that when I worked in the Carter Administration. I said, "No, the date on it was 1881, it's very old." The words at the very end of the dream: "Interactive caution."

♦ I can be impatient when I drive.

♦ Biting cuticles—unusual.

> **Prover #3 • Female • 42 years old**

Day 1
- Took it 7:00 p.m. evening of July 1. One hour later at 8:00 p.m. I got an itch—very itchy at the base of the right thumb.
- Great sleep that night. I usually get great dreams in a proving, I was really disappointed.
- Awake in the morning, but could not open eyes, felt stuck together. Went to manually open them with fingers and there was not any discharge, not puffy.
- Scratched the right thumb during the night and found red weals there in the a.m. Worse during day. Desire to put cold on it, which relieved the pain and itch but not redness. By 6:00 p.m. the itch had gone and the redness too.

Day 2
- I slept very well that night.

Day 3
- I did notice stress at work. I deal with low income women—we are short midwives and do not have enough to cover the hours, 100 hours for the week. I said, "No!" and was very adamant, I didn't care. I felt very guilty after this. A couple of people came up to me afterwards and praised me for being clear, but I still felt guilty, influencing them to stand up for themselves. I usually stick up for rights, so it was a reversal to feel guilty about this.

Day 10
- On the tenth day I got four new patients all in one day. I felt put against the wall, not ready for them, literally felt pushed against a wall. Normally I would be excited.
- Wasn't hungry, knew I should eat, but I did not feel hungry.
- Calmness overall—good sleeps.
- Convinced I was only placebo.
- I got a phone call from someone who thought I was able to fix a computer program. I asked how she knew me. I have a MAC and she had an IBM—we were virtual strangers. The computer business is like a foreign field. I felt why me? Then perplexed and then a desire to help, intense desire to help. A feeling of no idea of what to do. Not typical. I try to help but this is not in a field I know. I have no idea of what I am doing.

Comment:
Phone calls from people I had not heard from for 10–15 years, just found my phone number. Old friends calling.

Prover #4 • Female • 48 years old

Day 1
- Very restless during the day, hard to keep still or sit, not entirely unusual.
- Pain above eyes, intense stabbing pain.
- Feeling of expectation and excitement in the heart area.
- I had a few days vacation and I was staying away from home, but I wanted to keep in communication with family and friends, more than usual.
- Do not want to be quiet, resistant to any form of meditation. It went against what I wanted to do.
- The need to communicate is not from loneliness, but from a desire to hear and contact people.

Day 2
- A sense of this being a sweet remedy—it has to do with the sensation in my heart area. It reminds me of a time I was wearing this necklace of rose quartz for several weeks and was incredibly emotional about everything, with bursting into tears for no reason. Same feeling of very strong emotion here. But it is not a feeling of grief, more a feeling of sweet emotion. The "vibration" is like when one is excited as a child before their birthday, or a treat that is about to happen.
- Dream: Garden—walking in it—of the house I used to live in while I was in London. The neighbor next door allows me to buy her house and now I connect the two. My ex-husband is there and is happy as he can grow more flowers. A rose tree is broken and he mends it together again.
- Scab forms inside nostrils, especially the right. If I blow my nose it comes out—yellow and green and bloody. Forms every few hours in both, but the right especially, for a week.
- Dream: Of past friends—strong dreams, wake up at 4:00 a.m. Dream so strong I couldn't be bothered to write it down. But wake feeling disturbed—guilty in some way.
- Wake up every morning—very disturbed. Feeling of being guilty and grief, not pleasant.
- Nose continues bleeding easily, but not profusely if I blow it, and scabs are still forming.
- Stressful time of my life. Feel tired, but am working quite hard, so it may be normal.
- Dream: Having dinner with friends (three of whom I always dream of during a proving) and we are practicing a martial art. Water is dripping across the floor. I go to the toilet, but cannot urinate.
- Dream: Being in boat on the sea. I get off to see a friend or lover. When I return there is smoke and the sky is red, I am told my sister has died, I feel the deepest and most real sensation of grief. I wrap my arms around myself and am rocking back and forth racked with sobbing. It is like the few times in real life where I experienced profound grief. Although it is my sister who died, people bring me things from an ex-boyfriend, as though he had died.
- Many water connections in these dreams.
- Wake up feeling deeply sad.
- Dream: Of my son dying, woke depressed, with anxiety and grief. He is away working in Reno, I was so anxious to phone him, I was very disturbed and it haunted me all the day.

◆ I have an exaggerated sense of having to please other people more than myself. Duty and responsibility, to people, to animals. Lose sight of my own needs. Boundaries blurry.
◆ I went to stay at a friend's house and had to be careful to leave it fanatically clean. Need to be responsible, not put anybody out, completely abandoning my own needs, everyone else was going first, I had no idea of my own emotional needs.
◆ Dreams are disturbing and very vivid.
◆ Dream: Of my head being half a walnut shell as a skull and a cigarette butt in it, being squished into it by someone with their thumb. Woke with a terrible headache.
◆ Extremely thirsty.
◆ Feeling of being severely bitten by fleas—feels like I am covered with flea bites. Before going to sleep I do not know if it is real or delusion, but I feel them hopping all over, I could hear them crashing onto the pillow at night. I could not get to sleep. I think it is largely a sensation, formication?
◆ Sensitive to criticism.
◆ Disturbing and vivid dreams of father and ex-sweeties, the male element. Again, wake at about 4:00 a.m. and feel it is so vivid I will remember, but do not wake enough to write them down.
◆ Very connected to a kind of elemental or nature world (not totally unusual, but more so than usual). Feel connected to the plants and trees and flowers. Again, the sense this is a sweet, almost angelic remedy.
◆ More aware of being protected, not wanting to sound too hokey-pokey or "new age." It seems often I can be aware of my "guardian angels," or spirit guides, and know something on another level, more than my head wants to admit.
◆ Aware of being heavy, very, very, heavy, as though to sink through the bed. I felt a great sense of duty and responsibility, making list of lists of lists.
◆ Detail oriented to an anal degree.
◆ Just feeling very responsible that everyone should have everything they want.
◆ Struck that if they criticize me it is completely devastating.

General comments:
◆ I actually received the remedy a few days before I took it; I just held the remedy the first night and went to bed holding it in my hand (placebo). My hand got a really strong ache in it, put it in other hand and the pain would go to the other hand, every time I switched hands.
◆ Also prior to taking remedy I experienced: Just above eyes a pain, unusual.
◆ I felt tremendous agitation in chest and heart area like a very strong vibration, emotional feeling rather than physical.
◆ Expansion in the area of the heart chakra—a sense of expectation or excitement, like a feeling of being just so excited about something, like children get, about to burst.

> Prover #5 • Female • 40 years old

Day 1
◆ Took substance at 10:30 p.m. Images of gold, precious metals and gems in Persia. Jewelry.
◆ Sense of vibration in my mouth.
◆ Sneezing.
◆ Sumptuous, sensual images, desirous of beauty, beautiful things—melon, gentle, flowers.
◆ Desire for youth, to be young. Images of art metals. Wanting to stretch and smell the air.
◆ Awareness of my heart, the vibration now felt there.
◆ Ridiculous images, dancing bones, the 1950's.
◆ Dream: I am going to miss out on something.
◆ Dream: 7:30 a.m. Shopping for Christmas. Returning presents. Ultramodern store, ultimate technology.
◆ Dream: Advising a young girl to leave abusive relationship.
◆ Dream: Traveling with futuristic modes of transportation.
◆ Extremities: Numbing pains in index finger of left hand—as if smashed the finger. Numbing pain extends up arm when I raise arm over my head.
◆ Generalities: Pains in small spots: at left shoulder, in abdomen. Fresh air feels so good, so cool, so sweet.
◆ In meditation, focus of the mind narrows, the heart opens generously to cries from a goshawk, the body relaxes into stillness.
◆ 10:55 a.m. Stomach: no appetite at breakfast, finally ate just to eat at 10:30, and now I feel sick from it. Disagreeable stomach with head pain in one spot. Worse from heat. Wish I had not eaten.
◆ Extremity: Left foot, lower leg falling asleep from sitting.
◆ Clothesline broke, sad, almost cried over such a little thing.
◆ Greater ability to focus on and pursue small points of interest in studying. What has been feeling tedious and boring has become more valuable and more interesting.
◆ We need to operate from a place of enjoyment and pleasure.
◆ Abdominal pain in one spot over left ovary.
◆ Increased frequency of stool, three—four times already by 11:00 a.m. today, like a cleanse.
◆ Sneezing.
◆ Easily distracted from self-focus at lunch, desire to chit-chat with folks, wanting to connect.
◆ Inclined to play Lotto (numbers lottery), never thought of it before.
◆ Given gift from a friend of a tarot reading. During it I came up with the question, how do I resonate with this proving substance? Many indications that it is too soon to tell. What made an impression on me was the image of opening to new opportunities, good fortune; heart energy in abundance, with a petty line that puts the brakes on things. Afterwards I thought, it takes great discipline to have an open and compassionate heart. If the mind is not aligned to the heart's generosity, much could be wasted in the distraction of mind's judgments and/or conditioned—learned habits, draining the heart without replenishing.

Day 2

◆ Dream: Underground railroad, like in Civil War, at a miniature golf course where Japanese students are allowed to immigrate. An experienced counselor from Japan is there to persuade them to stay in Japan. The inexperienced counselor is available to give them advice if they wish to stay in United States.

◆ Dream: Trying to find someone who has moved. Coming to a street corner where I expected to find her address, there is a blockade. Visitors are being stopped and questioned before entering. There is an art opening there. I am concerned about being turned away but I am not.

◆ (Husband/partner) said I was talking in my sleep saying, "I'll just make it black." Making sounds like I was a pig in my sleep.

◆ 10:00 a.m. irritable, annoyed with minor circumstances; feeling my needs and rights are not being respected. They are not! I asked for what I wanted in the appropriate manner and was simply ignored (people coming to see the house at or within the time requested). Difficult letting it go. Critical, cutting thoughts in my mind of the people involved; peevish name-calling.

◆ Menses are late.

◆ Forgetful of calls to return, of observations I wanted to put in this journal.

◆ Impatient: I arrived five minutes late to an investors' group meeting, and no one, including the broker, had arrived yet. I left with an attitude, "Go in with these folks? Forget it!!"

◆ Bought a Lotto ticket! Thoughts enmeshed with brooding feelings about money, status, power, respect—not my everyday sort of musings.

◆ Very happy to be home, to be naked, to be at work on my current thesis, culling all the little ideas that may lead to larger gestalts. Before the remedy, it has been difficult to apply myself to this task.

◆ Headache after tai chi, maybe from standing long; in frontal sinuses, below eyes and over all of head.

◆ Sense of being dirty, ungrounded, scattered thinking. Not concentrating easily.

Day 3

◆ Dream: With my grandmother who is a large, thick-skinned animal, with huge skin tags which drag on the ground. I am swinging to see the ocean past the reeds and spy a large, strange bird. I point it out to my grandmother who turns to look and the bird rubs past her, sliming one of her hairy skin tags. Horses run to bite at it—where she has been slimed. She tries to escape into a narrow alley. It is the entrance to health club. I follow her wanting to help, they have all disappeared into the club. The manager comes up to me. T.W. is the manager! Suddenly there is word of an explosion. We move through the white tiled hallways deeper and deeper into the bowels of the earth. We come to the end, the scene of a cataclysm. Blood-dimmed water is everywhere. A woman, still alive and wailing with grief, is sitting on the carcass of my grandmother. She is holding two twin dead babies. I feel her pain; it is excruciating, but I have no feeling for my own loss, the loss of my grandmother.

♦ Menses started this morning. Usual slow start. Feeling more myself today, neither irritable nor impatient and not concerned with "the material world' as much as I have been the last couple of days.

♦ GM is selling the house—I remember being very annoyed by the wealthy and very young, beautiful women coming by to see the house. They have this look and feel of inbred wealth. Definitely felt an attitude in that. Conversation with a friend yesterday turned to the San Francisco scene of big money with its huge emphasis on style with incredible restrictions on what is and is not acceptable. I don't quite understand it. What has felt different with the proving is "get it for myself!"—about material things—rather than the "let it come, let it go" I am familiar with, with regard to material things, money, assets, resources.

♦ Another headache with exertion today, extends forehead to occiput.

Day 4

♦ 11:00 p.m. repeated the remedy. Images of green patina metal.

♦ After repeating the remedy last night, I felt very chilled, with numbness and tingling in my left arm and hand. Something of the sensation lingers this morning. Feels like something moving through my nervous system. This left side of mine, from scapula, down arm, and down back has been lit up by this remedy. There is old and mysterious stuff stored in this part of my body. The remedy seems to be shaking it up.

♦ Voice feels weak and congested this morning.

♦ Initially irritable and peevish on waking; (uterus congested from sleeping may be contributing). Feeling very well once up and moving.

♦ Very motivated to practice, do things, which are normally tedious.

♦ Some "mental congestion" from images of the movie last night, *Deadman*, an intense black and white film with a lot of death without conscience and then dying with conscious ceremony and honor.

♦ Stomach: Not much of an appetite. No desire for rich foods.

♦ Menses seem heavier, an easier flow than usual.

♦ Generalities: Cut myself and bled more than usual.

♦ Sexual energy went up. Playful and satisfying, open and genuine. It's great.

♦ Mood: One glass of wine, to celebrate my birthday, with dinner and I am thrown into a chaotic state of tears, seemingly causeless until suddenly I burst with the words, "I am so fed up with the world of buying and selling!!!" When will we wake up, and move beyond the lower aspects of materialism!! What is beyond?!!

Day 5

♦ New painting is full of bright colors in a wide range.

♦ Sat to mull and wonder and fell asleep. Not much thoughtfulness as I am used to. More energy for action than for musing.

Day 6

♦ Feeling very motivated to do all the piddly stuff, the boring stuff, get it done.

♦ Almost came to tears this morning when I couldn't find something I thought I had lost.

Day 8
- Questions of style and status. Is this still the proving?
- Menses lasting longer.
- Itching eruptions: Raised red single vesicles, like bites, maybe they are bites! Odd reaction, like blood blisters, bruising.
- Overwhelmed with thoughts of my ex-husband today. Obsession. I had to talk with him. Have not spoken in over a year. Nothing new between us, same old same old in talking with him. Just overwhelming urge to talk with him. Wishing I could have been more emotionally there for him in our relationship when we were together.

General comments:
After hearing what the substance was, prover commented:
- Coincidentally, I got into a conversation at a party with a woman who is an expert on roses so I thought to tell you about it. She said plants that are a flower that can survive anything are the old roses.
- Another coincidence is a woman I rent land from said the only thing she can grow is roses, I have often thought it would be a good remedy for her.

Prover #6 • Male • 50 years old

Day 1
- Took remedy 11:00 p.m. Considerably thirsty.
- Woke early, right knee throbs a bit.
- Mental activity.
- Day dream: On hill of snow. Dig to get sled.
- Low back stiff. Chilly in a.m.
- Flatulent. Stool odor.
- Stiff legs in a.m.

Day 2
- Difficulty rising. Slow to get up, but OK once up.

Day 3
- Dream: California.
- Repeat remedy 11:00 a.m.
- Dream: In a woman's housing. Celebrating a woman's special talents, especially her arms and legs. We are all served large clams to eat raw. I do not eat due to polluted waters. I go back to my dorm but I am not sure which room I am in.
- Distended. Flatulent (unusual).
- Slow rising. Sleep is unrefreshing.
- Dream: Talked to NH about remedy.
- Dream: Dogs in kitchen eating.

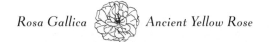
Rosa Gallica   Ancient Yellow Rose

Day 4
- Sleep unrefreshing. Slow to get going.
- No appetite in a.m.
- Did not eat till 2:00 p.m.
- Do not look forward to the day (unusual). Gloomy, not into work. Not motivated (unusual).
- Increased sexual interest.

Day 5
- Slept on abdomen (unusual) in a.m.
- Good energetic movement in meditation. Kundalini energy moving.
- Constipated (unusual).
- Good energy.
- Increased sexual interest.

Day 6
- Woke on abdomen. Right arm numb (unusual).
- Long walk resolved bowel problem.
- Increased sexual interest.

Day 7
- Slept well.
- Ate heartily. Appetite increased.
- Increased sexual interest. "Horny."
- Increased flatulence.
- At night, reading, I feel incapable. Wonder how I will teach. Too much to organize and prepare.
- Feel irritable and down. Would like to be alone.
- "Horny."
- Dream: Home converted into a school while I sleep. I woke to find classes in all the rooms filled with youngsters. Felt surprise.
- Dream: At end of dream with my wife I see a girl in a short plaid green jumper-type skirt and open-necked white blouse. I say to my wife, "Why don't you buy that outfit and put it on," and I'm thinking she will look very sexy and my thoughts turn amorous.

Day 8
- Woke with abdominal discomfort and flatulence.
- It is raining. This is the second time I notice with rain I feel down and insecure. Irritable and down from the weather. Usually I am impervious or I like it.
- Increased sexual interest.
- Dream: At a party I treat osteopathically several people. I treat one woman and we start to make love. I realize I need condoms. So I go to the store and inquire about the different types before I procure them. Felt people in the background laughing at my questions in the store and I feel embarrassed (would be very unusual for me).

Day 9
- Finding it hard to get out of bed.
- Decreased appetite on waking.
- Distended on waking.
- Wake with barely time to get to work. Usually my time for breakfast is 6:00–6:30 a.m., now, it is 7:00–7:15 a.m.
- Sexually aroused.

Day 10
- Hard waking.
- Good appetite.
- More tolerant than normal. Working with meditation teacher may have influenced this.
- Dream: I have to cross a body of water. I cross it myself in a makeshift craft. Then I come back for the others. Before we cross we go on a large boat that seems to fasten with other similar crafts like a boxcar on a train. Boats go out above and come back in below. It is a different direction than the boat I have already used. As we go out we see they are excavated extensively far below us.

Day 11
- Eruption on lip. Herpetic? Possibly. Inside lip (unusual), right side roof and right gums.

Day 12
- Mouth symptoms continue. Inflammation, pain, swelling inside lip, right side roof and right gums.

Day 15
- Mouth symptoms better.

> **Prover #7 • Female • 49 years old**

Day 1
- Dream: Go to hotel looking for a place to put up German exchange students. Large blonde woman is there with a small new baby. Then a man I know appears and shows us around this huge multiple room complex that they are sharing, basement suites, very plush. When we return upstairs, a small, petite woman with long, curly fiery-red hair comes to take the baby from her adoptive parents because they're Jewish and the woman says Jews can't raise his girl. I'm upset, screaming, horrified, and especially because the Jewish parents just seem to accept and even seem relieved about this, because she has been such a wild little girl.
- What I think is the theme for me in this dream, is a connectedness to this old place within me, to the little wild girl who is out of control. It may be at the core of what is going on between my son and me, where I alternate between being the little kid who was previously buried, and now just remembered for the first time in a long time, alternating with being the parent.
- Crick in my neck on the right side, not new, but more pronounced.
- Slight sore throat when I wake up.

Day 2
- Dream: In a big house, not like mine really, but it is mine in the dream. African student comes by to see it. Also, go to the international show, but in a different setting. Let's talk about international students.
- Bad headache starting around 7:00 p.m. Pounding at the back of my head. Felt like old premenstrual tension headaches. Lacked the dizziness and disorientation I have been feeling with more recent headaches. Needed to take two acetaminophen, then two ibuprofen before it finally eased about 9:00 p.m.

Day 3
- Awoke with my left ear plugged, could not hear out of it. I had a few problems with this last week, but never before. Ear drops felt very cold and uncomfortable. Used eardrops twice but they did nothing to relieve. My ear continued to be completely blocked and hot until about 5:00 p.m. At about 8:00 p.m. I was sitting eating dinner when my left ear felt odd. When I reached up, I found big gobs of ear wax had just come out. My ear continued to feel hot but was clear. Never happened before.
- Good energy, able to focus on work.
- Less than usual interest in food. Ate small amount of sweets without craving.
- Some nausea with ear symptoms.
- Bowel movement fast in morning. Different in that stool floated.

Day 4
- Feeling irritable—sensitive to noise, impatient with kids.
- Left ear still clear, but I hear some crackling/popping in right ear.
- Decided to keep appointment with person who used a syringe to clear wax from right ear.

- Eyes bugging me—stinging and tired.
- Little snacking. Continue to feel little interest in food although I eat just small amounts.
- Same fast morning bowel movement.
- Started menses, a little early? not sure. Feel unusually asymptomatic, other than headache a few days ago. How nice, I even continue to have pretty good energy.
- Difficulty remembering dreams, in part because I seem to be sleeping so heavily. For the third night I did not get up to urinate and felt very groggy in the morning.
- Dream: Remembered some part of a dream about a foreign student but then lost it.

Day 5
- A very emotional day. I missed a meeting at work and could feel my back tense as I felt irritable about being uninformed. Also was confused and emotional at a specific woman about not including me in the meeting. Felt very on the outside when I met with one colleague, and very "fringey" with the writer's group meeting. I was unable to say much in either case, and felt like I was on the edge of tears, hypersensitive and tense all day.
- I left the writer's group meeting crying about this boy I worked with, the most intense reaction churns ups so much within me, I do not want to be around him because of the feeling. In the car coming home, I cried and had memories of how I was at that age, a rebellious teenager/young adult—angry, life was hard. I identified strongly with the kids in the writer's group and even felt some kind of attraction to the wildness and intensity of feeling in one of the young men who was smart, but rebellious. Strong reaction, almost afraid of him. It put me in touch with that younger part of me that emerges less in my happier, stable adult life, but I missed those feelings. Later, talking with friends, I put these feelings together with the other dream, about the woman and baby—appreciating the fire—juxtaposing B. and the kids and my life now as calmness versus the earlier fire.
- Remarkably "grounded" for having a heavy period.
- Appetite and stool observation the same i.e. little interest in food although I eat just small amounts and have bowel movement fast in morning.
- Menses: Heavy flow without other symptoms. Some stirrings.
- Still sleeping heavily and having trouble recalling dreams.
- Dream: Again, I think dream was something about students. Do I really dream so much about work?

Day 6
- Feel good—a clear, productive day.
- My period is very minimal, really over already. Easiest period in two years, one day period, must be my remedy for menopause. No premenstrual syndrome, no headache.

Day 7
- I am beginning to think that either I am in a good place and this remedy is not affecting me, or this is "my" remedy. I have just finished the easiest period I can remember having in over two years—one quick headache and nothing else. No dizziness (cure), no incredible fatigue (cure), no bloat or heaviness in my body (cure). Emotionally I felt vulnerable, but in a healthy way. I feel healthy, clear-headed, pretty, vital. Good day at

work and with the kids, especially going to the movies with my son. Feel very relaxed, peaceful and self-contained. It's great.

◆ Continue to have little interest in food, no real cravings or hunger driving me. I had been getting hunger crazed like when I was pregnant, but that feeling is gone. Wandered around supermarket looking for something appetizing without much luck.

◆ It was hot today and I was aware of having some body odor, very unusual for me, a problem I cannot remember having since I was an adolescent. Have a new deodorant, maybe I should switch and see if it is still a problem.

◆ Angry that son came home after curfew. Felt like I let him know how I felt fairly clearly, and then let go of it.

Day 8

◆ Dream: As a family we are up in the mountains and need to drive back to town to eat. In a large kind of bakery/deli, and I cannot find anything to eat. I finally find a chicken kabob like in Zanzibar. When leaving, we discovered husband left something behind, so we go back up the mountain in two cars. I am with our son and we hit ice. I look back to see if husband is in his car and is all right. Finally, we come to a town and there is a festival happening. Native Americans are drumming for Hare Krishnas and I have the nice realization of the merging of cultures.

◆ Had a difficult time talking to son about responsibility—his coming home late and getting a "D" grade in biology because he is behind, etc. I have felt like I am having a hard time letting this "be," and unlike most heart-to-hearts, I only felt frustrated. I sense that he will not accept any responsibility and I want his motivation to change to be internal rather than external. I was very tense then hurt as was he. I do feel empathy, especially when B. tried to monitor me. Again, I am identifying too much.

◆ Husband returned and felt distant. I seemed more content to be on my own. Noticed that when we made love I started spotting a little. Still feel more grounded.

Day 9

◆ Irritable with husband and kids. Seem to want more, but I am not sure what.

◆ Energy still good. Appetite still low. Planning to do diabetic diet.

◆ More spotting.

◆ Dream: At a banquet for work. Lost the details.

◆ Also had a quick nightmare that woke me in the middle of the night, scared me, but I fell back asleep quickly.

Day 10

◆ Still quick to be irritable and frustrated at home, not so much at work, although I certainly was when a coworker said she would "tell me what to do." Is this teenage rebellion I am feeling? In trying to grasp a pattern to this remedy, I keep coming up with old "teenage" patterns for me—critical and frustrated and judgmental at home but pretty confident and competent in work relationships.

◆ Also, my menstrual cycle seemed to revert to older patterns as well as my energy. Still some spotting.

- Lots of tension with husband, but B. seemed to confirm that his demeanor is slow, depressed, etc., very unlike him, and I get very intolerant.
- Little appetite until late afternoon.

Day 11
- Again aware of my critical self at home. I am trying to lighten up.
- Felt energetic and creative at work, also very good about colleague stuff which is unusual. I find I am reaching out more there.
- Still spotting.

Day 12
- Dream: In a carriage passing through streets of Russia. Have the impression that I have been in a boring, protected place and now enter a very vivid area, lots of people dressed in furs, market, etc. Someone brushes my hair out wildly and I feel a little invaded. Later in a house with friends. Looking in rather bare rooms in a long hall. In one room is a man I recognize, who is sharing the house for awhile. Then something about being with husband, who has a long ponytail again, and we are in a raft or canoe. We get out and I need a tampon, go to look for one and I see S. in the distance with toilet paper. I need to follow some older man down stairs piled high with garbage, etc. to an underground to find her. Suddenly, we are in a more interesting but very poor area and a large troupe of dancers, perhaps Russian, weave their way past and I feel joyful.
- Thinking of all this, I am beginning to think that what I am dealing with now is different than I thought. I was seeing youth, versus older. Now, I think it is about active versus passive. The source of my irritation for days has been passivity, on husband's and son's parts especially.

Day 13
- Dream: At my book club gathering I need to call home, but I cannot remember my phone number. I ask for help, but no one knows it either. I am very upset because I know more than half of the people there, and cannot believe they don't know my number. I end up feeling very hurt and insecure and angry.

Day 14
- Vagina "sore."
- Dream: Awoke at 6:00 a.m. from a dream/nightmare: I leave a friend's house on my bike and get lost, and end up in a back dirt road at a house. I am attacked by an older man, no one I know or can connect with anyone. He is skinny, balding, mean and creepy. He is trying to rape me and I am throwing food at him. I get away and try to tell someone about him.
- Dream: A teaching dream in which I am in a theater trying to show a film. First I do a little pre-lesson, but no one seems too interested. Then I try to set up the film but I do not know how to run the machine, a cross between a VCR and a film projector. Finally someone comes to help me out.

Day 15
♦ Dream: Bad hotel dream.

Day 17
♦ Dream: I'm on a bus after a very long trip, we pull into the station and I can see my husband sitting on the grass waiting for me. As we get off some of the people pass through a room and then the rest of us are stopped, we have to wait. Because the others have already gone through, I object and finally defy the person in charge in order to get to my husband.

Day 18
♦ Dream: A party/bar scene with friend and others. We are first in an upper open room with a huge window looking at the sunset. Then we are in a crowd, and suddenly, huge missiles rise out of the trees and the crowd is cheering, but I am aware the idea is to destroy the U.S.

General comments:
♦ I also had irritability, every day a great deal of irritability during the day, especially mornings.
♦ My eyes have been very irritated and I have never before had allergy symptoms of the eyes. I haven't even been able to wear my contacts.
♦ Many nights couldn't remember my dreams, slept very heavily.
♦ Lots of food in dreams, but no appetite when I was awake.
♦ There was a lot of joy and enjoyment in the dreams.
♦ Dream: In big house with African students, Russian gypsies, Hare Krishnas.
♦ Focused a lot on what was going on between son and I. Much more anger and arguing than usual.
♦ As a theme I think of independence, struggle for independence.
♦ Twice I missed appointments, a meeting and a lunch date. Never happens normally for me.

Prover #8 • Male • 15 years old

Day 1
- I was in a very philosophical mood today.
- I got a rash on the inside of my legs.
- Stomach upset and a lot of gas.
- Was really tired.
- Dream: A game I was playing called *Diablo*.

Day 2
- I don't know if it was the heat or what, but I was incredibly hot and lethargic, and just generally slow all day long.
- Still have the rash on my legs.
- Headache in the morning but it went away.

Day 4
- One word described me today, lazy. My energy level was really low, and I had a hard time doing my homework.
- For some reason, I also felt really creative today.

Day 5
- Continued craving for smoothies is the only thing I can see as abnormal.
- Oh, I felt very competitive.
- Dream: Going to debate camp and solving really long and hard math problems.

Day 6
- Today I felt very restless and my energy level was really high. I felt awfully cooped up when I was forced to stay inside and do my homework.
- Dream: A really frightening dream about humongous spiders that were chasing me in a swimming pool.

Day 7
- I felt really low and depressed today, which is not normal for me on Fridays.
- I woke up really early, which for me is also unusual.
- Hiccups numerous times today.

Day 8
- I was really excited today. My brother had a soccer game, and I was just all over cheering for him.
- A continued obsessiveness with smoothies.
- A need to be around people and be sociable with everyone.

Day 9
◆ I woke up really early this morning to go paint-balling, then at the last minute, it all fell through. This kind of dragged on me for the rest of the day.
◆ I was very lethargic and got little physical exercise today, although I played a lot of computer with a friend.

Day 10
◆ If I summed it up in one word today, the word would be "angry." I just felt plain pissed off at the world, and was a real smart ass to my teachers at school.

Day 11
◆ I was really jittery and nervous today for some reason.
◆ I had a big test in one of my classes and I was really psyched up about it, which is not normal for me. Usually I am calm and collected about big tests.
◆ Dream: I was flying.

Day 12
◆ Incredible craving for pizza that lasted all day long. I just could not get it out of my head.

Day 13
◆ Honestly, I cannot think of a single thing that was at all out of the ordinary today. Except maybe that the whole day was just too ordinary, nothing exciting or anything.

Day 14
◆ Today was my day of sleep. I was so tired that I slept right through my alarm, and missed the first period.
◆ Also, I was very argumentative today. I got in a big fight with my parents and stormed out of the house for a couple of hours just to cool off.

Day 15
◆ I am completely obsessed with this computer game my friend has, and have been playing it constantly.
◆ I had a lot of mood shifts today. I went from happy to excited, to pissed, to sad, and back to happy.

Day 16
◆ Good mood today, lots of energy, and had a lot of fun.
◆ Weird rash on my legs for a couple of hours, then it went away. Smooth, red, blotchy rash.

Day 17
◆ Talk about highs and lows. I went from having absolute zero energy, kind of dozing, to having tons of extra energy and playing lots of basketball. It was kind of weird to feel so different so fast.
◆ I was in a good mood, though a little bored today.

Day 18
- Today was horrible. I got into one of the biggest fights I have ever been in with my parents. I got so angry—the angriest I can ever remember being—that I started screaming, cussing, and breaking things. Whew!

Day 19
- Today was cool. I got every class I wanted, and got really happy. The day just seemed to whiz by. Nothing abnormal.

Day 20
- Just the opposite of yesterday, today seemed to stretch on forever.
- I got the hiccups today four times, that was weird for me.
- Extremely tired.

General Comments:
- Took remedy three times.
- No hay fever. It WENT away (cure).
- Dream: Of spiders, and then I saw a black widow spider on our porch.
- Angry at parents with big fights, power struggles, tears. Screaming and breaking things, couldn't control my anger a couple of times. (REALLY not normal, this is the first time in my life I had felt and expressed real anger.)
- Running around and screaming and breaking things. Have never been that angry with it so close to the surface.
- Headaches and upset stomach like I might throw up.
- Energy level up and down a lot.
- Stressed out a lot.
- Stomach upset a lot at the beginning.
- Craving for pizza.
- Really into making smoothes: strawberries, bananas.
- I also had a baking session and made muffins.
- Fights with parents (many).
- Nausea after drinking orange juice the day before.
- Bloody noses (usual for me) before remedy, but not during.
- Lots of mood swings. Had a crying bout for about 30 minutes. This is not normal for me.
- Energy level was exceedingly low for me at times.
- Had a bad headache after crying.
- Thought I might throw up a couple of times.
- Stomach was upset again.
- I did not want to go to school. Felt very tired.
- Fell back asleep after taking shower.
- Came home from school feeling sick. A lot of dizziness, a headache and an upset stomach. By the end of the day, I felt much better.
- At times everything was pretty flat.

Prover #9 • Female • 39 years old

Day 1
- I felt unusually anxious this morning, possible at least partly attributable to the personal growth seminar I was taking. Like I had too much caffeine. Edgy and a bit impatient. Definitely more than normal. Feeling overwhelmed—impatience—hurried like I had coffee energy. Lots of energy, wired, but no stamina.
- Left calf muscles ached in the afternoon and evening, a dull, generalized ache in the bulk of the calf muscle.
- I slept a bit restlessly, up for a while about 2:00 a.m.
- Dream: I remember just the essence of the dream, I felt hurried.

Day 2
- I definitely feel anxious and impatient, especially in the morning. Irritable, short-fused.
- Distant from my immediate surroundings and interactions.

Day 3
- Slightly impatient, especially with my daughter this morning.
- Took second dose of remedy at night.

Day 4
- Felt hurried and worried this morning. These feelings are very particular to the morning. Usually subsides by 11:00 a.m.–12:00 p.m. Worried about all the things to do, but not very energetic.
- Stomachache midday and afternoon, especially after drinking water.
- Felt like I was going to have diarrhea, but did not. Not nauseous, just general pain in abdomen.
- I had some pain in my stomach and left calf.
- Pain also in muscles of arm, some aching.
- Soft stool.

Day 5
- Restless sleep. Awakened at 2:00 a.m. to find my cat looking down at me from a high window (ready to jump down on me). I got up to get him and found his whole hind end was covered with diarrhea/stool. Washed us both off.
- Dream: Dream of snakes but do not remember any details except that I was not scared, as I normally would be. No fear, which is unusual. I do not like snakes and I am afraid of rattlesnakes.
- Again the hurried feeling in the morning. Like I had already had my caffeinated tea. Feel more energetic, like I want to get out and run, or ride my bike, but when I do, I do not feel like I have as much stamina as usual.
- More nausea after drinking water in the middle of the day.

Day 6
- Bloody nose, left side, while making love.
- Diarrhea in a.m.
- Dream: Woman and I in a big four-wheel drive vehicle. Road muddy, like waist deep. I pull onto muddy road and two cars stop in front of me. I pull around and one of my front tires comes off but we keep on going and make it through the rest of the way on three wheels. I feel excited, relieved and proud to have done it.

Day 7
- Calmer today. Traveling by plane most of the day to Homeopathy Case Conference.
- Feeling like something is in both my eyes. Keep blinking them and rubbing, but mainly just blinking. They seem irritated, but not sore or painful. Lasted all day.
- Thirstier. Usually do not drink water during the day. Drinking more.
- Belly hurts. A little nauseous after drinking water, very soon after, and it is short-lived.
- Pain in muscles under left shoulder blade, worse turning head to right.

Day 8
- Same feeling in eyes, like dust or sand in them.
- Slight nausea after drinking water—immediately to ten minutes after. Subsides quickly.

Day 9
- Traveling home from conference, I decided to start a new "diet"—a completely different way of eating for myself. (I am <u>not</u> one to "do diets.")

General Comments:
- I also had a bloody nose three times, much more than usual.
- Went to Texas in the middle.
- A feeling like some thing in my eyes, irritated but not painful.
- Overall much hurriedness and impatience.
- Also I had a lesion on the arm before remedy—red, circular and itched a lot. I scratched it even though I don't usually let myself scratch itches. It seemed like it was healing and then erupted again into two pimples then like an ulcer before it scabbed over again.
- Reinjured eyes about two days ago and saw snakes—two snakes, I thought they were rattlesnakes, during a bike ride.
- Also during this time I completely changed my diet, for the first time maybe ever, eating a lot more protein and fruit, especially smoothies.

> **Prover #10 • Male • 45 years old**

Day 1
- High energy level until noon, then I felt very fatigued. At one point I thought I might faint. Drank water and faint feeling went away.
- Went to a workshop and did a conflict resolution exercise. I had great trouble coming up with an example of real life conflict with my partner.
- Desire bacon.

Day 2
- Decided to "call in sick" for work. I needed a clam, quiet, spacious day for myself. I totally "forgot" about being on call for work this day, until 6:00 p.m. when I was called in! I have not forgotten on call in 11 years of doing it.

Day 3
- Stayed home from work for fabricated reason.
- Vision "blurry" much of the day, as if my glasses were very dirty.
- Headache in forehead in evening.

Day 4
- Dream: I went to pick up my daughter at school and there was snow on the ground. I threw a snowball at a group and hit one of the children. I just walked away, left him crying there, pretending I did not throw it.

Day 5
- I hated my job today. Absolutely no tolerance for the usual sensory overload of the job.
- I recall that I dreamt heavily, but my sleep was disturbed and I do not recall the dreams.
- No more visual disturbances.

Day 6
- High energy. Learned how to roller-skate backwards.

Day 7
- Dream: I had done something that caused my ex-wife to not allow me to see my daughter anymore. She communicated this to me in letter. I read it in the dream and wept and wept. I woke up weeping, very unusual, never before.

Day 8
- No symptoms, no dreams. Repeated dose at bedtime.

Day 9
- Beautiful day. Normal energy. Great sleep. No symptoms.

Day 10
- Pain left low back. Woke up with it.

Day 11
- Wanted to bake. I rarely bake.

Day 12
- Happy, good energy. No dreams.

Day 13
- Very irritable, impatient, almost to tears.
- Took one hour nap after work! An unheard of length of nap.

Day 14
- More normal day at work. None of yesterday's irritations.

Day 15
- Wanted to stay home rather than go on a trip.
- Went to the mall shopping and had a good time. I hate the mall normally.

Day 16
- Six mile hike and my body held up well. Even though I am in better shape than ever before, I had real trouble with quadriceps muscles, which got so stiff and painful walking a long (one mile), steep descent, that I had to walk stiff-legged.
- Do I have some poison oak on my body? I am not allergic to it.

Day 17
- Yes, I have poison oak for the first time in my life!! Several small eruptions on left ankle, left thigh, right wrist, and right cheek.

Day 18
- Quadriceps muscles very sore after weekend backpacking.
- Scalp itchy.
- Constipated.
- Vivid dreaming, but little recall.

Day 20
- Poison oak continues to spread in numerous small clusters.

General comments:
- I had visual disturbance as if glasses were dirty and could not see very well. Had to pull off the road on the way to town and clean the glasses as if they were smudged, but they weren't.

- Emotional state was all related to work, really irritable at work, wanting to get the hell out of there. Oversensitive to stimuli there. I have stressful work, tolerance for work was low.
- I even played hooky from work. Felt guilty about that. I have not done that for years.
- I totally "forgot" about being on call that day. Then, later, I thought I was on call, but somehow the beeper and phone were both off, so I was just unreachable and embarrassed next day to go in and find out that someone had to go in for me at 3:00 a.m. for a case. Both these things have never happened to me before.
- Dreams disturbing.
- Hay fever.
- Sleep very deep and then also terrible sleep. Sleeping has been upset.

Prover #11 • Female • 46 years old

- Increased psychic communication with my significant other.
- Increased intuitive abilities at work.
- My study abilities were very focused.

General comments:
- Saw no change in my self. Before this had taken a 200C of new remedy and feel this remedy had started to act and continued to act through proving.
- Vivid dream recollection, but nothing that has not happened to me before.

Prover #12 • Female • 40 years old

Day 1
- Tired, eyes feel puffy.
- Thirsty. Craving salt.
- I know I have to sleep but restless before going to bed.
- Pain in right breast towards heart on going to sleep.
- Pain in right ear.

Day 2
- Tired, do not want to go to work at all.
- Ate a bag of potato chips, salt and crunchy, satisfying.
- Neck ache to shoulder, feels like it is going to snap.

Day 5
- Pain in ear and eye, blurring in eye on right side.
- Pain in the right temple at the eyebrow.

Day 8
- My good friend's birthday. Looking forward to partying and getting silly.
- Thinking about how easy it would be to start smoking again. Yuk! So many people smoke where I work.
- Not very hungry all day. Eat salad for dinner and drink too much.
- Bladder feels full all night. Dribble every 15–20 minutes. Finally fell asleep.
- Sour smelling perspiration.

Day 9
- Dream: Old man fixing a vacuum cleaner. I was upset because I could fix it, but I was eating cheese on bread, so I decided to keep eating and not help.

Day 10
- Thinking about traveling to sunny beaches and hanging out.
- I feel like being outdoors, getting hands dirty. I force myself to garden, weed, etc., but once I am doing it, it is fine.
- Legs feel heavy. Overwhelming sense of being tired, sluggish, with legs heavy.

Day 11
- Thinking about my mom, sadness about her getting old and working so hard still.
- Thinking a lot about family lately, and how I am very lucky to have an easier lifestyle regarding marriage, owning a home, creative work.
- Dream: Walking down cobblestone path to work with a friend. We are late. Walking past a car dealership, she wants to look at cars, but it was late, we had to hurry.

Day 13
- Dream: Inside a bar? or movie theater? I leave speakers in corner. I want to go back to get them, feeling frustrated at not getting speakers on burgundy seats from back of bar.

Day 14
- I am frustrated by a co-worker's laziness in helping to buy a wedding gift, but I do not confront her. The more I think about it, the more tense I become. She must sense it, and offers to go buy the card. Ha ha.

Day 15
- Good mood at work, but feel like I am always organizing the fun stuff at work.
- Big party tonight. I am proud of myself for not drinking too much. But smoked a lot of cigarettes and some pot.
- Restless, could not sleep until 3:30–4:00 a.m.

Day 16
- Went to friend's wedding. Felt good about being married.
- Sleepy in late afternoon. Took a nap 5:00–6:00 p.m.
- Constipated at 9:00 p.m. (from red meat?).
- In bed at 8:30 p.m. Looking forward to sleeping in.

Day 17
- Kept thinking about dental work, worrying about getting old teeth and bones. Feeling old and crumbly in the bones.
- Nervous, not finishing sentences.
- More perspiration than usual, but I tend to perspire more before menses.

Day 18
- Big dentist day. Being fitted for partial bridge. Anxious to get this over with.
- Very tired late afternoon.
- Crave mashed potatoes.

Day 21
- Very tired. Legs feel rubbery.
- Did not feel like going home after work because C. is visiting. He is a schizophrenic. Sometimes I am afraid of him.

Day 22
- I sigh a lot during day.
- Aching tooth, lower right side. Lasts maybe for one or two minutes.
- I get thirsty late afternoon. Feel like smoking a cigarette!
- Big party at night. Good time. Feeling social and humorous.

Day 23
- Woke up hungry, really hungry with stomach growl. Drank tea. No hunger until 10:30 a.m.
- I want to be alone. Party in afternoon, but I do not feel like going.
- Sadness about my mother growing old and still working hard. What is it going to be like when they die?
- Snapped at F. at party for being sarcastic with me. Drank three glasses wine 3:00 p.m.–5:00 p.m. Extremely tired. Went home to bed but did not sleep.
- Started period on time. Middle backache.
- Yellow mucous, cough.
- Hot while sleeping, but still want covers on.

Day 24
- Slept till 8:30 a.m. Could have slept more.

Day 25
- Teeth on right side ache. Back molars.
- Beginning of sore throat.
- Restless before going to bed. Drank coffee at 4:00 p.m.
- Cold at night.

General comments:
- Wanted to sleep in, hard to get up.
- Not wanting to go to work. Changed work schedules during proving so that I could come to work later.
- Irritable. I had a hard time going to work.
- I couldn't remember dreams three times.
- Craving cigarettes. Stopped smoking long ago and usually averse to smoking. Smoked on two occasions.
- Very restless at night.
- Some constipation.
- Salt and crunchy craving.
- Ears felt plugged.
- Got poison oak in two spots that took a long time to develop. It goes away and comes back.
- Psychic stuff. At work, working on something, and people came up and asked about things I was working on, at that exact time.
- Opened up a pair of jeans and found $20 in jeans at Salvation Army. Had needed $20 earlier and then what I bought cost exactly $20.
- Worried about parents dying.
- Irritability, more in afternoon.
- Eyes! Symptoms sometimes with glasses. Blurry.
- Right sided pain.
- Dreams, red, dark.
- Thinking about mother and women a lot.
- Ears waxy.
- Feeling—putting myself in other people's shoes.
- Not hungry most of the time.

Prover #13 • Female • 48 years old

Day 1

♦ It was Mothers' Day yesterday. As I was letting the pellets dissolve last night I experienced a bitter taste for about five minutes.

♦ Shortly after, I felt an aching, steady pain behind my right ear on the mastoid process lasting five minutes.

♦ Dream: Fragments. In an apartment, not mine, some family presence, sister? A middle-aged man, tall, lanky, longish dark hair with dandruff, in some relationship. We are getting together again. He lies beside me and I embrace him, signaling to sister we are indeed together. The feeling is that I am accepting him even though he is seedy and conceited. Though I like to clean people's scalps, I know it is not good to do his—that would bind us together—so I maintain an inner independence, though I let others see we are together.

♦ Got up early, had lots of energy in morning, got some cleaning done in a.m. with energy slump around 2:00 p.m.

♦ I came home and felt a real slump—tired, did not want to go to the Lomi Lomi class, but did it and it was lovely.

♦ Nose was itchier, felt more allergic to pollens.

♦ Throat intermittently itchy.

♦ Hungry for something in a.m. but not knowing what. I had cereal.

♦ Had early lunch. I eat when anxious or not knowing what to do next—for the activity.

♦ Abdomen feels flabby to me today.

♦ Rectum: Stool a bit difficult expelling at first, then okay.

♦ Muscles in right hip, tightness all day.

♦ Legs feel tight, in back too.

♦ Slept well, do not recall dreams.

♦ Daughter C. was very tired today and last night says her ears felt plugged, neck sore.

Day 2

♦ Do not feel like writing this, would rather go to sleep.

♦ Easy, steady mood most of the day, except when I could not find my wallet. Mild self-recrimination.

♦ I have been thinking, since doing this journal, of how much love I actually do express. I am not sure that it is a lot, especially to my husband, funnily enough.

♦ Energy good, again felt tired in late afternoon, laid down after supper for 20 minutes.

♦ More allergic reaction to pollen today and to horse.

♦ Throat itchier.

♦ Wanted salads today, did not finish supper, not that hungry.

♦ Spot on cheek I have had for two–three months seems a bit worse, slightly bigger, more scabby.

Day 3
♦ Main concern is finances. Not fear so much, as aware that things need to change if we are to keep daughter at a certain school.
♦ Again a little tired after supper.
♦ Feels like the herpes blister that just healed up is starting again. Unusual for it to reappear so soon.
♦ Woke up and for the first time in months, years? I wanted to lie on my stomach, which I did. When I turned my head to right side, and flexed right leg, (external rotation), and released tension in my shoulders, my shoulders really let go. The pain I had had in my rhomboids, since weed whacking more than a week before the proving started, went away.

Day 4
♦ More involved with plans to increase income. Will propose teaching part time at school.
♦ A lot of love for my daughters.
♦ Husband and I disagree on so many little things. Sometimes it bothers me, mostly because I genuinely like him, as well as all the deep loving feelings. It can be exasperating, though, and he seems to have a negative response to life—sees what does not work, what is not there.
♦ Enjoyed massage—abdomen felt bloated, almost numb over small intestines, uterus. I wonder if some of that feeling is from the C-section incision.
♦ Had diarrhea this a.m. after eating cantaloupe, a metallic smell.
♦ Itchy spots in forehead. More sun spot/irritations on right side of forehead for a few hours in a.m.
♦ Went into steam room before massage—very rapidly began to sweat—unusual for me.
♦ Allergic reaction to pony for first time. (I have been over these allergies for two years, and did not have them as a child.)

Day 5
♦ Continue similar patterns: fairly positive, but easily irritated.
♦ Decisions keep presenting—Do I really want to apply to teach at Waldorf? Do I really not want to do a play this summer? What is the balance between being open to the best possibility and spreading myself too thin and doing too many things?
♦ Tiredness again at 2:00 p.m. to 3:30 p.m.
♦ Not drinking enough. Do not feel thirsty except for mild hot black tea with sugar.
♦ Stool still runny. Is this a bug or the remedy?
♦ Allergies seem worse, itchy nose, throat, sneezing.
♦ Neck still a little tight, feels good from brisk walking, but tight from not doing stretches.

Day 6
♦ Not motivated to do housework.
♦ Feel a bit hazy—not sharply focused mentally.
♦ First roses blooming, I felt such joy.

◆ Pain under right ribs in liver, gallbladder area several times today. Pains short duration—four to fifteen seconds. Not a steady pain, not a throb, but increases and decreases in intensity.
◆ Stool still runny. No metallic smell.
◆ Began menses this a.m. four days early. Not much flow, clotting—unusual for me.
◆ Dream: "Bill Moyers"—I was driving to some border or crossing. On the way, road was torn up on right side. There was some delay. As I was coming back to the car Bill Moyers came up to me—very friendly, affectionate, wanted sex. He accused me of being dishonest about it, i.e. I should. I did not have an affair, but enjoyed the feeling.

Day 7
◆ Too groggy from allergies.
◆ Angry outburst when I bumped my head, "Sick of doing things wrong, hurting myself."
◆ Tired from allergies, but when I lay down 15–20 minutes, I can get up and carry on.
◆ At work, air conditioning helped allergies, felt good.
◆ Massive sneeze attacks this a.m. Washing out my sinuses with saline spray.
◆ Food does not excite me, but I still feel hungry at mealtime and snack at 5:00 p.m.
◆ Menses flow slightly less than normal.
◆ Tired. Went to sleep early.

Day 8
◆ Emotions somewhat wistful. Life is going by, things not yet done.
◆ Nostalgia.
◆ Energy: Wanted to move my body this a.m. Turned on television to an exercise program.
◆ Stomach: Reach for carbohydrates when I feel my body needing raw veggies. Habit? Weird.
◆ Thirstier at work and drank water.
◆ I have been noticing how I seem to be thickening—pulling down into body. I do not look stretched and elongated, nor do I feel it.
◆ The scab flaked off of spot on cheek tonight. Another dry area underneath.
◆ Perspired a lot today. Sour odor in spite of deodorant.

Day 9
◆ Very tired—allergies.
◆ Too tired to write.
◆ Eyes extremely itchy.

Day 10
◆ Feel "thick" mentally, groggy.
◆ Allergies bad.
◆ Left eye extremely itchy.
◆ Cannot write. Do not want to.

Day 11
- Excited: Encouraged and inspired about the school meeting last night.
- Allergies so bad I could hardly open my left eye. M. put me on Apis 3X today. My eye was swollen.
- Took a Claritin (Antihistamine) at 11:30 a.m. By 6:00 p.m. I was feeling normal.
- I am disappointed at letting this journal go. Another great beginning, not so great follow through.
- Last day of menses.

Day 16
- Took another Claritin. Eyes better, still feel the affects of the allergies.
- Went to counseling. First experienced a sadness that was not mine. I could actually feel myself feel my grandmother's sadness, knowing it was hers. Very odd, but unmistakable. This is the first emotional connection I have felt to her since I can remember. I remember her, but have not been able to feel anything.
- Dreams unremembered, but know there are people in them.

Day 17
- A holiday. Do not feel like doing anything. I read, lay around.
- Still tired.
- I have the energy to write in this journal, but I cannot be bothered. Not motivated.
- Conflict and ambivalence with kids about them staying overnight with friends.

Day 18
- Feel pretty good today, but still do not want to do anything. Shopping is the only chore I did.
- Do not want to be active. Rested.
- Had a half cup coffee today and yesterday. Sniffed remedy.

Day 19
- Have been reading a book, *Onions to Pearls* — "Consciousness is all there is. You are not the doer." A strong effect on me, though my heart has not leaped to it. My mind is meeting it. I am not thinking about it, bit I am letting it percolate.
- "Everything is perfect as it is." Hmmm.
- Took Claritin again. Some help. Eyes were itchy but bearable.
- Cat allergy has kicked in. Had a slight asthmatic feel, wheezing to get a breath, slight but definite. I have never had that with allergies, before, or ever, unless it was maybe at age thirteen with mono and bad cough.
- Very thirsty at night.
- Skin seems dry.

Day 20
- I feel odd. Dissociated? Not quite.
- Unenthusiastic.

- Feel like I might have some difficulty sticking to myself. Who is this?
- Feel tired, like I need a tonic, vitamins.
- I want sweets and foods that I do not really want when I eat them, but they are easy, as in habitual. For example, bagel and cheese at lunch instead of salad, which I did want, but I do not feel like making it.
- Thirstier today. Drinking water feels so good. Why don't I think of it?
- Scab on right knee. For a scrape, it developed a substantial scab and is slow to heal. It is tight, and cracks, and pulls when I kneel.
- I am finally able to write this up, but I am still mentally scattered, unmotivated. A sense of watching life happen. I have felt disconnected from Spirit and sense of humor for four to five days now.

Day 25
- It is unlike me to be so unreliable. This is five days later that I am filling this in. I always keep a commitment like this, and now I do not even seem to be bothered by the fact that I will have to fess up in front of everyone that I did not bother to do this regularly every night.
- Very thirsty at night.
- Embarrassed at not having picked up new glasses, have left them there for three weeks now.

Day 26
- Not much time for reflection today. Seemed pretty well focused and got things done.
- Energy was good. Managed to go through till 11:30 p.m.—late for me.
- Allergies bothering me: Eyes itch, nose sneezing and throat sore.
- I do not feel good when I eat pasta or bagels or toast, but I still do it.
- I realize I am out of touch with my belly. I do not feel the fat on it from inside.
- Dream unremembered.
- Skin dry.

Day 27
- Mind is still adjusting/absorbing that book. It did seem to disconnect me from a sense of joy and yet I think some realization is happening in me. Perceiving consciousness everywhere again.
- Good energy.
- I think I eat too much.
- A clear white or yellow energy seemed to emanate from my liver, an energy that seemed like neutral anger. My right leg was also energized, it felt warm. The right side of my abdomen and thorax was affected.
- Skin on my legs is so dry—shiny, flaky looking.

Day 29
- Another day not recorded—what is this, a latent teen rebellion?

Day 30
◆ Discouraged that I do not do a better job of organizing housekeeping.
◆ Noticed had gained a lot of weight over the last three years, 12–15 pounds. Suddenly it does not feel good. I decide to cut out sweets, but at the open house, I eat some goodies.
◆ Did not sleep well last night. Woke at 2:00 a.m. with allergies. Very thirsty, sore throat.

Day 31
◆ Some "resentment" fantasies.
◆ Feel sad and disappointed that one student is not passing the course. I resist making it my responsibility.
◆ Eyes a little itchy.
◆ Throat gets sore and dry at night.
◆ Wanted sweets today after lunch and dinner.
◆ Neck muscles tight, and upper back.
◆ Began menses early again, light flow.

General Comments:
◆ Initially forgot to take remedy and became surprised, irritated remorseful.
◆ I didn't like getting up in the morning.
◆ Lying around.
◆ I got exasperated a lot.
◆ Dream: Traveling in a car driving to Williams to some teaching or workshop event. Roadwork, big trench across road. I see someone in a four-wheel drive go up on a curb area and drive around the trench. I decide I can do that. I get my bicycle out of the car. Agree to meet up with family in Williams if they do not pass me on the road and pick me up. Dr. D. G. is in a car behind us, also stuck, going to the same place. Next I am with a girl who is both my daughters at once, in a car, and I am driving. I have taken a habitual turn off and am looking for the road back to the highway I need to be on. I am mildly irritated at my absent-mindedness.
◆ Dream: Communal living place with barriers in front and back, but alarm went off when to leave.
◆ Sweets craving, thirsty at night and got water.
◆ Minimal interest in sex.
◆ Irritable at forgetting details.
◆ Read book. It was totally bleak and was totally flat. Had to recover for a few days—joys leaked out of me.
◆ Tinnitus in left ear hasn't been as noticeable as usual.
◆ Uninterested in food, buying, cooking food. So many meals. I thought we should all go on a fast.
◆ Symptoms on right side.
◆ Fell on abdomen and scraped right knee.
◆ Pain in liver: pulsing.
◆ Allergy symptoms really bad, especially swollen conjunctivae. Apis helped, but so bad had to take antihistamines.

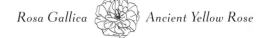

Rosa Gallica   *Ancient Yellow Rose*

Prover #14 • Female • 48 years old

[Turned in journal, didn't come to meeting, despite prior agreement!!]

Day 1
- Sleepy day. Almost dropped off to sleep at work by midday.

Day 2
- Dream: Taking someone in an airplane, somewhere, seemed like it was my job to transport a student.
- I slept well, felt rested.
- Daytime: Felt craving to be in nature, resentful of being cooped up inside.
- Rushed feeling, stressed out.
- Some unusual bouts of anxiety today, felt cut off from others, alienation.

Day 3
- Dream: Working with someone in the forest service and had a heap of papers to go through about a family with lots of bad problems and things against them. Woke some emotional disturbance, lack of equanimity.

Day 4
- Less irritation and anger at work today than last week. More acceptance.
- Feeling calmer, less reactive.

Day 5
- Awoke with dream: Working on a computer to help this family function. Ominous tones and gory feeling as I awoke.

Day 7
- Big fatigue midday, and earlier.

Days 8–11
- Days of no dreams, no physical symptoms but feeling more judgmental, critical.

Day 12
Dream: In a house out in the country, wanted to walk in woods, afraid something would happen to me. A little ways out a man appeared with intention to do me harm. I looked in his eye and became fierce like a wild animal, he backed away. I ran back home. When I returned home, later in the week, he was there with a family member, as her lover. I was freaked, awoke feeling frightened and vulnerable.

Day 17
- Tired, could sleep after work.

Days 18–26
- I notice the prevalence of disturbing dreams related to survival. Something keeps happening that is related to a death-life situation.
- I also am remembering more dreams.

> **Prover #15 • Male • 36 years old**

Day 1
- Took the remedy but was suffering so many cold symptoms I felt it confused the study.

Days 3–5
- Felt sharp burning pain in left inguinal area, about two inches from hernia scar, especially when twisting torso or sitting down. Possibly lymph activity during common cold which lasted Day 1 through Day 10.

Day 18
- Took remedy again.

Days 19–22
- Felt same sharp burning pain in left inguinal area, about two inches from hernia scar, especially when twisting torso or sitting down. In both cases the pain gradually decreased and disappeared.
- Left inguinal area pain twice again, but only for a few seconds.

Days 21–24
- Felt a surprising amount of anxiety, probably due to pressures concerning Christmas holiday.
- Felt frustrated that I had not completed tasks (shopping for gifts, sending greeting cards, etc.) and resented what I perceived as burdensome expectations by friends.
- Generalities: My situation not helped by an approaching departure date in five days when I will be relocating to another state, and lack of a present home due to a recent fire.

Days 25–29
- Feeling sentimental, nostalgic. I am looking at, seeing people, places and realizing it may be for the last time, or not again for a long time. A bittersweet feeling.

> **Prover #16 • Male • 38 years old**

Day 3
- Dreaming, but cannot seem to bring them into consciousness.
- Some stomach discomfort after eating, then totally relieved with eructation.

Day 4
- A lot of stirring in dreams, but I am not able to bring material to consciousness.
- Sleeping more on left side.

Day 5
- Sudden electric-like stabbing pain in left ear every half hour or so. Painful and then gone all in two seconds.
- Dream: Walking along rural path with my father. We come to a stream and a very clear pool of water. Within it are hundreds of crayfish on the bottom. We just observe them. Next we are in a small shack or shed. I notice a beautiful shedded skin of a snake. When I lifted it, there was a large snake which looked venomous. I grabbed it by the throat, as did my father. I want to kill it as I was afraid of being bitten. I choked it, my father let go. I stared into its eyes as its life went out. After it died I felt great guilt that I had to kill it. It lay limp on a table.

Day 9
- Pain in left ear continues.
- Right-sided neck tension and spasm.
- Dream: At a pit—told it is 1,400 feet deep—with two men, and it felt as though it was a punishment. One man says, "To hell with fear," and jumps in the pit. Then we are all falling in space bounding off the walls. Fear. We land at bottom and are okay. Then we are seated and being brought lavish food and pleasures.
- Dream: Walking down a staircase with my deceased grandfather. He is talking about gaining respect by doing what is not necessarily accepted by popular culture, for example, homeopathy. Feeling: Strange to be with him and know he is dead.

Day 10
- Dream: At social functions where two women asked me to attend a ball or something. I say yes to both, and then feel conflicted as to who I should go with, and that I may hurt one's feelings. Could not understand why I said yes to both.

Day 11
- Painful ear but only every two to three hours. Like a "Q-tip" that has gone in too far.
- Desire chocolate.
- I realize many dreams are at school setting I think is Hahnemann College. I am with other students that I am not familiar with, but we are together, unified (maybe the other homeopath provers of this proving—interesting). In many scenarios, hard to remember.
- One dream scenario I do remember is being with a group of students with Nancy and

Roger. We are trying to push a tree down. I say, "Why do we have to do work for you when we should be studying homeopathy." I rebel and leave the group, and go on my own.

Day 12
◆ Dream: A poisonous lizard spitting some kind of poison. Maybe a small Gila monster.

Day 19
◆ Ear pain better. Persisted two and a half weeks.
◆ Frequent urination at night, two to three times.
◆ Dream: Walk into a church office. No one is there in front. Lots of money for charity on desk, no one watching it. It could easily be stolen, I think. Not that I would steal it. I walk farther into church and find a woman in there. I ask her for pamphlets about relationships and she gives them to me. I have no shirt on and I am just aware of it. (It is unusual I would be in a church and asking for advice and especially entering with being only half dressed.) I then go home. I hold my son, although he is not my real life son, and I realize that I am for the first time angry and indignant that she, without any permission or request, was inseminated by another man in order to have this child. I yell at her and ask her why. She is very aloof and casual, and said something about how a friend thought it would be charitable.

Day 22
◆ Three days of left-sided heart pain, like the muscle of the heart had a mild spasm. Periodically.
◆ Dream: Things to do. The child, boy, does not feel like my own. (He is probably one and a half years old in dream). I wonder why am I only now bringing this up. I feel betrayed. I am next walking in neighborhood and two cats are in my path.
◆ A lot of dreams are "vague" in classrooms with classmates from past. Various themes.

Day 23
◆ On waking at night I have had the awareness of not knowing who I am, like my self is less tangible and I have to pull myself together. It is not unpleasant, just a little strange.
◆ Appetite increased last two weeks. I am hungry a lot and will eat and want more. Gained two to three pounds last few weeks.
◆ Sleep: I change positions frequently throughout the night. Whole proving this has been going on.

Day 25
◆ Dream: With Roger and Nancy. Roger drops a burrito on the ground and a snake eats it. Looks like a colorful Rattler.

Day 26
◆ Situation: My first lover calls me after a 15 year period of time. Bizarre. As I spoke to her, old feelings dredged up. She always withheld herself from me and I was never able to see her as her whole self. It would drive me crazy, she always had secrets from me. I longed to totally connect with her and be in her secret world. I loved her and wanted her

so much, but I never fully connected. We broke and my heart ached for years.
- Dream: Old friend, broken relationship (male) comes back. He brings me many sheep and many wrapped gifts.
- Neighbor brings me a gift of very expensive golf clubs. I do not know this neighbor. I do not play golf. Why golf clubs?

Day 27
- The issue of broken relations came up strongly in Lac Leoninum for me. This time the feeling is of secrets and unspoken completion or lack of completion. Yet seemingly "unreconnectable" relations with people disappearing out of my life with no resolve. This feeling is up for me since proving remedy. Not sure what to make of it.
- Feeling: unresolved, irreconcilable relationships due to withheld (secrets) communication, and then going separate ways.
- Two weeks later: Old friend writes me a letter which says that maybe the reason I attract people that withhold from me is because I immediately withhold myself from them.

Day 28
- Dream: Hiding away in a little room with a woman friend and making love to her. I kiss her lips and they distinctly taste like salt (Natrum muriaticum). I am passionately connected with her. I notice my two children are in the room saying, "Dad, when are we going home?" I think, "My god, they are going to tell their mother," then I feel guilt. No guilt up to that point. In real life this woman used to dance in a topless bar or something. She had an interesting bent on sex, like men want it more if they have to pay.
- Dream: My sister dies in this dream and I am devastated. She is there present in the scene, although I know she is dead. I want to be away from relatives that want to console me. I pull away. Go on my own. They are dressed up, and I do not want to be and I do not dress up, but unsure, self-conscious. My sister warns me that my true inner state will begin to torment me if I do not change. She says that she is okay with death, looking out into blue sky and white clouds with a seascape. I am not sure what she means that I have to change about myself. Feeling: Grief, incomplete.

Day 29
- Head pain, right temporal region, worse cough. Like being hit with a hammer.
- Left ear pain which is periodic and sudden. Like a "Q-tip" in deep ear.
- Cough with thick green expectoration, worse after eating.

Day 30
- Head pain right temporal region, one spot. When I cough it is like being struck with a hammer. Extreme pain. Must hold head in order to manage pain. The jerking of head during cough would take three to five minutes to recover from.
- Strong desire for chocolate.
- Cough worse after eating, thick mucous, green.
- Low energy.
- No desire to exercise.

ROSA ST. FRANCIS

Rose of St. Francis

ROSA ST. FRANCIS [ROSA ST F.]
Rose of St. Francis

Rosa canina assisiensis
Family: Rosaceae
Miasm: Cancer

This proving began when my dear friend and fellow homeopath, Dr. Bruno Galeazzi, expertly guided me through the holiest sites of Assisi, Italy, home of St. Francis. Francis, a devoted man of God in the thirteenth century, committed himself to a life of humility, poverty, and service. It was his vision that created a popular religious revival and he himself has inspired the Western imagination for more than seven hundred years. In the garden of the little chapel where Francis spent much of his prayer life, and where many of his followers took their vows, Dr. Galeazzi recounted the legend of Rosa St. Francis. It was then and there that I was inspired to make these roses, so in touch with the spirit of St. Francis, into a homeopathic remedy for healing. We spent the better part of a day looking for the nuns, who alone harvest these rose petals, but they had all disappeared into the chapels for prayer. Since I was scheduled to leave Italy the next day, Bruno took on the pursuit of these roses. One year later, the little package of dried blooms and leaves arrived at my door.

The proving of Rosa St. Francis has many themes in common with the proving of Rosa gallica but with a surprising number of additions. After bringing together all of the themes, those working on this project (entirely unaware of the details of St. Francis' life) discovered that there was an uncanny parallel between the motifs in the Rosa St. Francis proving and the motifs of St. Francis' personal history. In order to show this parallel, the themes will be listed twice, once in the legend and once in Francis' biography. The explanation for the mystifying similarity between the two goes beyond the scope of this write-up. However, what we do know is that the mythology of roses in general, and the rare physical characteristics of Rosa Saint Francis in particular, has inspired people to see this plant as having a unique relationship to the man, Francis. For millions, Portiuncula, the only place where this variety grows, is considered holy ground. Pilgrims gathering for centuries at this site, which Francis called "the gate of heaven," come to pray and meditate. For them, Rosa St. Francis is a tangible sign of this saint's passion for God and his life of miraculous transformation.

Blooming in the courtyard of Portiuncula, a humble chapel in the "green heart" of Italy, Rosa St. Francis stands three to four feet tall, with yellow petals, its leaves liberally spotted or "marked" with dark purple stains. Classified by botanists as a variety of Rosa canina, which typically has sharp "canine-like" thorns, this rosebush is thorn-less. These utterly unique rose bushes have continued to grow in an unbroken line on this small patch of earth for almost a century. (**GARDENS/NATURE**)

The story of Rosa St. Francis takes place long after Francis' own personal transformation from aspiring knight to monk. Like many Christian mystics, Francis viewed his body and its earthly desires as a barrier to complete union with God. As the legend goes, Francis, in an attempt to conquer these desires, throws himself into a thorny bush. (**EMBARRASSMENT/INADEQUACY**) Out of tenderness for the saint's suffering, (**LOVE/COMPASSION**) the bush begins a dramatic alteration, dropping its thorns and beginning to bloom, (**TRANSFORMATION**) only its leaves are forever stained with Francis' blood. (**BLOOD/LACERATIONS**) Then angels urge him to enter the nearby chapel. There he has a vision of Jesus and Mary. (**SPIRITUAL TEACHERS/MENTORS**) Jesus asks Francis what he desires. Francis replies: "I wish that everyone who comes into this place, would receive forgivness of sin and peace of soul." (**DESIRE TO HELP OTHERS**) Francis goes to Rome to ask Pope Honorius to recognize Portiuncula as a holy site and grant indulgences to those who visit it. (**CLARITY/INSIGHT**) Up to this point only the Holy Land and Santiago de Compostela were considered places worthy of pilgrimage status. (**CHALLENGING AUTHORITY**) After hearing the vision, the Pope, in an unprecedented act, grants Francis' request and sanctions the chapel as sacred ground. From that point in time until today an unending stream of pilgrims seeking forgiveness come to Portiuncula to reap the benefits of this indulgence.

The theme of transformation, so central to the miracle in the legend, binds this rose to the life of the saint who, from birth to death, goes through one dramatic change after another. It begins in 1182 when his mother has her newly born son baptized as Giovanni Bernardone. His father, a well-known cloth merchant away at the time of his son's birth, disagrees with his wife's choice of names and in an action that would be radical for its time, has his son's baptismal name changed to Francesco—the Frenchman—Francis.

His father, having aspirations for his son to become a man of culture, tutors Francis in the finer things of life. Francis ambitiously embraces his father's ideals, becoming a ladies man, frivolous with money, living a life filled with music, laughter, gallantry, and beauty. With a romantic notion of chivalry and the fight for justice, Francis, at the age of twenty, enters a "commoners" revolution with the neighboring city, Perugia. Immediately taken captive, he spends a year as a prisoner of war. Suffering with a severe illness, his father ransoms him, but Francis struggles almost two years more with ill health. At one point, delirious and on the brink of death he receives a message: "All that which now seems sweet and lovely will become intolerable and bitter, but all that you used to avoid will turn itself to great sweetness and exceeding joy" (Gasnick, 37). In *The Focus of Freedom* Romano Guardini reports:

> This experience affected him deeply. The old, carefree self-assurance left him. Gradually he convalesced, but the disquiet remained. . . . he rose and went out . . . to commune with nature. . . . He followed a secret oscillation that determined his entire life; one pole lay in the city, the other in nature. (**GARDENS/NATURE**) He sought the life-giving powers of the earth to renew his strength. . . . but there was no response. (Gasnick, 50)

Francis once again throws himself into his former life, repeatedly saying, "I know that one day I will be a great prince." Impatient for this transformation to take place, Francis dressed himself in all his finery and set off for knighthood, only to give everything to a poor knight shortly before he was supposed to leave. He had received another message, like the first, that made these dreams of knighthood appear foolish. The entire city mocked him, his father grew furious at his son. Not knowing what to do, Francis immerses himself again in the old life (50). (**CONFUSION**)

Yet, signs of Francis' gradual conversion continue. As Thomas de Celano, his biographer writes, one day while riding with his friends he passes a leper who comes suddenly out of the woods. The man was in a terrible state of human disintegration with ulcers and open sores everywhere and he smelled horribly. Francis, to the horror of his companions, hesitates but a moment, then holds the leprous hand and kisses it (de Celano, 27). (**LOVING FEELINGS/COMPASSION**)

Francis' father, appalled by his son's behavior and with a reputation to protect, insists another stint in the army will bring him around. On hearing this, Francis takes off to live in some nearby caves. Guardini describes the final stages of his conversion:

> One day he [Francis] invites his friends to dinner. They make him king of the feast. At the end of the meal the group stormed through the night, their song and tumult echoing in the streets. . . . Then suddenly it happened, God touched his heart: [As

the Legend of the Three Companions describes] "Behold, on the instant the Lord visited him, such great sweetness filled his heart that he could neither move nor speak, and could feel or perceive nothing but sweetness." The companions noticed that he was no longer with them; they returned "and saw with amazement how he had changed into a completely different person. . . ." (**TRANSFORMATION**) He soon receives a vision of the Crucified Christ telling him, "Go therefore and repair my house." (**CLARITY/INSIGHT**) (Gasnick, 51)

With no sense of the scope of this vision, Francis returns to town to steal some of his father's cloth, intending to sell it and use the proceeds to give to the poor priest of a nearby church. When discovered, his father locks Francis in the cellar in chains. Wanting to humiliate his son back to his senses, Francis' father brings him to court demanding restitution. There the tables are turned, Francis disowns his father, removes all the trappings of his former life, including the clothes on his back, and before the entire community walks away naked. (**CHALLENGING AUTHORITY**)

Francis assumes a hermit's habit and turns his attention to nursing victims of leprosy. (**DESIRE TO HELP OTHERS**) He then repairs San Damiano, San Pietro, and Portiuncula, churches in the hills surrounding Assisi. Yet, it is when Francis turns barefoot preacher that his conversion from Giovanni Bernardone to Saint Francis is complete. His joy and passion soon attract a dozen like-minded men of noble birth. (**SPIRITUAL MENTOR/TEACHER**). He called these men Little Brothers and they joined Francis' vision of preaching the pure love of God while living a life of poverty, humility, and care for all creation.

Francis' message centered on a radical love for all beings. His kindness for the poor knew no bounds; Brother Thomas describes: " . . . the soul of Francis melted toward the poor. . . . He was known to beg a garment from a rich person only to gleefully give it to the next poor person who passed by. Pourrat, in *Christian Spirituality,* writes: "It was often noticed that when he had just been praying his eyes would fill with blood because he had wept so much and so bitterly" for those who suffered in this world. (Gasnick, 92).

His love for creation became legendary. Given this gentle man's spirit, it is easy to imagine the stories come to life. In one, Francis picks up worms off the road and places them to the side so that they will not be trod upon. In another, Francis prepares honey and wine for the bees in winter so they would not suffer and die from the cold (Celano, 78). He cherished flowers in this same simple and devoted manner. It is said that when he came upon a large grouping of them he would stop and admire them for their beauty and then preach to them exhorting them to praise God. Phyllis McGinley in *Kind Men and Beasts* describes his more concrete political actions on behalf of all creatures:

> He felt so strongly for the mistreated animals of his day, for the snared birds and beaten horses and hungry dogs, that he went to the burghers, to the governors, finally to the emperor, begging for a law against their abuse. . . . He demanded that farmers be forced to treat their cattle humanely. . . . He wanted towns and corporations to take time off from levying taxes and scatter crumbs, instead, on the frozen roads. He pleaded for hostels where strays could be fed and housed, and he raged against the caging of larks. (Gasnick, 81) (**CARE FOR ANIMALS**)

Francis' radical vision of love for all, creates a religious renewal for common folk throughout the empire. For those joining his little band of brothers, Francis insists on a few simple, yet profound rules. (**ORDER/DISCIPLINE/ORGANIZATION**) "Let the brothers . . . take heed not to make any place their own and maintain it against anybody else. And let whoever may approach them, whether friend or foe or thief or robber, be received kindly (Gasnick, 43)." Francis understands that the moment you own something you begin to feel you must protect it from another.

Francis intends for each of the brethren to draw away in nature in order to renew their spirit (**CALMNESS/SERENITY**) and intensify their experience of God's love. However, they were not meant to remain there, each was expected to teach and preach this word of love, actively living it out. The beneficiaries were the poor and the outcast. Francis continues to model the life of a knight, yet now his "Lady" is poverty, and those in need, he treats as if they were kings.

In spite of his renunciation of a private life, one of the most profound and beautiful aspects of Francis' story is his relationship with Clare. As a teen, Clare knew Francis as a slightly mad neighbor whose reputation was built around his rebellion against his father's mercenary ways. Then one day she hears him preach and a light pierces her young heart, she is altered forever. They begin to have long talks and finally it is decided; she will take the vows of poverty, chastity and obedience at Portiuncula. She becomes the first of the "Poor Ladies of the Lord," turning from a life of pampered luxury toward a life of total surrender to God and loving service to the poor. Mirroring Francis' own conversion, Clare sees herself spiritually married to Francis through her exclusive vow to Christ. Though she stays within the enclosures of the convent and sees Francis only rarely, the two are faithful until the end—"Do not believe," said Francis, "that I do not love her with a perfect love"—and between them they invigorated not only Italy but also Christian Europe. They kindled, as Remy de Gourmont has said, "a new poetry, a new art, a renewed religion" (Gasnick, 73). (**OLD ACQUAINTANCES/ LOVERS**)

Francis, like the Buddha and Jesus, experiences affliction by demons and devils. For him, these often come as carnal temptations. Similar to other mystics of his time, Francis experiences his mortal flesh as an enemy worthy of contempt, preventing him from fulfilling his desire for complete union with God and God's will. He calls his body "Brother Ass" and either ignores it or works to keep it under submission. (**EMBARRASSMENT/INADEQUACY**) This burning desire to rise above anything that separated him from God, by joining himself to the physical sufferings of Christ, expressed itself in the legend of the rose.

Struggling with his own limitations was not Francis' only challenge. Near the end of his brief life, Francis' little brotherhood, which had grown into a great religious order numbering in the thousands, began to be in distress. In *Crises in the Order*, John Moorman describes:

> The machinery that had proved adequate in the early days, when almost every question was decided by Francis personally, was now proving itself hopelessly inadequate. There was, for example, no means of testing the vocations . . . no training, no novitiate. . . . Many had never seen St. Francis and had only a vague idea of what he stood for or what his wishes were. . . . The whole thing was growing more haphazard and chaotic. . . . Francis felt himself losing grip. . . . he was not a great administrator, nor could he direct the affairs of a great religious order. (Gasnick, 94)

Francis was certain of his original vision but influential men within the brotherhood, who did not share his ideals, began to depart from the original Rule and intention of the Order. On many occasions, Francis expressed his rage, both verbally and physically, at these violations (**OPINIONATED**) but was "mocked and sneered and ignored" for his efforts (94). He witnessed his vision of a community ruled by humility, simplicity, and poverty eroded from within by his own brotherhood. Francis retreated into nature seeking strength in the wounds of Christ, praying that he might feel in his soul and body, the pain that Christ suffered, and the love which made it possible to bear such passion willingly. He doubled his "fervor and austerities" enduring, more intensely than usual, the effects of near starvation. (**FOOD/HUNGER**) Experiencing ecstatic visions during this time of struggle, he reportedly experienced in his own body, the wounds of Christ: "His hands and feet appeared as though pierced with nails . . . there was a wound in the right side, as if made by a lance, from which blood frequently flowed" (Gasnick,

100). (**BLOOD/LACERATIONS**) Many witnesses attest to seeing the marks of these wounds on his body, in spite of Francis' attempts to keep them hidden.

Most of what we know of St. Francis' life is a mixture of subjective and objective truth. Whether it is the marks of the stigmata on Francis' body, or the marks of his blood on the leaves of Rosa St. Francis, it is difficult to know where reality ends and imagination begins. The homeopathic proving itself, only further mystifies the belief that these flowers and St. Francis' life were transformed from a mutual encounter. The legend of Rosa St. Francis and the proving challenge us to contemplate the intimate connection between the spiritual and physical world. The rose bridges these two worlds and becomes a compelling symbol of transformation. May it be for those who seek it.

PRAYER OF ST. FRANCIS

Lord, make me an instrument of your peace,
Where there is hatred, let me sow love;
...where there is injury, pardon;
...where there is doubt, faith;
...where there is despair, hope;
...where there is darkness, light;
...where there is sadness, joy;

O Divine Master, grant that I may not so much seek
...to be consoled as to console;
...to be understood as to understand;
...to be loved as to love.

For it is in giving that we receive;
...it is in pardoning that we are pardoned;
...and it is in dying that we are born to eternal life.

Rosa St. Francis   *Rose of St. Francis*

Rosa St. Francis Themes

Rose of St. Francis

- *Transformation*
- *Blood/Lacerations*
- *Calmness/Serenity*
- *Clarity/Insight*
- *Confusion*
- *Care for Animals/Dogs*
- *Embarrassment/Inadequacy*
- *Opinionated*
- *Old Acquaintances/Lovers*
- *Desire to Help Others*
- *Gardens/Nature/Weather*
- *Old Ailments*
- *Challenging Authority*
- *Loving Feelings/Compassion*
- *Food/Hunger*
- *Spiritual Teachers/Mentors*
- *Order/Discipline/Organization*
- *Water*

Transformation

#1 I got a strong sense that there was a theme running through all my dreams—transformation.

#1 Dream: . . . She told me stories about how everyone had changed so much. People who were married, fell in love with someone else, and started a new life with the new person while still staying with the other. It wasn't hidden or clandestine. It wasn't like having an affair; the relationship just changed into something else. . . . I kept having similar conversations throughout the dream with other people. . . . They would tell me their whole story, which always involved relationships that suddenly changed into something totally different. . . . It suddenly became clear to me what was going on with all of these failed relationships—people just suddenly transformed and became someone else (but kept their appearance, name, identity). . . .

#1 Dream: . . . Then some people approached me and said that now was the time for my own transformation. I felt a bizarre sensation that I was no longer myself, I was changed into someone else. I resisted so hard. . . . Just as I was coming out of this dream, when I was partially awake, I had a very strong message—"This is it! This is the dream that says it all about the remedy." The word, which presented itself to me, was "transformation." I had the feeling that I was given a gift. It was a very powerful dream.

#1 Dream: Went to a weeklong seminar with my dad, who, in my dream had pancreatic cancer. . . . The conference was on the rapid changes that are seen in pancreatic cancer, i.e. the physiologic change seen in patients with this condition. During the week, my dad got sicker before my eyes, mirroring the lecture topics. . . .

#1 Dream: . . . The naked guy has now fallen to the ground and he is laying there, in my way, in a splayed out fashion. He then proceeded to turn into tree roots, flat against the ground. . . .

#3 My pre-proving state was very overwhelmed and anxious and <u>this</u> changed during the proving. . . . Second day of teachings with the Dalai Lama. Very calm throughout day, noticed easy flow of events today—no problems with traffic, crowds, obstructed seating—all of yesterday's inconveniences/irritations gone.

Irritability, impatience, nerves on edge, easily "flared up" before proving. . . . handling any difficulties with calmer approach (less excitable). (Strong contrast b/w pre- and post-proving states.)

#5 Dream: . . . I talked to my neighbor. . . . He looked different in some way. I realized that he shaved his beard. Then I realized it was someone else . . .

#5 Dream: A friend of mine came out as gay. . . .

#1 Dream: . . . I begin a romance with a guy. . . . He is very tough, wears a black leather jacket and has bleached blond spiky hair. He goes around talking tough to people. He ends up getting into a bad fight. . . . and gets hit in the head repeatedly. . . . When he comes to, he is not tough anymore but rather gentle. He is head-injured and sort of dull thinking, mellow and sweet. . . .

#6 Dream: . . . On the other beds many ill persons were waiting for an organ transplant. . . .

#1 Dream: . . . The maintenance crews came into our house, and put in a new blue carpet and were redoing the kitchen—new tiling on the counters. It looked nice. We weren't upset but surprised. They hadn't finished the transformation; they were in the middle of it.

#4 . . . Angry and upset when friend's son called and asked to stay at the house. It was our anniversary—had plans to go to dinner. Changed plans, ordered pizza and visited with him. It ended up being fun, hearing his different way of looking at things. It was like walking back in time, his facial expressions and smile similar to my old classmate (his father) but not as conservative. . . . I felt like a kid again. . . .

Blood/Lacerations

#6 Woke up at 6 a.m. with a pleasant sensation of internal heat; diffused in bones, around the mouth, on my head. It was as if the blood in the veins were warmer. . . .

#6 Dream: . . . I was lying on a bed and a nurse was putting a needle in my right arm for phleboclysis. . . . Then there were some problems with a patient that a doctor, dirty with blood, carried away with a white sheet. . . .

#1 Lots of mosquito bites, large red welts . . . I scratch 'til the skin breaks.

#1 I did an inordinate amount of suturing (in the ER)—complicated lacerations (fingertips, face, kids). I don't know what it means but it caught my attention.

#3 Dream: . . . ends with a dog (bloodhound) attacking me—I see little cuts on (the palm of) my hands, very minor, like scratches, and two of my cousins are there (one of whom is trying to give me a tetanus shot (!?) . . .

#4 Dream: . . . A phlebotomist arrives and is upset that I didn't introduce her as "Doctor."

#5 . . . Saw stars when I blew my nose, some blood in discharge. . . .

#6 Usually during the second day of menses I have copious, profuse hemorrhages, today NO! . . . Menses have ended, lasting only for three days, this time the flow has been scanty, (usually I have profuse hemorrhage).

Calmness/Serenity

#7 . . . I am calmer than usual about this slight quarrel with V.

#9 Wonderful feelings on waking. Serenity during the day.

#9 Dream: About the family—serene. . . .

#6 I spent the day with an interior calmness and quietness that usually I don't have. . . . Usually I have a go-ahead and combative character, now I feel docile, mild.

#6 . . . I passed the exam on dietetics and I felt much calm, no fear or anxiety (which usually happens in similar circumstances). Much clarity of mind.

#6 Used the color blue for eye make up (unusual); that color gave the sensation of tranquility and calmness.

#1 . . . The flight was especially bumpy, uncomfortable and scary. My body reacted the same way that it usually does when I'm in a small plane flung about by strong winds . . . but I noticed I was not as upset mentally. I easily talked myself into staying calm.

#3 . . . Very calm throughout day, noticed easy flow of events today—no problems with traffic, crowds, obstructed seating, all of yesterday's inconveniences and irritations are gone. . . . Calm—setbacks do elicit irritation/anxiety but this is very much attenuated.

#3 . . . Still very calm—handling any difficulties/conflict with calmer approach (less excitable). (Strong contrast b/w pre- and post-proving states.)

Clarity/Insight

#1 Dream: . . . when I was partially awake, I had a very strong message—"This is it! This is the dream that says it all about the remedy." The word, which presented itself to me, was "transformation." I had the feeling that I was given a gift. . . .

#7 We did special breathing session. Then did a visualization about our mission in this life and our ideal life. Very powerful. . . . [I realize] It's not my business if V. is rude. . . .

#7 Dream: . . . . and I knew he was going to injure her violently (I had seen the scene before).

#6 . . . Much clarity of mind.

#1 Dream: Plane crash on the tiny runway here in town. . . . I saw it vividly as if I was there.

#1 Dream: . . . It suddenly became clear to me what was going on. . . .

#2 Dream: I am under the care of the Dalai Lama. . . . I'm told that I'll be twenty-four percent safer if I stay with him.

#5 Sudden insight: I realized how much personality and emotions relate to illness and how little this is addressed in modern medical theory. I thought, "That's profound." It just dawned on me how little that gets addressed.

Confusion

#4 Dream: . . . I am supposed to talk about a writing assignment. Supposed to write 250 words on _____, nobody can think of what.

#4 Impairment of rational thinking. . . . Decrease in ability to understand nuances of what others are saying. . . . Decrease in logical function.

#5 Found out, to my shock and confusion, that my DEA number had been voided due to failure to complete application. They said they never received my application—I had filled it out a long time ago. . . .

#6 Dream: It was very confused. . . .

#5 Anxious about making plane. When I got out here there was some confusion in my pick up. My sister told me to meet her outside by the Southwest gate. I flew Southwest and went out to meet her but she wasn't there. . . .

#6 Dream: I was in a large hospital room with many metallic beds put there in confusion, higgledy-piggledy. . . . On the other beds many ill persons were waiting for an organ transplant. It looked like a garage, an assembly shop; some male nurses were throwing the organs, frozen, in vacuum-sealed packs. . . .

Care For Animals/Dogs

#5 . . . Worried about my dog, because I had hired this dog walker and I didn't know this guy. Maybe my house would be cleaned out, or my dog left alone.

#6 More cares for my cat, and for a person living nearby.

#5 Moved to tears by story on the radio of pet dog who kept getting in trouble. . . .

#7 Dream: I was a dog (Saint Bernard). I was behind a fence and felt very happy when they let me out.

#4 Dream: I am looking at dogs. A collie is forward. I say to Trish, "The hair is too long." A corgi comes forward and then a bijou (we have a bijou). The bijou is standing with his front legs up, wanting us to take him, but we don't want a second dog. He was kind of cute. The dog was appealing.

#3 Dream: . . . ends with a dog (bloodhound) attacking me. . . .

#4 Dream: A female patient in my bed, when returning I find her lifting her leg to pee on a closet door.

#5 . . . I went into the woods, and as I was coming out a dog came running out barking. . . .

Embarrassment/Inadequacy

#8 Dream: We decided for a tennis match even if I can't play tennis. At the beginning I felt inadequate about the situation, after I had overcome the embarrassment I enjoyed the situation and felt relief.

#5 . . . I had scheduled a tennis weekend with a friend of mine and I felt like I might not be able to play tennis. . . .

#5 Dream: My piano teacher had moved his piano into his kitchen. . . . I wasn't playing well, felt embarrassed.

#4 Dream: Everyone was supposed to raise their fingers indicating how many gods they believed in. I was supposed to count the number of fingers. I realized I was counting people instead of fingers. I felt a little foolish.

#5 Dream: . . . Was walking back through the streets of Manhattan in a familiar section where I used to live, hoping to find my bike. I suddenly was seized with fear that I was naked and embarrassing myself but was relieved to realize I had my underwear on. . . .

#5 Dream: I was playing golf (I played golf a long time ago but I almost never do now). . . . Didn't know if I could do it. Shocked this would be difficult. Someone said I had been playing well and I knew he was right. (I am terrible at golf. I didn't play very well).

Opinionated

#5 Dream: . . . They seemed more entranced by someone with a giant digital camera with a three to four foot video display screen. . . . I was annoyed at their distraction by the banalities of materialism.

#2 Dream: My daughter is wearing baggy, very old-fashioned clothes for her first day at work. Nylon pants like old ladies wear. I tell her she looks weird. . . .

#4 Dream: Go to see a house down in Dover Circle (VA). It's more open and I really like it but I think that the couch is on the wrong side of the room. . . .

#6 Dream: . . . I experienced anxiety in looking at the incompetence of the nurses while dealing with people. . . .

#4 Dream: A good woman student with no money gets a scholarship to a state university. The scholarship board monitored how she was doing. This seemed very intrusive. The school was far below her intellectually. She was doing them a favor by going there but she needed the money.

#1 Dream: . . . [N. and R.] are running a school. . . . We are all excited because we are going to open a clinic in town. . . . It is to be an abortion clinic. . . . N. and R. feel it is very important to have the media there. I don't think that it is a good idea and say, "The media and abortion don't mix."

#4 Dream: I'm labeled as a disgrace because they thought that I was killing everyone. I was simply trying to reduce the death and destruction.

Food/Hunger

#2 Very hungry, especially for carbohydrates. I ate my way through the kitchen. I ate a loaf of bread and cheese. . . .

#7 Very hungry the whole day. Desire to eat chocolate and ice cream, always hungry.

#2 Very hungry—voracious appetite continues. It's rather a nightmare. Feels compulsive, as I am not really hungry.

#2 Eating continued for about a week and then abated suddenly. One day I noticed that I had hardly eaten anything and didn't really feel like eating anything.

#1 . . . Very hungry—ate quickly. . . .

#3 Husband commented on sudden loud rumbling and growling of intestines (onset 5–10 minutes after remedy) and lasting several minutes.

#7 Was very hungry, craving bread and butter.

#7 I was very hungry after waking, better from eating more than usual. This hunger lasted for several days.

#7 Every day: much hunger.

#10 . . . More hunger after the first dose. . . Hunger in the evening. . . Hunger at lunch. . .

#1 . . . then got a hungry sensation in stomach—very hungry after half an hour. . . .

Gardens/Nature/Weather

#9 Ideas about the substance: A flower or flowering plant, yellow flower like a sunflower, without thorns.

#5 . . . That day the sun was very bright, too strong, and it seemed to bother me. It felt too strong for me, even with sunglasses; I wanted some clouds in the sky.

#2 . . . I got very interested in my garden, which is a huge space. Very determined. It's very difficult to do anything with it because it's so dry. Upset about the oak trees dying. Found out they had Oak Death. Spent a lot of time gardening and researching cures. I even gave them a remedy. I made a vegetable garden.

#1 . . . Accomplished a lot—got a lot of yard work done. . . . Thunderstorm with heavy rain and hail in afternoon. Came inside . . . . Otherwise, would have been outside doing yard work. Driven to do the whole front yard: raking, making piles, fertilizing the yard, cleaning up and throwing old stuff away. Cutting trees down, pulling weeds and clearing out driveway before it started pouring. As soon as it stopped I went outside again.

#1 . . . Worked in the garden after work, planting tomatoes, eggplant, and peppers. . . .

#1 . . . Immediately on taking remedy it started to sprinkle.

#5 . . . Coolness and wind was annoying. The wind was blowing me around on my bicycle, felt annoyed by it.

#5 Rain didn't seem to affect mood. It was raining hard. I wondered if it was the rain, but it didn't seem so. Energy good. . . .

#5 Sunny weather raised spirits. . . . (I really felt a lot better in sunny weather. I noticed my reaction to the weather more than usual which may have to do with the proving.)

#2 . . . I've been gardening a lot, which is unusual. . . .

#5 Dream: . . . There was an ice storm in June, odd. . . .

#7 . . . Stayed a bit in the sun because today the weather was beautiful.

#5 . . . Annoyed by damp, cloudy weather.

#7 . . . very hot weather. Went for a walk near the L. river. Intolerant of the sun because too hot. . . . Better at sunset.

#8 Ideas about the substance: A green grass, not a flower, thread-like, smooth, thorn-less, sour taste.

Old Acquaintances/Lovers

#7 Dream: . . . At one moment P. appears behind me and starts to caress my hair. . . . Finally I talk to him and tell him how badly and incorrectly he ended our relationship.

#5 Dream: . . . Thought I saw an old flame.

#1 Dream: Went to a weeklong seminar with my dad, who in my dream had pancreatic cancer. (In real life he died two years ago of colon cancer.)

#3 Dream: . . . Also an appearance of my aunt and her daughter—again these are family members that I'm estranged from. . . .

#7 Dream: About M., a lady who used to do the housekeeping at my mother's.

#1 Dream: . . . When I finally found the person who was going to tell me my schedule and show me where to go, it turned out that she was the ex of a good friend of mine. . . . .

#1 Dream: Initially I go to see my old friend, T. (who I actually didn't really see in the dream).

#3 Dream: An old friend from the university and I do homework . . .

#3 Dream: . . . two of my cousins are there—one of whom is trying to give me a tetanus shot (!?) in a crowded market place. . . .

#4. . . . It was like walking back in time, his facial expressions and smile similar to my old classmate (his father). . . .

#5 Dream: . . . I met another guy who used to live across the hall from me in college. . . .

Old Ailments

#8 . . . In the afternoon herpes on lips. It's the third time it happens —the last time was two or three years ago—now it is milder. (The herpetic eruption lasted for about ten days; it remained quite small and there hasn't been as much boring (pain) like the last time I had it.)

#7 . . . Muscular pain in left adductor of leg (exacerbation of an old trauma). . . .

#6 . . . herpes on right upper lip. . . . When younger I used to suffer from herpes on lips, but usually it was on left side.

#1 Tight feeling in right heel at insertion of Achilles tendon, upon taking first steps after sitting or lying down. Difficulty fully dorsiflexing foot—secondary to pain at Achilles tendon. Resolved with walking for about two minutes. (This is not a totally new symptom for me—I have had it off and on for the past year or so. Much more noticeable now—stronger.)

#3 Strange pulsing—vibration of right eardrum, not painful, per se. . . . (I've had problems with my right ear in the past from barotrauma due to traveling by air with a head cold but this particular sensation is totally new—previously experienced sharp shooting pains and/or blood rushing through ear on lying down.)

#4 Left big toe hurt briefly in evening. Past injury—usually a minor inconvenience. This time it was intense and at times I stumbled.

#5 Left ankle pain, site of old injury —transient. (This was a recurrence of an old symptom. Last September I had a really bad ankle sprain.) I woke up and my left ankle was just killing me.

Order/Discipline/Organization

#1 Dream: . . . I wrote this quote "military style discipline and order; didn't seem unreasonable."

#4 Dream: Trying to see if a computer program could make patient decisions for me quickly.

#1 Dream: I was involved in some campaign. . . . there were strict rules and I had to be up at 6 a.m.

#1 Dream: . . . There was a huge mansion. . . . everything in it is very clean, tidy, and in its place.

#4 Very tense getting out of town; leaving work, planning details of conference, trying to reach friend's son. Dilemma: didn't want to be late but needed to slow down to finish details. . . .

#4 . . . Felt hassled after dinner getting things organized.

#7 Dream: . . . We had to tidy up the place after meetings. . . .

#1 Dream: Working . . . at a place where we had to take two showers a day. They provided . . . towels. . . . I went to take my end of the day shower, looked in the bag and had no towel. . . . . There was a beautiful sack of plush aqua green towels on another table but he told me, "Those are only for the pool," so I couldn't use one.

#7 Dream: I was attending a workshop. . . . We were sitting in two lines in front of each other. . . . Then we [the people in the class] were all walking. . . . following each other in a row.

#4 Returned from vacation. Angry the house was a mess and daughter had not cleaned.

Challenging Authority

Proving Master: Prover #10, #8, and #7 took more than one dose of the remedy, . . . disregarded the indication to take more doses only if they didn't react to the previous one. #6 also wanted to take more than one dose, but was forbidden by the proving master because she already reacted to the first dose.

#2 I wrote very little with this remedy, but usually I love doing provings and write a book full. This time I just had a little piece of paper by my bed, and wrote five entries on this piece of paper. I don't know if it was resistance, or I couldn't be bothered, or something to do with the remedy.

#5 . . . In some ways pretty disabling for a while, it made me do something that I knew I shouldn't do, which may invalidate the data. . . . (treated neck pain with Bryonia).

#5 Dream: While shopping in a mini mart I seemed to be inadvertently stealing things. I didn't want to. I put things in my pockets and realized before anyone caught me that, if discovered, I could be accused of stealing. I would get in trouble. I was buying muffins, cheese, bread, newspaper and insisted on not using a shopping cart for some perverse reason, even though one was available.

#4 Dream: My son procrastinates in completing an assignment. There is a sheet telling him what to do in my car. I run outside to tell him. He is turning around in the station wagon with wood squares for sides. He shows it to a friend, who says, "It's only homework."

#4 Dream: . . . A phlebotomist arrives and is upset that I didn't introduce her as "Doctor." . . .

#4 Dream: A cell system of fomenting revolution. . . .

Desire to Help Others

#7 Dream: I was a doctor. . . . I felt a bit scared about meeting up with some bad people. But then all the staff and some nurses came out to help me. . . . Then I was in a hotel where my sister . . . was with a lover (a ranger who, on the surface, is kind), but I knew he was going to injure her violently. . . . I was trying to save her.

#6 Dream: . . . On the other beds many ill persons were waiting for an organ transplant. . . . I wanted to help the group of ill patients. . . .

#6 I felt fine when alone, standing still; but when the group needed me I was there to help.

#1 I was so struck with the movie *Simon Birch*. He knows that he was sent to this earth to do something special, everyone thinks he is weird and he ends up saving a bunch of children. . . .

#1 Dream: . . . I begin a romance with a guy. . . . he ends up getting into a bad fight. . . . and gets hit in the head repeatedly. . . . he is semi-conscious and I am stroking his cheek. . . .

#2 Upset about the oak trees dying. Found out they had oak death. Spent a lot of time . . . researching cures. I even gave them a remedy.

#4 Dream: Helping a kid get back home. . . .

#4 Dream: I'm labeled as a disgrace because they thought that I was killing everyone. I was simply trying to reduce the death & destruction.

#4 Dream: . . . an older guy is climbing up, he's having problems. I am helping him. . . .

#10 More disposed to . . . do something helpful for others.

Spiritual Teachers/Mentors

#1 Dream: . . . all of the people from the school/clinic are wandering around like zombies, bummed and disappointed. . . . R. [teacher] gives us a speech that lifts our spirits. . . .

#2 Dream: I am under the care of the Dalai Lama, peaceful setting like a monastery. I'm told that I'll be twenty-four per cent safer if I stay with him. It's not like me to dream in percentages. . . .

#2 Dream: Last night, having a wooden mala, had to be precisely curled up in a shoe and given to a Buddhist monk.

#3 [Attended] four days of teaching with the Dalai Lama.

#3 Dream: . . . Seeing crowds of Buddhist monks walking up and down sidewalk. . . .

#5 Dream: It has a religious component. Talking to a headmaster at school about my son, his behavior and grades.

Loving Feelings/Compassion

#10 More disposed to love others . . .

#7 Dream: . . . I was in the mountains and it was starting to snow, so I held my baby tight. . . . I have the sensation of reciprocal love.

#6 Great ability to tolerate other people, more love for other people, more maternal.

#6 I noticed more of a tendency to be "motherish" (more affective as a mother). . . . More full of cares for my daughter, desire to understand her emotions.

#6 More cares for my cat. . . . and for a person living next door that was suffering because her cat had escaped. . . .

#4 Dream: . . . when I grab him I feel a pistol (which I take from him). He insists on having it back. I feel compelled to give it back so I empty the clip. It turns out it was his son that was killed. His wife entreated me to give him back his gun.

#5 Dream: A friend of mine came out as gay. I remember feeling sad for him because I thought gay people have it hard in today's world.

#5 Moved to tears by story on the radio of pet dog who kept getting in trouble. The dog was very rambunctious and she lived on a farm. The dog managed to strangle itself at one point, get run over by a tractor, needed CPR at one point. The girl's father gave it mouth-to-mouth resuscitation. I was moved to tears by this story—the girl had this love for the little dog. . . .

#6 Dream: . . . [I] was taking in my arms a friend of mine that I met the afternoon before. . . .

#6 During the proving period I had been worried about a person living next door that was suffering because her cat had escaped, and the cat's name is Roseto (similarity with the name Roseto, Rose garden, of San Francis roses).

#1 That evening watched video, *Simon Birch*. I had tears running down my face virtually through the entire movie! Felt very sentimental and weepy. . . .

Rosa St. Francis   Rose of St. Francis

Water

#8 Dream: Sea—ocean—clear and beautiful water. After a short time the water started to became troubled, but I wasn't worried, on the contrary I was experiencing pleasant emotions. There were some rocks in the sea to which we could cling. . . .

#7 [Nap] . . . Impression of floating and blurred vision as if I were in the water. Sensation of transparent waves passing over me. I was inside the waves.

#7 . . . sensation of gurgling water in left ear, like a "*palo de agua*" (an empty piece of wood partly filled with sand that produces a sound similar to flowing water when tilted to one side or the other). . . .

#6 Dream: I found a pair of moccasins, black leather, inside a plastic bag soaked with water.

#4 Dream: . . . Was going to put something in trunk but it was flooded full of water. A hose had been in there and I couldn't close the trunk.

#7 Dream: . . . Then I was driving a car with a girlfriend, we were going to the sea. . . . Then I was in a hotel in a forest near the sea with R. and V. . . . Then I was lying in a cave over the sea.

#7 Dream: . . . we were preparing to do some water breathing. . . . Afternoon session of TB [breathing exercises] in water.

#6 In this period I felt a tranquillity and deepness like the profundity of the oceans.

#1 Dream: Working (unknown what kind of work) at a place where we had to take two showers a day. . . .

#4 Dream: . . . In reality, there is a big tidal estuary there, but in the dream the river is dry. As I'm walking back toward the house it is low tide and I can't see it. . . . The house had a waterfall with fish in it . . . .

#5 Dream: . . . Middle-age guys were surfing down some man-made wave water park in NYC. . . .

ROSA ST. FRANCIS...*Rose of St. Francis*

MIND	ACTIVITY; desire for, alternating with, lassitude
	ANGER, irascibility; business, about mistakes, over his
	disorder, about
	friends, towards
	trifles, at
	understood, when not
	ANSWER; snappishly
	ANXIETY; alternating with; cheerfulness
	business, about
	dreams, on waking from frightful
	family, about his
	friends at home, about
	weather, rainy, about
	work; inclination to work; anxiety with
	ATTACHMENT; strong; others, to
	AWARENESS heightened; time of awakening
	BENEVOLENCE
	CALMNESS
	CARES, worries; full of; dog, about
	full of; relatives, about
	CHEERFUL
	CLARITY of mind
	COMPANY; aversion to
	aloof
	CONCENTRATION active
	difficult
	CONFUSION of mind
	DELUSIONS, imaginations
	animals, tigers
	body, body parts; feet; separated from body, are
	internal tissues; she sees the
	child, children; feeling like a
	dirt, dirty; air is
	energy; full of, she is
	expanding; feels as though she is occupying the whole room
	floating; water, in
	life; simple, is
	waves, of; transparent waves passing over her
	DREAMS
	abused; being, too weak to defend himself
	accidents, of
	crash of plane
	accusations; wrongfully accused, someone is
	acquaintances, distant
	airplanes; flying in; plane goes into a loop, makes a 90-degree turn and lands on a street
	amorous; taking him up in my arms
	anger, angry

animals, of
   biting him
   dogs
     appealing
     attacked, by
     bitten by
     black
     frightened by black dog
     lazy, of
     Saint Bernard, a
     spiders
     tigers
anxious
   studied his part for a play, realized he had not
   relief
attacked, of being
   dogs, by
   he avoids attackers by pretending to read
   he reduces the perimeter to one entrance
audience
baby; she has had a baby and doesn't know who the father is
beard; neighbor shaved his
beautiful
beds; metallic, in hospital room, in disarray
bicycles
biting
   herself, flesh; brittle; like chalk
boasting
body surfing
body, body parts
   back; touching her, someone is
   hands being cut
   head; bald spot; enormous
   head; bald, chocolate, covered with
   head; onion, like an
   stomach as storage depot
boyfriend, of; old; jilted by
buildings; where one can talk and be heard from far away, in a
business, of; opening a business
   anxious about
cancer, of
cars, automobiles, of; driving to the sea
   trunk flooded with water
   wood squares for sides, with
ceremonies, of
changed
   someone else, into
cheated; being, of
colored
   blue
   green
complaining, about
computers, of; seeing if it could make decisions for me quickly
conferences; meetings

confusion; others observe his; with amusement
conversations
   car, in a
country; beautiful
   foreign
   foreign; Italy
criminals, thugs
dancing; man
   woman, with an older man
dead, woman leaves him for dead
death
   quickly, desires to die
   that he is to die
digital camera with large video display screen
disappointments
disgraced; accused of killing everyone
doctors; being, of
doors; complicated system of
   many
drugs; psychotropic drugs or drugs, hallucinogens
embarrassment
   has overcome and feels relief
enemies; enemy-friend tried to assassinate me but saw I could fly
errors, mistakes; making, of
escape, of
family, own
father is a famous Italian clothes designer
fights
flying; beanie cap with propeller, using a
foolish; feeling foolish
forest, of a
friends
   meeting of
   friends; old
frightful
golf; playing
groups, of;
   conferences, meetings
   he is lying near
help, helping
   child get back home, a
   people, unable to help others
homeopaths, of
homeopathy; tennis pro interested in
homosexual; friend is
hospitals, of
   hospital beds converging in the middle like washbasins
hotels, of; forest near the sea, in a
houses
   big; mansion
   new, moving into
   waterfall and fish in it; with a
housekeeper, of
hunter; with a bow and arrow

ice storm; June, in
inadequate, he feels
incompetence; of others
injuries
    hands; cut, being
jail, of; hanging paintings in a cell
late; being, of
library
losing; things
    keys
lost; being
lucid
many
materialism
meetings
metamorphosis, changing into someone else
mistakes, makes
moccasins, black leather, in plastic bag, soaked with water
monks, about; Buddhist; procession of
mountains, of; snowing
music
    concert
nakedness, about
neighbor, helpful
noise
    commotion
none
observing; rather than participating in her dreams
offending others
order; and military discipline
organ transplant; waiting for, ill persons are
outsider; being an
parties, of pleasure
paths
people, of
    changing; people are, tree roots, into
    assembled
    changing
    crowd
    influential persons
    seen for years, not
    unknown
phlebotomist
piano; moved into kitchen
    playing, in public
places; public; Italian
pleasant
political; rally; students fight for right to not take drugs in school
public campaign
pursued, of being
quarrels, strife
relationships, of
    changing
relatives

    estranged
religious
remembered; cannot be
revolution
rising; 6 am, at
robbers
romantic
rooms, of; crowded, had to crawl to get in
rules, strict
saving others; trying to save her mother
school, of
    headmaster talking about son
sea (see water)
searching
    treasure; for ancient secret
serene
sexual identity; ambiguous about one's
sexual; woman, he is enjoying being with a
shocked; about difficulty playing game
shopping, of
    mother, with
showers; bathing (people, bathing)
singing, of
speech; giving
    giving, a long
stealing; didn't want to
strange; things; a sense of
strangers, of
    foreigners, being among
sympathetic, of being
teaching job, seeking
theft; committed; of having; didn't want to
throwing; frozen vacuum-packed organs
thugs
towels; beautiful plush aqua green, desires
train; cooking rice on a
transformation, about
trap, being trapped
treasure, searching for.
treatment; medical, injection
underground; must go underground to enter
unsuccessful efforts
    frustration, anxious
urinating; woman; lifting her leg to urinate on closet door
vanishing; words
vengeance, of taking
venipuncture
vivid
    morning
    remember, could not
    vivid scenery
    walking, of
        Buddhist monks
    wallet

    wandering; familiar streets, getting lost
       streets, in
   water
      danger from
      danger from troubled water; despite danger feels serene
      rivers; dry, river is
      sea, of; became troubled
         cave, by the, lying in a
         clear and beautiful water
         driving in a car to the
         hotel in a forest near the
      waterfall and fish in the house.
      waves, of high
    women; bossy
      female patient in my bed
   work
   worms
      proliferating, despite attempts to eliminate
      tries to eliminate
      creeping
   zombies
EUPHORIA
   causeless
FEAR; robbers, about, while he's away from home
FEELINGS; wonderful, on waking
FORGETFULNESS
   things, of where he put
FRANTIC, frenzy; late, when
HELP; wants to, others
HORRIBLE *things, sad stories affect her profoundly*
HURRY, haste; eating; while
   time, for the appointed, to arrive
IMPATIENCE; trifles, about
INDIFFERENCE, apathy
INDUSTRIOUS, mania for work
   mania for work; outdoors
INSIGHTFUL
INTOLERANCE; others, of
IRRESOLUTION, indecision
IRRITABILITY
   evening, agg.
   business, about
   competitiveness of others, from
   controlled
   noise, from
   weakness; with
   weather, rainy or cloudy, in
   working, when
JESTING
JOY; sense of joy decreased
LOQUACITY
LOVE; feelings of love, coming towards her and from her
MIND; LOVE; general; humanity, for
MEMORY; loss of memory periodical

	MEMORY; weakness of, done, for what he has just
	MILDNESS
	MISTAKES, making
	time, in
	MOOD; agreeable
	changeable, variable
	even
	OPTIMISM
	PATIENCE
	QUIET; wants to be
	RESTLESSNESS, nervousness; night
	RUDENESS, yawn, to, but hard to stop
	SENSES; control imperfect
	SENTIMENTAL
	SNAPPISH; wife, with
	STRANGER, strangers; aversion to; house; in his
	SYMPATHETIC
	TALK; talking; talks hasty
	TENSION, mental
	evening, in
	THINKING; logical thinking, inability for
	THOUGHTS;
	control of thoughts lost
	disconnected
	distracted
	intrude and crowd around each other
	persistent, business, about
	profound
	wandering; studying, while
	TIME; passes too slowly, appearing longer
	sense of, clear, about the time of his awakening
	TRANQUILITY, serenity, calmness
	alternating with; irritability
	UNSYMPATHETIC; friends; towards
	WEARISOME
	WEEPING, tendency;
	easily
	morning
	sympathy with others
	WEEPING; tearful mood; general; desire to weep
HEAD	HEAT, brain
	HEAVINESS
	evening
	ITCHING; forehead
	PERSPIRATION; of scalp
	SWELLING; forehead
HEAD PAIN	LOCALIZATION; occiput; extending; neck, to
	sides; left
	temples; evening; agg.
	ACHING
EYE	ITCHING, particles in there, as if

	SWELLING
	TEARS; burning
	TIRED; sensation
EAR	DISCOLORATION; redness; right
	INFLAMMATION
	ITCHING; external ear
	PAIN; general; behind ear, left
	PULSATION; right
	yawn; while suppressing
	eardrum
	SWELLING; right
	WATER, sensation of; rushing into ears
HEARING	*IMPAIRED; noise; waterfall rushing, like*
NOSE	DISCHARGE; general; right; morning; waking, on
	morning
	burning
	clear
	watery; right
	OBSTRUCTION; morning; waking, on
	waking, on; right
	SNEEZING
	animals, from; horses, goats, llamas, from
FACE	DISCOLORATION; red; spots
	ERUPTIONS; herpes, lips
	upper
	pimples; nose; around, about
	HEAT; sensation of; cheeks
	lips
	SWELLING; cheeks; sensation of
MOUTH	DRYNESS
	thirst, with
	ERUPTIONS; herpes
	PAIN; General: tongue; drinks; warm, agg.
	SWELLING; cheeks, inside of; sensation of
	ULCERS; herpetic
TASTE	ALTERED; beer and cheese, for
	SOUR; beer tastes
	cheese tastes
TEETH	GRINDING; waking, with
	PAIN; general; neuralgic
	Incisors
	SENSATION; odd, when together
	SENSITIVE, tender
	brushing
	brushing left side, on
	incisors

THROAT   IRRITATION; Cough; tickling; throat, in
             ITCHING
             SWALLOWING; difficult

EXTERNAL THROAT
             TORTICOLLIS; drawn to, right

STOMACH   *APPETITE; constant*
                increased, hunger in general
                   morning
                   dinner
                   on waking
                wanting; morning
             ERUCTATIONS; general; eating; after
             GURGLING
             HARDNESS; pylorus, sensation of
             HEARTBURN
             NAUSEA; pain, during
             NOISES; rumbling
             PAIN
                general; fruit juice, after
                   lying down; amel.
                burning
                pressing; light, amel.
                sudden
             THIRST
                evening
                water; drinking; cold

ABDOMEN   *DISTENSION*; morning; waking, on
                noon
                diarrhea; amel.
                flatus, passing; amel.
                painful, stool; amel.
                walking; agg. in open air
             FLATULENCE
             FULLNESS, sensation of
                morning
             ITCHING; inguinal region; scratching; amel.
             PAIN; general; standing; amel.
                walking; agg.; while
                cramping, griping; stool;
                   agg.; after
                   agg.; before
                   before; hard

RECTUM   **CONSTIPATION** (cured symptom)
                general; flatulence, with
                   offensive
                hard stool, from
                   AM and PM
             DIARRHEA; morning
                painless

STOOL BALLS, like; small
HARD

BLADDER PAIN; burning, urination, during, after exertion
URINATION; frequent

URINE ODOR; strong

FEMALE GENITALIA
MENSES; scanty

SPEECH AND VOICE
VOICE; husky
 rough

RESPIRATION DIFFICULT
IMPEDED; obstructed, running, while
SUPERFICIAL; morning

COUGH BREATHING
EXERTION; agg.
TALKING; from
TICKLING; larynx; in from tickling in

BACK CONSTRICTION or band sensation; dorsal region; Scapula
CRACKING; cervical region
FORMICATION; dorsal region; scapulae
PAIN; general; motion; amel.; gentle
 sitting; agg.
 walking; agg.; while
 cervical region
  left
   turning head on
  right
  bending head; agg., left to
  descending stairs
  jar, agg.
  looking, up, on
  motion agg., head, of
  raising the arms
   the head
  turning head, left to
   right, to, amel.
  extending; dorsal
   downward
   lumbar region, left, to
 dorsal region
 lumbar region, left
  lumbago
  left
   standing; amel.
 spine
  aching; dorsal region; scapulae; between

drawing, cervical region
    dorsal region; scapulae; between
        right; between spine and right scapula
        walking, while
pinching, cervical region
sore, bruised, beaten; cervical region
PERSPIRATION; cervical region
STIFFNESS; cervical region, left
    turning head on, painful side to
motion; amel.

EXTREMITIES

AWKWARDNESS; hands; typing, when
  lower limbs; stumbling when walking
COLDNESS; upper limbs; hands; one-sided; one hot, other cold
CONSTRICTION; ankles
    walking; amel
CRACKING; joints; elbow
FORMICATION, crawling; lower limbs; crossing legs
  leg; extending; amel.
HEAT; upper limbs; elbow
    hand
    hand, left
      cold and pale, the other hot
    shoulder
RESTLESSNESS; sitting, during
STIFFNESS; morning
TINGLING, prickling; lower limbs; legs; crossing legs
TREMBLING; general; upper limbs; hands
    exercise, after
    morning
WEAKNESS; upper limbs; hands; exertion, after
    motion, on
    persistant
    trembling

EXTREMITY PAIN

GENERAL; upper limbs; elbow, left
    motion, amel.
    right, bending arm, when
      fully flexed, when
        motion; agg.
    lower limbs; hips; right; waking, on
      deep in bone
    lower limbs; knees; rest amel.
    walking; while
      legs; left
      foot; heel
ACHING; bones
  lower limbs; bones
BURNING; upper limbs; forearms
CUTTING; lower limbs; ankles; outer, lateral
SORE, bruised; upper limbs; elbows; motion; agg.
    wrists
      driving, during

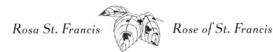

	SPRAINED, as if; upper limbs; motion agg.
	    elbows; left
	      right
	    lower limbs; toes; first, left

SLEEP	DISTURBED
	    heat, by
	PROLONGED
	REFRESHING
	SLEEPINESS; *heat; during*
	    reading agg
	SLEEPLESSNESS; general; evening; bed, after going to
	    night; latter part of night, in
	    midnight; before
	      after
	        one a.m. or two a.m., until
	        one thirty a.m. – two thirty a.m.
	        two a.m. or three a.m.; until
	        three a.m.
	        three a.m. – four a.m.; between
	        three a.m. – four-thirty a.m.; between
	        four a.m.; until
	        five a.m. or six a.m.; until
	WAKING; night
	    midnight; after;
	      frequent
	YAWNING; frequent

PERSPIRATION	MORNING; waking, on and after PROFUSE
SKIN	ITCHING; scratch, must, until it bleeds;

GENERALITIES	BATHING; desires, cold
	EATING; amel.; after
	ELECTRICITY; sensation of
	ENERGY; lots of
	FOOD and drinks; bread and butter; desires
	    chocolate; desires
	    cold drinks, water, desires
	    ice-cream; desires
	    peanut butter, desires
	HEAT; flushes of
	    sensation of
	      blood vessels, in
	      pleasant internal
	      waking, on
	    vital, lack of; waking, on
	INJURIES, blows, falls and bruises; ailments from, old
	LIGHT; sunlight; agg.
	    amel.
	MOTION; agg.
	SLUGGISHNESS of the body; morning

WEAKNESS; sit down; desire to
WEARINESS; tendency
  born tired, as if
WEATHER; cloudy; agg.
  hot; agg.
WOUNDS; bites
    itching
    mosquitoes

JOURNALS..Rosa St. Francis

EDITOR'S NOTE: *Punctuation, abbreviations, and individual stylistic nuances of the original journal entries have been preserved wherever possible.*

> **Prover # 1 • Female • 38 years old**

Overall impression:
- I didn't have a whole lot of mental symptoms. Generally had a lot of energy, more energy for productive work. More dreams than usual, and a few physical symptoms.

Day 0
- Took remedy at 10:30 a.m., sitting outside on the deck. Immediately on taking remedy it started to sprinkle.
- Felt an ache in occipital area down neck, then got a hungry sensation in stomach—very hungry after half an hour. Ate a bowl of cereal—burped a lot after eating.
- Lots of nervous energy—revved up, want to get things done, be productive. Have incredible amount of productive energy. Accomplished a lot—got a lot of yard work done. The day seemed very long—I did so much and the day just kept on lasting. It's now one a.m. and I'm tired.
- Thunderstorm with heavy rain and hail in afternoon. Came inside and studied. Got very sleepy while reading Kent's dissertation on Lycopodium—took power nap. Otherwise, would have been outside doing yard work. Driven to do the whole front yard: raking, making piles, fertilizing the yard, cleaning up and throwing old stuff away. Cutting trees down, pulling weeds and clearing out driveway before it started pouring. As soon as it stopped I went outside again.
- That evening watched video, *Simon Birch*. I had tears running down my face virtually through the entire movie! Felt very sentimental and weepy. I would have normally cried toward the end—it was unlike me to cry during the whole thing.
- Tears burned. (L > R) Eyes continued to burn (L > R) and were puffy. (They don't typically burn when I cry.)
- Dreams just before waking at about 7 a.m.

Day 1
- Dream: Working (unknown what kind of work) at a place where we had to take two showers a day. They provided the showers and a bag with shampoo and towels. We had a specific time to take our showers. The other people who worked there, were doctors I knew who work at Yuba City. I went to take my end of the day shower, looked in the bag and had no towel. I got very upset and went outside to talk to the bumbling guy who

fills the bags. He couldn't find a towel, but rather kept handing me something else, that he presented as if it were a towel, like underwear and a vest. There was a beautiful sack of plush aqua green towels on another table but he told me, "Those are only for the pool," so I couldn't use one. I was irate and went around complaining to everyone.
- The dog woke me at 7:30 a.m. to let her out, fell back asleep and woke at 8:00 a.m. Fairly awake, but so comfy I slept again. Fell into deep sleep, woke up exactly at 8:10 a.m., again fell into deep sleep. Woke at precisely 8:20 a.m., drifted back to sleep. Then a neighbor knocked on the door at 8:30 a.m. I thought it was unusual that times were so clear to me. Woke up thinking about all of the things I wanted to get done today.
- More thirsty than usual.

Day 2
- Made a point to jot down my dreams this morning—had a bunch of short dreams during my 15 minutes of snooze time. Wrote down very brief descriptions while half asleep—I'm not really sure what I meant but here goes.
- Dream: I was involved in some campaign and the goal was to please the public, there were strict rules and I had to be up at 6:00 a.m.
- Dream: Don't know what the dream was but I wrote this quote "military style discipline and order; didn't seem unreasonable."
- Dream: In a computer store looking at a titanium Macintosh laptop. The screen showed gorgeous photos and videos of beautiful and vivid scenery and video footage of many cultures from around the world.
- Dream: Plane crash on the tiny runway here in town. (It happened last Friday night—K. and I had heard a lot of ambulances and sirens but we didn't find out what happened until Monday morning.) I saw it vividly as if I was there.
- Still high energy level today at work. Think I'll take another dose, not sure if I'm having much in the way of symptoms—hard to know...
- Off and on a clear watery nasal discharge from right nare.

Day 3
- Not much that I noticed today—after lunch while walking back to work, had unusually intense lower abdomen bloating and fullness. It was painful. Felt as if my intestines were balloons, < walking, eased considerably when I stood still. Lasted about 15–20 minutes.
- Pain between shoulder blades in rhomboids. R → L which felt a bit like a pulling sensation and tingling feeling in the muscles, right side more than left; felt it yesterday twice and today three to four times, each lasting for about ten minutes.
- Energy level for productive work high. Worked in the garden after work, planting tomatoes, eggplant and peppers. Felt chatty today with my patients. I will take another dose before bed tonight.

Day 4
- K.'s birthday. Energy level not quite as high today.
- Intrascapular tingling/tightness today, more on right side. Became painful and aching

late afternoon after a motorcycle ride. Sore and tingling through until bedtime.
- Early evening while outside, may have been bitten by an insect, not sure. I didn't see or feel it. Large itchy welt on forehead just right of center—3 cm x 1 cm, red, raised, and itchy. Right ear helix, itchy, red, and swollen. The intensity of the redness and swelling decreased but the raised skin is present four hours later.
- Continue being more thirsty than usual. Eating meals faster (usually a very slow eater). I feel like I've been talking faster since taking the remedy. (K. says she hasn't noticed.) I have a speedy feeling, revved up—wanting to get things done.

Day 5
- Started period today, on schedule, no strong symptoms or unusual changes.

Day 6
- Noticed my period is less painful than usual, very fleeting uterine cramping almost imperceptible—usually have cramps on the first day only and I'll usually need to take 40 mg ibuprofen—especially if working.
- Walking home from work, 6 p.m., mouth so dry it hurt, difficulty swallowing (more difficult than painful).
- Usually prefer room temperature or cool drinks, now I want cold drinks.
- Usually wash my hands in hot (very warm) water. Now I use cool water.

Day 7
- Today went camping with K., rode motorcycles two hundred miles, felt great.
- Still have persistent tingling/pulling sensation, medial to right scapula. (It occurs almost always while walking.)
- Dream: (Vivid early morning dream.) I was working where I do now and was assigned to go to another facility once a month, as the "Woman's Health Specialist" to perform colposcopies because they didn't have anyone who could do them. (When I first started this job five years ago, there was a sign: "Women's Health Specialist" outside my office.) When I arrived, I discovered the facility was a huge University medical center. It didn't make sense that they would need my services but I went along with it. I was walking in a sea of people—many of them doctors, all of them very smart-looking people in a hurry to get somewhere. Oprah Winfrey and a cameraman walked up to a person I didn't know, who was walking next to me. She started congratulating her for being voted in as the new "something or other" at the school. I walked on, as if I knew where I was going, but really had no idea. When I finally found the person who was going to tell me my schedule and show me where to go, it turned out that she was the ex of a good friend of mine. I didn't know that she was going to be the person showing me around but I was pleasantly surprised. It was great to see her. (In the dream she looked like the psychiatrist on ER.) She told me I was only scheduled to see K.H., (in real life, a family doctor I know who worked for the Indian Health Service in A.) who recently became the Chief of Internal Medicine at the medical center after leaving IHS. K.H. wanted to consult with me because she had questions about her mammogram. I was excited to see her, but knew I wouldn't know the answers to her mammogram questions. Besides, I was there

to do colposcopies. We went to find her. I was behind my friend and I didn't see where she went. I was upset and I didn't feel qualified to answer the questions. I was going to have to refer her on. I ended up making a wrong turn and found myself in a parking lot by some shops in a strip mall, where there was loud music and much commotion. People sitting on the wall nearby, smoking pot, and some naked guy singing bad, loud, heavy metal music. I realize I am in the wrong place and turned around to find my friend but discover that the way back is up a very steep hill. I couldn't seem to get there. The naked guy has now fallen to the ground and he is laying there in my way in a splayed out fashion. He then proceeded to turn into tree roots, flat against the ground. I used him for leverage to climb out. I started sweating. It was difficult getting out and I was beginning to worry that I wouldn't make it. I woke up scared and bewildered.

Day 8
◆ Great day camping! Went for a long hike down into a canyon. I felt very exhausted. I had to stop on the way out of the canyon. It was really noticeable. I wouldn't usually feel that exhausted. I sweated more than usual—on my head, the back of my neck, and around my waist where I was wearing a fanny pack.

Day 9
◆ Broke camp, packed up, had breakfast at the lodge. Very hungry—ate quickly. Rode the motorcycles home—very fun. Felt great. Much less afraid on the bike—more comfortable.
◆ Lots of mosquito bites, large red welts, very itchy, and hot. Hard to stop scratching once I start—all over legs and arms. I scratch 'til the skin breaks.
◆ Calves and quads sore from yesterday's hike. (Not any worse than I would expect from a hike like this.)

Day 10
◆ Dream: Initially I go to see my old friend, T. (who I actually didn't really see in the dream). I'm aware it's been a long time since I'd seen her last. There was a huge mansion. It is cold and sparse and everything in it is very clean, tidy, and in its place. There were many people there, all family and close friends of T.'s. I was talking with a woman, whom I didn't know, but who was linked to all of the people there. She started sharing a lot of personal information about herself and others at the gathering. She told me stories about how everyone had changed so much. People who were married, fell in love with someone else, and started a new life with the new person while still staying with the other. It wasn't hidden or clandestine. It wasn't like having an affair; the relationship just changed into something else. She gave the example of one woman, still married to her husband who had uncharacteristically started to beat her, who was also seeing a woman; she was certain that "she has sperm," even though she knew that she was a woman now. She was bragging about this other woman. I kept having similar conversations throughout the dream with other people. They felt like counseling sessions. They would tell me their whole story, which always involved relationships that suddenly changed into something totally different. Everyone wanted my attention, wanted to talk to me. There was

a graduation ceremony going on as well; one of the sisters was graduating. During the ceremony there was a lot of commotion and everyone congregated in one part of the building. I decided that this was all too weird and I would go get the keys to the car and leave. I went to the room where I knew that I left my keys. I looked on the pillow where they had been and they were not there. I looked all over and could not find them. There were lazy dogs lying on the pillows obstructing my search but they were not mean or growling, just physically in the way. Even though I couldn't find the keys, I headed for the front door to get outside, thinking maybe I could figure out a way to get into my car. As I was approaching the big glass door leading outside, a maid or servant said, "Oh no dear, you can't leave, you can never leave." I was disbelieving and scared and upset. I got frantic trying to get out. Then some people approached me and said that now was the time for my own transformation. I felt a bizarre sensation that I was no longer myself, I was changed into someone else. I resisted so hard. I was looking for a pen to write down, "Why can't I leave?" but the words would not materialize. Either the pen wouldn't write or they would fade as soon as I wrote them. I felt desperately that if I could write it down, it would be my ticket out. People began to smile patronizingly and shake their heads as if to say, "Poor dear, she'll learn, she should just give up trying to get out." I was so upset and frustrated and scared. I tried to bite someone who came close and tried to put his arm around my shoulder. His flesh was like brittle chalk. When I bit him it came right off in my mouth. It didn't hurt him at all. Then I bit myself and the same thing happened. I knew I was trapped forever. It suddenly became clear to me what was going on with all of these failed relationships—people just suddenly transformed and became someone else (but kept their appearance, name, identity). I experienced it as a very powerful dream.

♦ Just as I was coming out of this dream, when I was partially awake, I had a very strong message—"This is it! This is the dream that says it all about the remedy." The word, which presented itself to me, was "transformation." I had the feeling that I was given a gift. It was a very powerful dream.

♦ When I awoke I was sweaty and hot and noticed the ache/pull to the medial of my right shoulder blade. I also had a runny nose on right side, left side plugged up.

♦ Following that dream I had another: K. and I were at work one day. The maintenance crews came into our house, and put in a new blue carpet and were redoing the kitchen—new tiling on the counters. It looked nice. We weren't upset but surprised. They hadn't finished the transformation; they were in the middle of it.

♦ Right rhomboid tightness while walking to and from work again today.

♦ Very productive around house after work.

Day 11
♦ Tight feeling in right heel at insertion of Achilles tendon, upon taking first steps after sitting or lying down. Difficulty fully dorsiflexing foot—secondary to pain at Achilles tendon. Resolved with walking for about two minutes. (This is not a totally new symptom for me—I have had it off and on for the past year or so. Much more noticeable now—stronger.)

♦ Dream: Went to a weeklong seminar with my dad, who in my dream had pancreatic cancer. (In real life he died two years ago of colon cancer.) The conference was on the rapid changes that are seen in pancreatic cancer, i.e. the physiologic change seen in patients with this condition. During the week, my dad got sicker before my eyes, mirroring the lecture topics. I felt sadness and loss and I woke up missing him a lot.

Day 13
♦ Dream: N. and R. (homeopathic practitioners and teachers of mine) are running a school. The class is a bit larger but included the same people as in real life. We are all excited because we are going to open a clinic in town—there is no clinic like it anywhere nearby. It is to be an abortion clinic. We are gearing up for opening day, and we have a big gathering (a party to celebrate and invite the community). N. and R. feel it is very important to have the media there. I don't think that it is a good idea and I say, "The media and abortion don't mix." A lot of people come and there are speeches. A sort of low–level pandemonium breaks out because some rowdy people are protesting. Somehow I begin a romance with a guy who is initially a stranger, but later in the dream is a member of the class. He is very tough, wears a black leather jacket, and has bleached blonde spiky hair. He goes around talking tough to people. He ends up getting into a bad fight during the ruckus and gets hit in the head repeatedly. He and I escape into a car and sit there quietly until the brouhaha dies down. He is semi–conscious and I am stroking his cheek. When he comes to, he is not tough anymore but rather gentle. He is head–injured and sort of dull thinking, mellow, and sweet. After the "party" is over, all of the people from the school/clinic are wandering around like zombies, bummed and disappointed. We eventually gather in some building by the helipad and R. gives us a speech that lifts our spirits. We decide to get on the helicopter and try to put it all back together. The blonde guy comes over to me and asks if I am going to join everyone back in Philadelphia (where the school is). I had been thinking that I wasn't going to continue, but when he asks me, I say, "Yes," and give him a big hug. Everyone is glad. (This last part is very dramatic and schmaltzy, like the end of an old corny movie.)

Day 14
♦ Working this weekend. Long draining day in ER today—grumpy and exhausted when I get home.
♦ Right–sided runny nose with sneezing—8 a.m. to 1 p.m. Watery and burning, not red.
♦ Tender to pressure at right heel posteriorly, just distal to Achilles insertion. No pain with walking or at rest, only if I push on it.

Day 15
♦ Still have tender spot on back of right foot below Achilles insertion.
♦ Another long day at work, too busy to notice any symptoms.
♦ One thing that really stood out about my weekend in the ER was that I did an inordinate amount of suturing (in the ER)— complicated lacerations (fingertips, face, kids). I don't know what it means but it caught my attention.

Day 16
♦ Dull ache in head, bilateral between temples, around 8 p.m.; cheeks feel hot and puffy.
♦ Irritated throat with tickle producing a cough—short sharp cough originating at the anterior mid-neck/throat—relieves tickle for only a few seconds. Also achy feeling in bones of pelvis, legs.
♦ Again, felt very sentimental when the basketball team I was rooting for qualified to go on to the final round. I wasn't crying but welled up and was more emotional than I usually would have been.

Day 17
♦ Feeling achy today—my bones ache. Lumbar–sacral area, cervicothoracic joint, legs (shaft of bones, not joints).
♦ Also sore throat continued all day since last night. Ticklish cough, very irritating. Worse from talking, worse flow of air (breathing with open mouth). Somewhat low energy, had to go in room and sit down while I was waiting for patients to be screened or for labs to come back.
♦ Usual strong craving for sweets has diminished since taking the remedy.
♦ Tender spot on anterior tongue, left of center—feels like a sore but looks only like a slightly enlarged papilla—pale, no redness. Pain < hot liquids.

Day 18
♦ No longer achy feeling—I feel like I'm getting over this thing that feels like a viral infection, except my throat remains scratchy and irritative, cough persists. Voice is slightly gravelly today.
♦ Flew this morning, on one leg of the trip I was in a small hopper plane that carries about 12 people total. I don't like small planes (or any planes really). The flight was especially bumpy, uncomfortable, and scary. My body reacted the same way that it usually does when I'm in a small plane flung about by strong winds (sweaty palms, jaws clenched, muscles in legs and arms contracted, and general tenseness) but I noticed I was not as upset mentally. I easily talked myself into staying calm.

General comments.
♦ I got a strong sense that there was a theme running through all my dreams—transformation. It was also in a pre–proving dream before I took the remedy.
♦ The pain between shoulder blades in rhomboids ran throughout the proving.

Impressions of the remedy:
♦ I felt like it was going to be an insect—caterpillar to a butterfly—something that transformed. Also, my desire to do things—work. Busy like an insect—industriousness.

| Prover #2 • Female • 53 years old |

General Observation:
◆ I wrote very little with this remedy, but usually I love doing provings and write a bookful. This time I just had a little piece of paper by my bed, and wrote five entries on this piece of paper. I don't know if it was resistance, or I couldn't be bothered, or something to do with the remedy.

Day 0
◆ Dose one. Took the bottle and held it in hand before taking. Felt light-headed, especially the top part of head from the eyes up, slight headache in both temples. Took the first dose and immediately had a dull ache in both calves.
◆ Dream: My daughter is wearing baggy, very old-fashioned clothes for her first day at work. Nylon pants like old ladies wear. I tell her she looks weird. She says something to me, which I don't remember except that it was trivial and not of a serious nature. I worked myself up. I was sobbing deeply, as a result of what she said, although I knew it was nothing. I woke myself up by the sound of myself sobbing deeply. I felt really sad, though for no reason I could find. It was coming out of a really deep grief.

Day 1
◆ Dose two.
◆ Mind very active, very impatient for people to answer me. Impatient with family and what I feel is warranted. I was annoyed by people being slow and dozy. Not efficient.

Day 2
◆ Very hungry; especially for carbohydrates. I ate my way through the kitchen. I ate a loaf of bread and cheese and… I got very interested in my garden, which is a huge space. Very determined. It's very difficult to do anything with because it's so dry. Upset about the oak trees dying. Found out they had Oak Death. Spent a lot of time gardening and researching cures. I even gave them a remedy. I made a vegetable garden.

Day 3
◆ Very hungry—voracious appetite continues. It's rather a nightmare. Feels compulsive, as I am not really hungry.
◆ Dream: I am under the care of the Dalai Lama, peaceful setting like a monastery. I'm told that I'll be twenty-four percent safer if I stay with him. It's not like me to dream in percentages. That felt quite good.

General Comments:
◆ Day three was the last time I wrote notes. Filled in notes later.
◆ Eating continued for about a week and then abated suddenly. One day I noticed that I had hardly eaten anything and didn't really feel like eating anything.
◆ Noticed an "efficient" frame of mind, mentally. Got things done that I had been

putting off. I sat down and said, "Ok, I'm going to do work that had piled up."
- In some ways felt very lethargic. I hadn't phoned any friends, very antisocial, withdrawn and miserable. I didn't write that down because I didn't like that side. I wrote down efficient because it felt more positive.
- Felt physically lazy although I've been gardening a lot, which is unusual (not strenuously, more just putting seeds in seed boxes).
- Generally feeling between being efficient and snappy or judgmental. Feel like curling under a sheet, sleeping, not doing anything.
- Feel a bit discontent in a vague way, not quite happy. Subtle. I felt like there were things I could be angry about but there's a part of me that's not getting to me, more a kind of heavy lethargy.
- No particular physical symptoms, in the last week or so, no dreams.

Night before Prover's Meeting:
- Dream: Last night, having a wooden mala, had to be precisely curled up in a shoe and given to a Buddhist monk.

Prover # 3 • Female • 34 years old

Overall my impression is that the remedy played itself out quickly. It was almost like a blip on the screen. I thought about re-dosing... the proving coincided with four days of teaching with the Dalai Lama. My pre-proving state was very overwhelmed and anxious and <u>this</u> changed during the proving.

Day 0
- Dose one at bedtime. A few minutes later, after taking the remedy, I experienced a strong pain in right forearm—like a pulled muscle with burning sensation that intensified over the next few minutes, then abated—elbow joint felt "wrenched," < extending arm straight—no change from rubbing or heat. A few minutes after elbow <u>pain</u> subsided, low back pain (sharp) and stiffness while lying in bed—localized to small of back, > stretching. It is almost as if remedy went directly to those areas that were overused during the day and drastically intensified sensations that normally would have gone unnoticed.
- Husband commented on sudden loud rumbling and growling of intestines (onset 5–10 minutes after remedy) and lasting several minutes.

Day 1
- Second day of teachings with the Dalai Lama. Very calm throughout day, noticed easy flow of events today—no problems with traffic, crowds, obstructed seating—all of yesterday's inconveniences/irritations gone. Irritability, impatience, nerves on edge, easily "flared up" before proving.

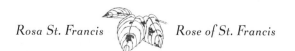

♦ Right elbow stiff, felt sprained/wrenched on waking—stiff on full extension with some soreness and sharp local pain at inner aspect on full flexion. Stiffness throughout day, < full extension. Around 5 p.m. noticed similar stiffness in left elbow joint on full extension, (came and went through evening).

♦ Dreamt most of the night,—very vivid and ongoing with multiple subplots (most of which I don't remember clearly)—like a soap opera.

♦ Dream: Starts with an old friend from the university and I doing homework when I realize I've misplaced my wallet and checkbook (they looked just like mine). I begin searching for them in various places—apparently retracing my steps carefully. This was the lengthiest segment of the dream and the clearest. Main feeling is frustration and anxiety as I search. (Pretty typical of responses I've had in real life to this same situation.) As I'm searching it becomes clear that I'm in a city in Italy. It is crowded, full of people (Italians, very expressive, loud and melodramatic). They're just talking and distracting me from my search—these are the "subplots"—a jilted Italian boyfriend who shows up again trying to impress me; my father (a famous Italian designer?!?) being awarded an Oscar posthumously. These aren't so clear because even in my dream I'm aware that they are distracting me from my main objective, i.e. finding my wallet. I'm not interacting with them really, just watching and moving on with my search. I do remember finding my things eventually—with great relief. Dream ends with a dog (bloodhound) attacking me—I see little cuts on (the palm of) my hands, very minor, like scratches, and two of my cousins are there—one of whom is trying to give me a tetanus shot (!?) in a crowded market place—here too I feel almost like a detached observer (bemused). (None of the places in the dream are familiar to me. I thought the location was interesting, no desire to go to Italy. Looked like those wide-open streets—streetlamps very ornate—a palazzo. I didn't know any of the people except for my two cousins and old school friend. I'm estranged from all three of them. The friend is someone who wouldn't be there for me if I were in need. With regard to my cousins—if they walked into the room right now, I would feel a lot of antipathy and anger toward them. Family problems, convoluted reasons. In the dream, the antipathy did not materialize. No anger, just strange. Also the location of Italy is strange. I have no connection to that country. (No strong feeling/connection/reaction to people in the dream.)

Day 2

♦ Day three of teachings with Dalai Lama. Hot, tired, and sunburned. Calm—setbacks do elicit irritation/anxiety but this is very much attenuated.

♦ Stool, hard, round, pieces a.m. and p.m. Soft stool was symptom prior to proving.

♦ Very slight stiffness in right elbow, only apparent with full forced extension (with weight).

♦ Dreamt most of the night but too tired to remember dreams in detail (interrupted by episodes of deep sleep), again there was an element of searching (not sure for what)—searching through old antique kitchen utensils. Also an appearance of my aunt and her daughter—again these are family members that I'm estranged from. No strong feeling to dreams, more detached.

Day 3
- Day four of teachings with His Holiness. Still very calm—handling any difficulties/conflict with calmer approach (less excitable). (Strong contrast b/w pre- and post-proving states.)
- Stool, still firmer and better formed.
- Some awareness of dreaming but unable to recollect much on waking, except seeing crowds of Buddhist monks walking up and down sidewalk (definitely related to teachings!!).

Day 4
- Calmer overall, yet work-related anxiety surfacing again—overwhelmed feeling not as predominant as before.
- 7:30 p.m. very sharp pains in epigastrium—sudden (no relation to meal time) with some associated nausea, < deep pressure, > lying still, light pressure.
- Stool firm/hard, preceded and followed by mild abdominal cramping.

Day 5
- Generally calmer—irritability easier to control—less reactive to unexpected events/delays etc.
- Stool, still firm/formed.

Day 7
- Stool in evening very hard—constipation most of the day.

Day 8
- Continuing to remain calm overall—I occasionally get overwhelmed feeling with work or teaching but it fades quickly.
- Strange pulsing—vibration of right eardrum → not painful, per se.
  - brief duration.
  - nothing makes it worse or better.
  - happened 15 + times throughout the day.
  - no obvious triggers (head position, etc.).

(I've had problems with my right ear in the past from barotrauma due to traveling by air with a head cold but this particular sensation is totally new—previously experienced sharp shooting pains and/or blood rushing through ear on lying down.)

Day 9
- Ear pulsing, surge/vibration several times over the course of the day (less often than yesterday). Right ear only, brief.

Day 10
- Calm overall. Same symptom of pulsing in ear but less frequently than yesterday.

Day 11
- Symptom of pulsing/vibrating in ear continued but much less frequently—about three to four times throughout the day.

Day 14
- Same calmness overall. If irritated, can keep it in check, it passes quickly. (Very different from my pre–proving state.)

Day 15
- Overwhelmed feeling surfaced again today, almost as strong as during pre–proving phase—anxious feeling in pit of stomach and great anxiety over work left to be done—however easier to deal with feeling than before. Less distracting and could work through it and get things done.
- Pulsing/vibrating of right eardrum in late afternoon, three to four times. Sometimes associated with suppressed yawn, which may have initiated it today. Brief duration.

Day 16
- Low-level anxiety regarding work but more manageable than before proving.
- No ear symptoms today.

Day 17
- Very good mood—calm and relaxed. One occurrence of surge/vibration in ear late in evening when suppressing a yawn.

Day 18
- Apathetic, lack of motivation—difficulty concentrating on work. Not as pronounced as during pre–proving phase.

Day 19
- Calmer today—less apathy but more irritable with delays, loud noises → these moments are fleeting.

Day 20
- Calm state of mind—little anxiety or irritability—these pass quickly.

Prover #4 • Male • 49 years old

Day 0
- Difficult discussion with wife about developing a private practice. Talked about homeopathy and life goals.
- Dose one.

Day 1
- Awoke at 7:30 a.m. then went back to sleep. Awoke grinding teeth. Ordinary day, ran errands.
- Wife observes:
- Impairment of rational thinking.
    - ↑ in anger to the point of impairing communication.
    - ↑ in distance.
    - ↓ in emotional connection to others.
    - ↓ in ability to understand nuances of what others are saying.
    - ↓ in logical function.
- Don't know if I agree. I was not in a good space. There was a ↓ in a sense of joy.

Day 2
- Good mood. Good day. Met friends I haven't seen in awhile. Spent time outside.
- Lay awake in bed at 11:30 p.m., woke up at 12:30 a.m., 1:30 a.m., and 4:50 a.m.
- Dream: A female patient in my bed, when returning, I find her lifting her leg to pee on a closet door. A phlebotomist arrives and is upset that I didn't introduce her as "Doctor."
- Dream: Joining a health club. Need a lock. There is a number to call and get one instantly. Decide to not join part with a steam bath. I am supposed to talk about a writing assignment. Supposed to write 250 words on _____, nobody can think of what.
- Dream: I am looking at dogs. A collie is forward. I say to Trish, "The hair is too long." A corgi comes forward and then a bijou (we have a bijou). The bijou is standing with his front legs up, wanting us to take him, but we don't want a second dog. He was kind of cute. The dog was appealing.
- Whacked weeds—weakness and tremor in hands.

Day 3
- Woke up at 1:15 a.m. and 3:00 a.m.
- Mood more even.
- Morning, tremor in hands. Lack of control while typing. Some weakness persisted throughout the day. Worse when using hands.
- Dream: Trying to see if a computer program could make patient decisions for me quickly.
- Mood pretty good. Confused as to whether or not to take another dose.

Day 4
- Mood good.
- Mild soreness in the wrists.
- Woke up at 3:30 a.m. and 6:00 a.m.
- Dream: A cell system of fomenting revolution. Enemy-friend tried to assassinate me but saw I could fly and realized the folly. It was kind of cool.
- Dream: I'm enjoying being with a woman. My companion wants to have sex with her and I say ok, but he wants her to actually choose him.

Day 5
- Irritated at work, informed of out of state Medicaid patient with criminal problems. Frenetic when late. A bad day, aware of feeling ...
- Slept through the night, woke feeling cold but it was 72° (usually prefer cool).
- Dream: On a plane flight, it goes in a loop and makes a 90° turn due to a problem. Lands on a street. One person tells me his name. It was interesting. Another gets donuts. I ask what kind of donuts do they have in Germany. Feeling of curiosity.
- Minor teeth grinding upon waking.

Day 6
- Evening, very tense.
- The son of a friend shows up unannounced, saying he has no place to live. Operating without information. I have plans to leave town the next day. Really furious at the situation and my friends. Didn't want a stranger in our house. Intense feelings. I said, "This is not our problem." Really angry.

Day 7
- Very tense getting out of town; leaving work, planning details of conference, trying to reach friend's son. Dilemma—didn't want to be late, but needed to slow down to finish details. Got out of town and through the desert—mellow at the little hotel.
- Teeth feel funny together.
- Sleep, up and down, partially due to heat. It had been a hot day.
- Dream: I'm in a building where you could talk and be heard a long way away. Tried it a couple of times. Went to the other side of highway (like a highway from Chicago to St. Augustine—used to drive it thinking you could be heard in several places). I was heard several places in the building. Ready to go somewhere. Had just heard a concert. Two other people had to go, we put six people in a car like a Ford Granada. Was going to put something in trunk but it was flooded full of water. A hose had been in there and I couldn't close the trunk.

Day 8
- A pretty good day in the desert. Snappy with wife a few times while cruising around the desert. Felt hassled after dinner getting things organized.
- Dream: Everyone was supposed to raise their fingers indicating how many gods they believed in. I was supposed to count the number of fingers. I realized I was counting people instead of fingers. I felt a little foolish.

Day 9
- Woke up at 2:54 a.m. and 4:15 a.m.
- Dream: Helping a kid get back home. He expected to be ripped off because a black person with black teeth had previously been given a job without the boss knowing it and this made the boss unhappy. Boss tried to cheat black guy, who charged the boss more and gave the money to the kid. I dropped the kid off at one home and he was supposed to go to his home from there. I waited to watch him but he saw us. He was going to the bathroom. He made a noise. I was afraid he'd wake the family.
- Dream: A good woman student with no money gets a scholarship to a state university. The scholarship board monitored how she was doing. This seemed very intrusive. The school was far below her intellectually. She was doing them a favor by going there but she needed the money.

Day 10
- Returned from vacation. Angry the house was a mess and daughter had not cleaned. Angry and upset when friend's son called and asked to stay out the house. It was our anniversary—had plans to go to dinner. Changed plans, ordered pizza, and visited with him. It ended up being fun, hearing his different way of looking at things. It was like walking back in time, his facial expressions and smile similar to my old classmate (his father) but not as conservative. Enjoyed hearing his perspectives on his parents and us—he's counter-cultural. I felt like a kid again. He stayed a week. I wasn't happy with the way it happened but it was ok.

Day 11
- Left big toe hurt briefly in evening. Past injury—usually a minor inconvenience. This time it was intense and at times I stumbled. My wrist was also slightly sore.
- Woke up 2:20 a.m. and 4:30 a.m.
- Dream: A woman with an older man dancing and she leaves him dead.
- Dream: My son procrastinates in completing an assignment. There is a sheet telling him what to do in my car. I run outside to tell him. He is turning around in the station wagon with wood squares for sides. He shows it to a friend, who says, "It's only homework."
- Dream: Someone around my friend's age is calling my home. I mention it to my companion. There is a semi-romantic tinge to our relationship and she says that she has dated the caller in the past. She says, "No big deal," and "I'm a woman with no wood." (I took it to mean in the Chinese medical sense—no initiative or anger, no liver.)
- Dream: I just fixed up the house and bought another because of the view. The new one was very funky with a two–bedroom area that you couldn't get to because stairway access was too crowded, had to crawl up a corner to get in because the rooms came together so closely.

Day 12
- Wrists slightly sore while driving.

Day 13
- Dream: Go to see a house down in Dover Circle (VA). It's more open and I really like it but I think that the couch is on the wrong side of the room. In reality, there is a big tidal estuary there, but in the dream, the river is dry. As I'm walking back toward the house it is low tide and I can't see it. I realize I haven't seen the bedroom and I wonder how much to offer. Going to California. The house had a waterfall with fish in it (similar to the one at the University of Pennsylvania).
- Dose two.

Day 14
- Dream: It has a religious component. Talking to a headmaster at school about my son, his behavior and grades.

Day 15
- Dream: Off and on about the proving and the idea of metal came up. (I had heard about metal from the pharmacy when ordering the remedy.)

Day 16
- Dream: Took my remedy. I'm under attack. I reduce the perimeter so that there is only one entrance. To enter you must go in and then underground. The enemy gets inside. I have only one arrow. I try to get more but I have to avoid the attackers. I pretend to be reading a book about the American drug scene in the library in a carol. We succeed but we couldn't have succeeded without decreasing the perimeter. My homeopath enters and says that I may not have symptoms since I've been on steroids.

Day 17
- Dream: I'm labeled as a disgrace because they thought that I was killing everyone. I was simply trying to reduce the death and destruction. They were trying to kill me because they didn't believe me. One of the hunters was using a bow and arrow. I know I'm going to die because they are out to get me. I'm worried that the arrow will go in the wrong way. I want to die quickly and was trying to catch the arrow so I could make sure the arrowhead went straight to my heart rather than hitting the ribs. I felt misunderstood and quite worried that I wouldn't be able to catch the arrow and get the job done and would go through a lot of pain.
- Dream: I'm involved in a horse race and someone was killed. A lot of people are trying to kill the person they think is responsible, but he is not responsible. People are shooting but I only have a BB gun (which does not work). He/I/we get away using a Beanie cap with a propeller that lets us fly. We land in a store or hotel, then fly over a body of water like Hampton Roads, Gig Harbor. On the other side, an older guy is climbing up, he's having problems. I am helping him up but when I grab him I feel a pistol (which I take from him). He insists on having it back. I feel compelled to give it back, so I empty the clip. It turns out it was his son that was killed. His wife entreats me to give him back his gun.

Day 18
- I got irritated trying to work out a lease for office space. Landlord wanted tax returns.
- Dream: About work and office.

General comments:
- Grinding teeth. Didn't record it every day, but was aware of them being together and touching. There was a sense of something.
- Really bad tremor in hands went away after a day but there continued to be a subtle feeling. I knew my wrists were there. There was a sense of something. I called it weakness but it wasn't really. There are still times when I know they're there, but I wouldn't notice it now if it hadn't have happened. I would probably ignore it if I hadn't had that experience of the really bad tremor and I'm trying to pay attention to what's going on.

| Prover # 5 • Male • 44 years old |

Overall impressions:
- Pretty severe physical reaction, which I'll get to. In some ways pretty disabling for a while, it made me do something that I knew I shouldn't do, which may invalidate the data. The problem I had was a severe left-sided neck cramp and a pinching pain in my neck that was much worse if I moved it at all. Left, < any jarring, laying on it. I had scheduled a tennis weekend with a friend of mine and I felt like I might not be able to play tennis. We had reservations at a place in the mountains. He was coming from far away so I tried to treat it by taking Bryonia, and then repeated the remedy.
- I remembered a lot of dreams, which was unusual. I didn't notice a lot of themes, but didn't think about it either. Very weird dreams, wrote as many as I could. Couldn't pick out any affective component, but some of them had to do with what was going on in my life.
- On the mental/emotional level nothing that profound. I'd been under some stress at work, lot of ups and downs, which was related to normal things.
- Some things happened, some befallments...
- I started on the assumption that I would be coming out here in the middle of June (wrong weekend), so I only have 17 days of proving.

Day 0
- A little tense in a.m. but somewhat fatigued. Mentally retyping resume. Anxiety about job, relationship issue. A little sluggish, but had good energy during run.
- Took nap during afternoon, sleepy, felt better later. Awoke with right nostril blocked. Saw stars when I blew my nose, some blood in discharge. A little itchy in evening.
- Hungry in middle of day. Overate in a.m., felt bloated towards midday.
- A little congested breathing while running.

- Right leg a little stiff in a.m., better on moving around. Right elbow slightly sore on deep flex. Toenail injury less painful.
- Dream: My piano teacher had moved his piano into his kitchen. His girlfriend was being surprisingly pushy—I wasn't playing well, felt embarrassed.
- Took remedy in evening before going to bed.

Day 1
- Energy low in early a.m., picked up in middle of day. Sleepy in a.m., nap helped.
- Sneezing and nasal congestion. (Typical for month of May: allergies, a lot of pollens in the air. May's a bad month. Not as bad as earlier in the month.)
- Felt slight shallowness in my breathing in a.m.
- A little muscle stiffness in the a.m.—right elbow cracking noise.

Day 2
- Felt good in the morning, sharp, attentive—got tired as day went on—felt a little depression in evening. Energy good all day until I returned from work—felt better after dinner. Annoyed by damp, cloudy weather.
- Pain in left side of neck in afternoon, made me want to move it—stiffness, worse motion. I couldn't get rid of it. Never before.
- Intermittent sneezing, nasal congestion.
- Hungry in evening—craved peanut butter and jelly.
- A bit flatulent today. Urine seemed stronger smelling than normal.
- Right thigh continues to feel a little heavy and weak. A little stiff in a.m.—stopped run.
- Dream: (Some of these were just flash dreams). I dreamed of a chocolate covered bald man's head. It just was a weird thing, like an onion.
- Dream: I was looking for a teaching job—(I am actually looking for some teaching). I talked to my neighbor who knew more about it than I thought—was very helpful. He looked different in some way. I realized that he shaved his beard. Then I realized it was someone else when I saw him with his beard.
- Dream: While shopping in a mini-mart I seemed to be inadvertently stealing things. I didn't want to. I put things in my pockets and realized, before anyone caught me, that if discovered I could be accused of stealing. I would get in trouble. I was buying muffins, cheese, bread, newspaper and insisted on not using a shopping cart for some perverse reason, even though one was available.

Day 3
- Worried about neck pain and the weather for coming two days. I was scheduled to go to Vermont for a tennis weekend. Excited about trip but worried about whether I'd be able to play tennis. Took some Bryonia hypericum—felt a little better the next day. Worried about my dog, because I had hired this dog walker and I didn't know this guy. Maybe my house would be cleaned out, or my dog left alone.
- Energy good.
- Nose intermittently stuffy. Some jarring.

- A lot of flatulence.
- Urinating more often than usual. Seemed like I have just urinated and I had to go again even though I hadn't had much to drink.
- Pain in neck experienced as an acute twinge—had to cock head to right. (The pain was on the left. I was guarding it, unconsciously. It was this really bad pinching pain, and if I turned the wrong way, it would be like a spasm of pain. I felt like I might pass out it was so intense, and was afraid that if I tried to play tennis and jerked, I could be in bad shape. It seemed to be behind the ear. It felt tender when pressed in. It was sore—(rhomboid trapezius). Pain in neck worse motion, jarring, going downstairs, lifting head, running. Neck still very sore, very bad—stiff and painful. Neck sore to deep compression. Tilting head to right or looking right helped a little. It felt like a pinched nerve, or something pinching in there. I thought maybe I should go to a chiropractor because the facets of the spinal column were pressing on a nerve. When I played tennis that evening, I was guarding it quite a bit, it seemed stiff, I couldn't reach high or look up. The results of the game were not good. It seemed to be behind the left ear too. I was pleased that I was able to play tennis, but afterwards it felt bad again, it seized up and I tried Bryonia that night.
- A little restless that night, woke up very early at 4 a.m. to use bathroom.

Day 4
- A little irritable in the evening, annoyed with myself about tennis toward the end of the day—good energy in morning.
- Pain still experienced behind left ear, seemed to be more in the neck than left ear.
- I thought I felt a cold sore but nothing was there, a strange bump in my cheek.
- Craving for cold drinks, copious amounts. A little dyspeptic after dinner—fish and vegetables. A little upset stomach—pain after drinking fruit juice.
- Neck still painful. More mobile, felt much better in a.m., but worse again as day wore on and I move it.
- Perspiration copious but very active.
- Sleep frequent waking.
- Dream: Wandering streets of NYC, familiar to me but I managed to get lost and wandered into a school library, people were loitering, hanging out like people do in the summer in NY, and observing my confusion with amusement. Hard to get out—door system was complicated. I was wandering through the doors, there were a lot of doors, and I couldn't get out. I was finally able to negotiate this complicated door system. I locked up my bike and worried it would be stolen. Middle-age guys were surfing down some man-made wave, water park in NYC. I wanted to go, but no one would lend me a board, so I tried bodysurfing in my underwear. Was walking back through the streets of Manhattan in a familiar section where I used to live, hoping to find my bike. I suddenly was seized with fear that I was naked and embarrassing myself but was relieved to realize I had my underwear on. Nobody seemed to notice. I finally found my bike. Some guy was looking over bikes and muttering something as if he was planning to steal one. So I cozied in there and took my bike. I met another guy who used to live across the hall from me in college. I even remembered his name. Hadn't thought of his name for years.

He didn't recognize me. He asked me out of the blue if I would be his roommate. I didn't want to reveal to him I knew who he was. I asked him if he was a grad student and he said yes. I declined his offer. Then to my relief, I found my bicycle.
◆ Dream: A friend of mine came out as gay. I remember feeling sad for him because I thought gay people have it hard in today's world.

Day 5
◆ Moved to tears by story on the radio of a pet dog who kept getting in trouble. The dog was very rambunctious and she lived on a farm. The dog managed to strangle itself at one point, get run over by a tractor, and needed CPR. The girl's father gave it mouth-to-mouth resuscitation. I was moved to tears by this story—the girl had this love for the little dog. Otherwise, mood good that day. Impatient with traffic. Sunny weather raised spirits. I felt sleepy in the afternoon. (I really felt a lot better in sunny weather. I noticed my reaction to the weather more than usual which may have to do with the proving.)
◆ Sneezing in the evening after encounter with goats, llamas, and horses.
◆ Felt a little dyspeptic in the morning—stomachache after sweet drink—brief.
◆ Left ankle pain, site of old injury—transient. (This was a recurrence of an old symptom. Last September I had a really bad ankle sprain.) I woke up and my left ankle was just killing me. I was almost limping around. It was worse when I first got up, worse when walking, but if I kept walking long enough it seemed to get better. It was much worse running, I couldn't run. My neck still hurt quite a bit, worse jarring/movement/running—especially downhill.
◆ Perspiration, profuse, exercised a lot.

Day 6
◆ Took the remedy again. Just back from Vermont and thought I might have antidoted it by taking the Bryonia.
◆ Felt unmotivated and sluggish in the afternoon. Positive and optimistic in the morning. Reflective in evening. Annoyed by people that day—averse to company.
◆ Good energy. Sun helped improve my spirits and energy level.
◆ Intermittent sneezing, no runny nose. A little postnasal drip in the evening, (I sometimes get that.)
◆ Thirsty for cold drinks.
◆ Some coughing while playing squash, air seemed dirty.
◆ Neck still painful, less sharp, more of a dull ache, worse motion, jarring, twisting to left. Ankle still a little weak and painful.
◆ Dream: Tennis pro was not too keen on regular medicine, was into homeopathy. I was surprised at the coincidence. I said, "Oh really?"

Day 7
◆ Anxious in a.m. about date—felt let down afterwards. Sad, annoyed at my friend—very competitive playing pool and obnoxious.
◆ Had energy in the morning, went for a long run and felt very good—got tired last 5 miles. Unusual, because most of March and April I felt washed out, recovering from a flu.

- Sneezing in a.m.
- Diarrhea in the woods while trail running. (Sometimes when I go out for long runs I have loose bowels and I head out to the woods. I was in an area that was semi-rural, suburban and woods. I went into the woods, and as I was coming out a dog came running out barking. The owner came out and said, "I never saw anyone running out of the woods." But I was afraid when I came out that he'd have his shotgun. I felt embarrassed, nervous, and a little afraid he might want to make a big beef about it. I don't know if it was his property. As I was running, my neck was hurting in the beginning, and then better the longer I ran.)
- Stiff after run. Perspiration, heavy while running.
- Slept well.

Day 8
- A little cranky at having to go to work. Felt better in the evening. Encouraged by patient's positive response to Aurum.
- Felt worn out and stiff—stopped run.
- Sneezing off and on during the day.
- Still have pain in my neck behind ear, a little better. A little lower back pain. Right leg heavy and weak.
- Dream: Dream of bald spot getting huge—I was shocked and mortified at how large it was. One of those friar tuck enormous bald spots.
- Slept well. Awoke at 4:30 a.m. to pee.
- Many phone calls from personal ad, got to be too much.

Day 9
- A little listless in the morning, more upbeat in evening. Found job listing that was of interest. A little impatient during the day.
- Energy high—had a good run. Coolness and wind was annoying. The wind was blowing me around on my bicycle, felt annoyed by it.
- Pain behind ear still present, better. A little lower backache while running. Left neckache still present.
- Desired pasta.
- A little flatulent.
- Awoke early in morning, 6:30 a.m.—slept until 7:30 a.m.

Day 10
- My moods were changeable today—optimism alternating with anxiety. Energy good in a.m., felt sluggish in the afternoon.
- Sneezing. Nose and eyes felt a little itchy, as if there were particles in there.
- Neck pain still present but a little better.
- Dream: My brother's stomach is a storage depot for_____considering alternative. Patient wanted to take me out to a show after our session. Wandering the streets of NYC, Harlem—fear of muggers. I was in my bare feet. I had a lot of wandering streets dreams.
- Pimple, right cheek near nare, in a.m.

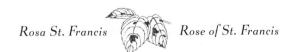

Day 11
- Felt tense and stressed in the morning, very indecisive. Thinking about job possibilities and consulting work, it was stressing me out.
- Neck pain still present, but better.
- Dream: I was invited to speak with another doctor at a high school. Some students had organized a rally to fight for their right to not have to take drugs in school. The other doctor was more soft-spoken but better able to win their attention—I was frustrated. I began speaking about how they might solve their problems with homeopathy but they began filtering out of the room until no one was left, so I had to stop speaking. I was annoyed. They seemed very disorganized, not even the other doctor could get their attention any longer. They seemed more entranced by someone with a giant digital camera with a three to four foot video display screen. He was using the camera to take a 360 shot of the group. I was annoyed at their distraction by the banalities of materialism.

Day 12
- Depressed, weepy in early morning, not sure why. Felt well in the late morning—after about 11 a.m., moody the rest of the day.
- Rain didn't seem to affect mood. It was raining hard. I wondered if it was the rain, but it didn't seem so. Energy good—felt better after exercise.
- Thirsty in evening.
- Had a burning pain at the beginning of urination after work out.
- Left ankle pain in morning, better motion—worse after running. Neck still a little stiff and sore. That really bad left ankle pain had disappeared completely after two days. Then I had it again this morning...
- Dream: Bought a new house and moved in too early. Former owner came back angry. Realtor screwed me. I vowed to get back at him. There was an ice storm in June, odd. Met someone I liked while at the movies. Thought I saw an old flame.

Day 13
- Mood up and down during the day. Concentration poor in morning, better in the evening. Energy good. Sunshine ameliorated mood in afternoon.
- Left ankle pain and stiffness much worse after run yesterday. Had to stop run. Neck pain almost totally gone. Right dorsal thigh pain, tightness. Left anterior thigh stiffness. Right elbow painful when fully flexed.
- Chafed my back with backpack while running.

Day 14
- Found out, to my anger and shock and confusion, that my DEA number had been voided due to failure to complete application. They said they never received my application—I had filled it out a long time ago and forgot about it. I called to get the updated certificate and they said they never got my application, so they voided it. I was very annoyed and wondered what am I going to do about. Anxious about this all day. Also realized that I got the dates wrong about the conference. I felt shock and was angry with myself, scrambling for ideas—agitation. I was annoyed with myself. Am I going to be able to go?

Or skip this? How can I quickly remedy the situation? I realize I have a friend who had Rapid Rewards so I asked if he would trade mileage. I didn't have to pay anything but I had to reschedule all my patients. I had things scheduled for every day—it was a hectic time.
◆ Sleepy during day. Hard to stop yawning with psychotic patient. I usually don't see people with this level of psychosis. I rarely yawn because it's rude. Sleepy in evening.
◆ Abrasion in back. Neck pain almost totally gone. Surprisingly, left ankle pain 99% better.
◆ Woke up early—5 a.m.—anxious, restless, had trouble getting back to bed so I got up.
◆ Chaffing from running with backpack on mid-spine.

Day 15
◆ Sudden insight: I realized how much personality and emotions relate to illness and how little this is addressed in modern medical theory. I thought, "That's profound." It just dawned on me how little that gets addressed.
◆ Energy fair. Felt good during morning. Obsessed about job, anxiety. Bright sun, felt a bit too strong for me. That day the sun was very bright, too strong, and it seemed to bother me. It felt too strong for me, even with sunglasses, I wanted some clouds in the sky.
◆ Sneezing during day.
◆ Thirsty during day, usually for cold drinks.
◆ Right leg still a little heavy when running. Right ankle tight. Neck pain very slight.
◆ Dream: I was playing golf (I played golf a long time ago but I almost never do now). I was at the 16th hole with these people, we accidentally skipped the 17th hole and we had to go back. I had to chip the ball into a basket-like metal contraption, and it would run out through a pipe onto the green, like miniature golf. Didn't know if I could do it. Shocked this would be difficult. Someone said I had been playing well and I knew he was right. (I am terrible at golf. I didn't play very well.)

Day 16
◆ Felt tired, fuzzy-headed in the morning, concentration not good. Anxiety in a.m.—restless. A terrible time concentrating—better in afternoon.
◆ Aching pain left ankle, just the inside, in the evening. Transient aching in right elbow while running, then went away. Aching, heaviness in left ankle while running. Left neck pain better.
◆ Woke up early in the morning. Slept okay.

Day 17
◆ A little anxious about trip. Mood good. Went on job interview, I thought it went ok. I wasn't sure. One person had some philosophical disagreements but later she seemed to understand. Anxious about making plane. When I got out here there was some confusion in my pick up. My sister told me to meet her outside by the Southwest gate. I flew Southwest and went out to meet her but she wasn't there. Eventually she found me. I thought all of the terminals were together and wasn't noticing where the Southwest terminal was. Even though we both got there at 9:00 it took 45 minutes for her to find me.
◆ Good energy, p.m. well.
◆ Nose runny on plane.
◆ Flatulence on plane.

| Prover #6 • Female • 45 years old |

Day 0
- I feel well, the day has passed as usual.
- At 11:00 p.m. I took the remedy, first dose.

Day 1
- Woke up at 6 a.m. with a pleasant sensation of internal heat, diffused in bones, around the mouth, on my head. It was as if the blood in the veins were warmer. The sensation lasted for ten – fifteen minutes.
- I spent the day with an interior calmness and quietness that I usually don't have.
- First day of menses.

Day 2
- 9:30 a.m. pleasant warmth inside my head, heat is between skull and brain, and around my mouth.
- 11:30 a.m.–12:30 p.m. gastric acridity (heartburn), burning in esophagus.
- 12:30 p.m. right hand cold, left hot.
- Usually I have a go-ahead and combative character, now I feel docile, mild.
- Usually I'm a chilly person, now I feel an internal warmth, not disturbing as in flushes, but diffused.
- The strong pain in my left elbow, wrist and shoulder joints are no longer localized in precise points, but seem to be more diffuse and milder. Pain in left elbow has dissolved, joint movements have improved.
- 5:30 p.m. sensation of heat in shoulder, elbow, and hand joints.
- Usually during the second day of menses I have copious, profuse hemorrhages, today NO!

Day 3
- Dreams: I found a pair of moccasins, black leather, inside a plastic bag soaked with water.
- 11:30 a.m. again warm sensation inside my head. 2 p.m. hands very, very hot, almost pulsating, throbbing from heat.
- During the entire day I almost never perceived pain in my left elbow.

Day 4
- Dream: I was in a large hospital room with many metallic beds put there in confusion, higgledy-piggledy. I was lying on a bed and a nurse was needling a vein in my right arm for phleboclysis. On the other beds, many ill persons were waiting for an organ transplant. It looked like a garage, an assembly shop; some male nurses were throwing the organs, frozen, in vacuum-sealed packs. Then there was some problems with a patient that a doctor, dirty with blood, carried away with a white sheet. I experienced anxiety in looking at the incompetence of the nurses while dealing with people. I wanted to help the group of ill patients, but was incapacitated to act. I was always observing the scene from my bed and feeling anguish.

- 2:30 p.m. the same strong heat on my hands.
- 5:30 p.m. until 7:00 p.m. gastric acidity, heartburn.
- 8:00 p.m. heat inside my head.
- Menses have ended, lasting only three days, this time the flow has been scanty, (usually I have profuse hemorrhages).
- Today, very little pain in elbow.

Day 5
- Slept badly, sleep very disturbed, but I don't remember any dreams.
- 3:00 p.m. and 9:00 p.m. very hot hands.
- 6:00 p.m. gastric acidity, heartburn.

Day 6
- Awake between 2:00 a.m. and 5:00 a.m., then I fell asleep (usually I wake up at 5:00 a.m. and don't sleep until morning).
- 11:30 a.m. right hand icy cold and left hand warm. 3:00 p.m. warm hands. Compared with the first days, now heat in my hands is less intense and lasts less.
- 12:00 p.m. and 7:00 p.m. heartburn.
- Today I never felt pain in my left elbow, I can feel it only if I turn the joint a certain way.

Day 7
- I feel calm and quiet.
- 11:00 a.m. hand and head hot, pleasant internal warmth of meninges.
- 3:00 p.m. I passed the exam on dietetics and felt very calm, no fear or anxiety, which usually happens in similar circumstances. Much clarity of mind.

Day 8
- I woke up at 7:00 a.m. with a strong pain in my left elbow. I tried to move it and felt a very painful cracking of the joint, then the pain soothed.
- 9:30 a.m. and 2:30 a.m. hands very, very hot.

Day 9
- Dream: I saw a spider hanging from his cobweb that clung to a wall lamp. I can't remember where I was and can't remember anything else.
- 4:30 p.m. only palm of hands hot, not the whole hand as before.
- 7:00 p.m. and 10:00 p.m. heartburn.

Day 10
- Dream: I was behind the scene in a theater and had great anxiety because I realized at the last minute that I hadn't studied my part.
- 11:00 a.m. internal heat in my mouth, but much less than the first few days.
- 3:30 p.m. hot hands, only palms.
- 7:00 p.m. heartburn.

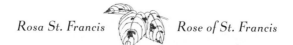

Day 11
- 4:00 p.m. and 5:00 p.m. palm of hands hot.
- I start to feel again the usual pain in my left elbow. It was painful from late afternoon (5 p.m.) till time to sleep, mainly during torsion of the joint.

Day 12
- 11:00 a.m., 3:00 p.m. and 11:00 p.m. hot hands.
- 7:00 p.m. some heartburn.
- Today I felt very little pain in my left elbow.

Day 13
- 11:00 a.m. and 6:00 p.m. hot hands.
- 7:00 p.m. some heartburn.
- I noticed that during the last few days I don't feel pain in left elbow during the day, but during the evenings there's aggravation until morning. When I wake up it's painful and I feel better after motion; it hurts a little all the day until evening, then it gets worse again.

Day 14
- 11:00 a.m. heartburn.
- 12:00 p.m. hot hands.
- 9:00 p.m. pain in left elbow, I hadn't felt pain all the day.
- During this period I sleep well, it's a restful sleep. This morning I slept until 8:00 a.m., it hasn't happened for months. I used to wake up between 6:00 a.m. and 7:00 a.m. Tonight I slept 8 hours.

Day 15
- 9:30 a.m. and 3:00 p.m. hot hands.
- 7:00 p.m. heartburn.
- Dream: It was very confused, I can remember taking in my arms a friend of mine that I met the afternoon before. Then I saw him in a street and I was very distant. He was talking with another person sitting in a car.

Day 16
- 9:30 a.m. hot hands.
- 11:00 a.m. and 6:00 p.m. heartburn.
- This morning I had pain in my neck, right side, like torticollis, drawing pain like a cord, less elastic than usual. I was impeded to turn my head to the left. It lasted all day.
- 5:00 p.m. mild, left-sided migraine, lasted until time to sleep.

Day 17
- 11:00 a.m. hot hands.

Day 18
- 4:30 p.m. and 7:00 p.m. hot hands.

Day 19
◆ 12:00 p.m. and 7:00 p.m. heartburn.

Day 20
◆ 6:00 p.m. hot hands.
◆ This morning herpes on right upper lip, but I think it's a consequence of anger that I had four days ago. When I was younger I suffered from herpes on lips, but usually it was on left side.

During the entire proving period:
◆ Calm and quiet.
◆ Desire to stand still, sitting.
◆ Had the sensation of not having feet, cold feet.
◆ Sensation of heat in waves, as if heat flows in waves over me.
◆ Used the color blue for eye make up (unusual); that color gave the sensation of tranquility and calmness.
◆ Docile, mild.
◆ Great ability to tolerate other people, more love for other people, more maternal.
◆ More full of cares for my daughter, desire to understand her emotions.
◆ More cares for my cat, and for a person living nearby.

Other comments:
◆ During the first few days I felt a diffused sensation of heat, in bones, around the mouth, on my head and joints. (It came back for several days.) In the last days, I only had hot hands.
◆ Great joint elasticity.
◆ I have the impression that the remedy acts on stomach, uterus, joints, and small blood vessels.
◆ Diarrhea for several days, 7:30 a.m. and 8:00 a.m.; watery, painless.
◆ After the first week: sensitive teeth, superior and inferior incisors, electric sensation.
◆ A lot of heartburn before eating, at 11:30 a.m. and 7:00 p.m. One to two hours after eating: stony hard stomach, like a stone on stomach.
◆ Craving for ice cream.

General impressions:
◆ In this period I felt a tranquility and deepness like the profundity of the oceans.
◆ For the entire proving period I never felt my feet (not a physical but psychological insensibility).
◆ I felt a desire for living in a group, like in a colony of animals.
◆ I felt fine when alone, standing still; but when the group needed me I was there to help.
◆ I noticed more of a tendency to be "motherish" (more affective as a mother), very worried and full of cares for my daughters.
◆ Sensation of internal heat.

- For years I used to not remember dreams, during the proving I dreamt a lot:
    about a spider which I throw away.
    about new shoes that I find soaked with water.
    about a person living next door.
    about anxiety before reciting a poem in public.
    about many metallic beds in a large hospital room. A nurse puts a needle for phleboclysis in my arm and looks at the other patients. The male nurses were throwing frozen organ for substitution to the other patients. I felt anguish to be in a crazy place and anxiety as I looked at the incompetence of the nurses while dealing with people. I wanted to help the group of ill persons, but was incapacitated to act.

Ideas about the substance:
An animal, not a rigid remedy, a mammal of the cold oceans, perhaps a penguin because they don't have feet. A docile, mild animal that lives in groups.

Further notes referred after the provers' meeting:
- During the proving period I had been worried about a person living next door that was suffering because her cat had escaped. The cat's name is Roseto (similarity with the name Roseto, Rose garden, of Saint Francis roses).
- On July 1 I took the second dose of the remedy. (I wanted to take the second and third doses during the proving, but after consultation with the proving master he suggested that I not take further doses.) After the dose, no more pain in left elbow, tendons and joints, but there was a return of headaches, old symptom, on forehead, like left-sided migraine, over the ear extending to the nape of the neck; gnawing, tearing pain. The pain started over the head and extended to the nape of the neck.
- Menses lasted two days.
- Persistent palm of hands hot.
- Diarrhea is better, creamy stool.

Prover #7 • Female • 28 years old

Proving Master: Prover #10, #8 and #7 took more than one dose of the remedy, inappropriately, as they already reacted to the first dose, but they wanted to take more than one dose and disregarded the indication to take more doses only if they didn't react to the previous one. Prover #6 also wanted to take more than one dose, but was forbidden by the proving master because she already reacted to the first dose and followed his instructions.

During the proving period prover #7 attended a seminar about respiration—breathing exercises.

Day 0
- Morning bowel a bit better.
- TB session very relaxing. Afternoon breathing to expand consciousness to the upper chakras. Night party. Danced a lot. Had a fight with V. because he told me in a rude manner that I should cook for him.
- Took the remedy (first dose) at 1:30 a.m. Shower.
- Felt angry with V. when going to bed because he went there before me and turned the lights off. When I arrived, I needed to write something. I asked, "Can I turn the light on for a bit?" He answered rudely, "I'd prefer you don't." I felt really bad. I lay under the sheets and try to elaborate with a mental "the work… ." It's not my business if V. is rude. I fell asleep very quietly. I am calmer than usual about this slight quarrel with V.

Day 1
- Woke up first time at 7:15 a.m. to pee. Can't remember any dreams, went back to bed and slept until 9:30 a.m. Got up feeling very rested. Good mood.
- Had breakfast (tea + bread + jam) quite hungry, more than usual. Intestines working better. (Constipation was a strong symptom before proving.) Menstrual cycle in reduction.
- 10:30 a.m. went to the K. to meet other people in the course. I feel very attached to them. It's been a great week. Today is rainy so I stay at home, tidy up and read a little bit. 12:00 p.m. received shiatsu treatment. Made me feel very relaxed. I don't have any unusual feeling or physical symptoms.
- 3:40 p.m. fell asleep, napped. While half asleep, I saw a tiger walking quietly. Impression of floating plus blurred vision as if I were in the water. Sensation of transparent waves passing over me. I was inside the waves. (All this occurred during the nap.)
- Spoke till late with people in the course. Took remedy (second dose) at 1:20 a.m. Went to bed laid near V., I had the impression of expansion, of occupying all the room and full of energy. After turning on my belly, that sensation disappeared and I fell asleep.

Day 2
- Woke up at 7:30 a.m.
- Dream: Don't remember the dream clearly. Just that I was lying near a group of people. I was near F. and he was touching my back.
- Got up at 8 a.m. Feeling air in my belly, swelling tension and flatulence. Have to evacuate gas.
- 6 p.m. TB session. Felt electricity in my whole body at the end of the session. Toward 7 p.m. I experienced a sensation of diminished hearing with the sound of waterfalls in both ears. Lasted 10 minutes.
- When bending forward with knee crossed felt very strong tingling in both legs. Stopped when returning upright.
- 8 p.m. did another TB session, afterwards I felt very energized. Then we danced a bit. Good mood.
- Midnight: took the third dose of the remedy. Went to bed near V., fell asleep without being aware of the moment.

Day 3
- Woke up at 7 a.m., feeling good, slept very well.
- Dream: About M., a lady who used to do the housekeeping at my mother's.
- Morning session of TB, 45 minutes sitting. My breathing is becoming more fluid.
- At 1 p.m. ate lunch. Stayed a bit in the sun because today the weather was beautiful.
- Afternoon session of TB, it's difficult for me to breathe fully with chest + abdomen. It was very relaxing though.
- 8 p.m. sensation of gurgling water in left ear, like a "*palo de agua*" (an empty piece of wood partly filled with sand that produces a sound similar to flowing water when tilted to one side or the other), lasted two to three minutes.

Day 4
- Dream: I was in a supermarket with my mother. We were buying newspapers and magazines. We realized we had bought some things in common. The shop was almost closing. Then I was driving a car with a girlfriend, we were going to the sea, and on the way we met some Swiss girls. Then I was in a hotel in a forest near the sea with R. and V.
- I'm very hungry at lunch.
- Afternoon TB session. I feel light-headed and peaceful after it. Went to bed at 12 a.m.

Day 5
- Did usual 5 rides. During TB group session at 9 p.m. felt a lot of energy.
- Intense pain, like a knife, in left ankle (outer malleolus) for less than one minute, while breathing.
- Went to bed 12 a.m., slept very peacefully.

Day 6
- Woke up at 8 a.m. When brushing my teeth they feel very sensitive on left side, upper and lower.

Day 7
- Teeth not sensitive when brushing.
- 8 p.m. head heavy, lasted 10 minutes.

Day 8
- Woke up at 7 a.m., know I dreamt but can't remember.
- Morning had my first client in TB, session went well.
- Lunch, very hungry.
- Afternoon TB session, while breathing—pain right ankle lasted a few minutes.
- At dinner still very hungry. Ate rice. Studied for exam.

Day 9
- We did special breathing session. Then a visualization about our mission in this life and our ideal life. Very powerful. Afternoon session of TB in water. Evening ate with all the people of the course. Danced till 2 a.m.

Day 10
- Teeth sensitive when brushing on left side of the mouth. Pain is like caries in the teeth, there is hypersensitivity.
- Nice journey back, but motorway blocked and needed to go all the way around by the lake. Took me 5 hours.

Day 11
- Very hungry the whole day. Desire to eat chocolate and ice cream, always hungry.
- 2 p.m. while driving to L. pain in left low back, > standing, < sitting in the car. By 4 p.m. when I came back and got out of the car no more back pain. Legs feel tired. At dinner it was difficult to stay still, sitting in the same position, desire to move legs.

Day 12
- Dream: I was in the mountains with the TB course. We were staying on a train in which we were cooking rice. Then I was lying in a cave over the sea. V. was asking me if I loved him and I was answering no. Then I was in a big house with some participants in a course. I started to do the 100 breaths and in that moment P. introduced me to them, making me angry.
- Woke up at 10 a.m. very relaxed.
- Teeth very sensitive when brushing, but not sensitive to cool or warm.
- Very hungry all day.
- At the airport, head heavy (only 15 minutes before boarding).

Day 13
- Dream: I was a dog (Saint Bernard—big domestic dogs that usually live in the Swiss mountains). I was behind a fence and felt very happy when they let me out.
- Woke up at 9:30 a.m., did five rides and one hundred breaths. Don't feel tired.
- Teeth still sensitive when brushing, left side.
- Bowel function good.
- Very hungry. Ate only fruit at lunch.
- While walking around in P. very intolerant to warm weather. Feel little energy when walking up the stairs.
- Evening went to a conference.
- Very hungry at dinner.
- Brushing teeth, sensitive upper left.
- Went to bed 12:10 a.m.

Day 14
- Dream: Included all the people of TB (this is usual for me to have dreams in which I am together with people from a seminar I'm taking). I was attending a new course with them including J., R., and C. We had to tidy up the place after meetings. J. was also there.
- 9:00 a.m. went to meeting in P., I feel very good. Not hungry at all, even though I didn't have breakfast.

- Went to visit my grandmother by car, 2 hours drive out of P. Muscular pain in left adductor of leg (exacerbation of an old trauma), I can feel it when I move purposely.
- Went to bed 12 a.m. Don't feel tired at all.

Day 15
- Dream: I am with all the Dutch and Italian people of the TB course, J. answered me badly, making me cry. At one point I was in a private hospital in A., but it looked like my grandmother's flat. We were lying or sitting on some beds. Every bed converged in its middle like a washbasin, in the middle was the hole.
- During the day felt well—very hot weather. Went for a walk near the L. river. Intolerant of the sun because too hot, much weariness and desire to sleep in the afternoon. Better at sunset.
- Was very hungry, craving bread and butter.
- Went to bed at 11:15 p.m.

Day 16
- Dream: I was attending a workshop with J. There were lots of people. We were sitting in two lines in front of each other. At one moment P. appears behind me and starts to caress my hair. I react in a brusque manner telling him to leave me alone. He insists. Finally, I talk to him and tell him how badly and incorrectly he ended our relationship. Then he goes away suddenly.
- The day was very hot (36°C) and I didn't have any energy and felt just like lying on a bed in the shade. Drove car to P., really hot there too.
- Ate oysters and sashimi. After dinner had a long walk through P.
- At 2:00 p.m., gas in bowels, with abdominal distress and a lot of abdominal swelling. At 4 p.m. discomfort in bowels plus a lot of gas with bad smell. 6:30 p.m. diarrhea (once only) had less swelling of abdomen. Felt better after discharge.

Day 17
- Dream: I was following the TB course. I had to go there everyday by car from P. That day I went on the wrong motorway and arrived late to the course. I was upset by that. Then we were all walking in P., following each other in a row.
- Bowel ok.
- Weather very warm. Evening did lesson and met people I hadn't seen for long. Ate a bit and went to bed at 11 p.m.

Day 18
- Dream: I was still attending the TB course. There were B. and V., we were preparing to do some water breathing. We had to do everything in a hurry. V. told me, "Let's make love." I hesitated because I was not sure to love him, but suddenly it was already time to go.
- Teeth not sensitive anymore.
- Very hungry all morning. Feel bloated, much gas in bowels, better after stool and passing air.
- Today is a day off and I feel very relaxed. 11 a.m. reading a book, Joy while lying near

the pool during the afternoon. When I got up had pain in right knee while walking, stopped after sitting and the pain didn't come back again.

Day 19
◆ Dream: I just had a baby, don't know who the father is. I am in the mountains and it is starting to snow, so I held my baby tight. He cried in my mother's arms and stopped crying when he was in my arms. Then I was in a big hall attending a meeting given by people from South America.
◆ During the day, bloated bowels, gas.
◆ At the supermarket an African man approached me with the excuse that he wanted some easy food, then an Italian heard that I spoke English and was wanting to see me again to practice… very insistent. I was perplexed by them showing interest in me.
◆ 5 p.m. went to see a patient with MS to speak about Kousmine method.

Day 20
◆ Dream: I was a doctor who had to hang some paintings in a jail cell during the night. I felt a bit scared about meeting up with some bad people. But then all the staff and some nurses came out to help me and came in the room with me. Then I was in a hotel where my sister (who was in reality my mother) was with a lover (a ranger who, on the surface, is kind), but I knew he was going to injure her violently (I had seen the scene before). I was trying to communicate with my hands about him, but my mother didn't believe me. I was trying to save her. Then I went to K. but F. was not there. There were a lot of nice people and we did all the TB training and exercises. My sister A. came there too.
◆ Lots of wind in the bowels the whole day.
◆ Brushing teeth is not sensitive anymore.
◆ Went to bed at 2 a.m. Difficulty falling asleep.

Day 21
◆ Dream: V. was in the dream, but I don't remember anything more. Woke up at 6:40 a.m. before the alarm rang, feeling well.
◆ While driving to V., on motorway feel sleepy. Still air in the bowel, abdomen distended.

General Comments:
◆ I have the sensation of reciprocal love.

After the first dose:
◆ I was very hungry after waking, better from eating more than usual. This hunger lasted for several days.
◆ Better bowels, better stools. Constipation was a strong symptom before proving.
◆ Much weariness, meaning more relaxed.
◆ Slept in the afternoon.
◆ Sensitive teeth.

After the second dose:
- In the morning, abdomen full of air, swelling tension, and flatulence.
- Noises in the ears like water, like falls.
- Formication when crossing legs, better extending them.
- Low back pain, left side, < when sitting in the car.
- Desire to move legs, while sitting.
- Every day: sensitive teeth (after the 18th day no more teeth pain).
- Every day: much hunger.
- Intolerant of hot weather, much weariness and desire to sleep in the afternoon.

Ideas about the substance:
- An animal, a mammal, gentle.

> Prover #8 • Female • 31 years old

Day 0
- Dream: I was with a group of friends (that I couldn't recognize) in a garden of a holiday house. We decided to have a tennis match even if I can't play tennis. At the beginning I felt inadequate about the situation, after I had overcome the embarrassment I enjoyed the situation and felt relief.
- Dream: Sea—ocean—clear and beautiful water. After a short time the water started to became troubled, but I wasn't worried, on the contrary I was experiencing pleasant emotions. There were some rocks in the sea to which we could cling. Some persons were with me: my boyfriend, my sisters and some of their friends; the latter were the only ones experiencing negative sensations.
- A bit nervous and tired all the day (in the evening I took the first dose of the remedy).

Day 1
- I feel so tired! Really tired. This morning I must put much strain to take my eyes open; how I wish I could close them and rest! Nervous because I couldn't rest as I was at work. (This effect lasts for three days, from the third day I get better.) Mood good enough.

Day 2
- Same story. I'm really tired: physically and mentally! From morning till evening.

Day 3
- Morning fine, also the mood and felt less tired. In the afternoon general nervousness, and tiredness has arrived. In the evening I take the second dose of the remedy.

Day 4
◆ Much tired and also nervous, irritable. Slight improvement during the afternoon. Weariness, but less compared with the first dose. Annoyed by others. During a nap in the afternoon I dreamt (that's unusual for me, to dream during naps): small worms, I wanted to eliminate them, but they continued to proliferate.

Day 5
◆ Everything is normal. Almost fine. In the afternoon herpes on lips. It's the third time it happens—the last time was two or three years ago—now it is milder. (The herpetic eruption lasted for about ten days; it remained quite small and there hasn't been as much boring (pain) like the last time I had it.)
◆ I don't remember the dreams and don't have those annoying feelings during the day.

Day 18
◆ In the last two to three days I started again to "feel" my dreams during the day. I hadn't realized this in the beginning, but I actually didn't feel this sensation for the last ten days; before the proving I felt this sensation every day.

During the last period of time
◆ Menses copious (usually scanty).
◆ Seven days after second dose: hot hands.
◆ Annoyed by others
◆ Empty memory (weakness of memory) for names of persons and things, for some days.

Ideas about the substance:
◆ A green grass, not a flower, thread-like, smooth, thorn-less, sour taste.

Prover #9 • Male • 39 years old

Day 1
◆ Dream: About the family—serene (positive dream, occurred toward morning).
◆ On waking, slight pain in the bones. I had pains from the neck to the dorsal region, like when you sit for long and there's cracking in your joints.
◆ During the morning, more positive, apex toward lunchtime, culminating in causeless euphoria from extreme gaiety. I have been telling jokes until evening.
◆ During the morning more allergy, worse at lunchtime. No burning in stomach. (Strong symptom before proving.)

Day 2
◆ No burning in stomach. Euphoric, hyperactive.

- On waking, pain at the right hip joint.
- Again euphoria and hyperactivity all day.

Day 3
- Itching in the inguinal region, scratching ameliorates but not for long.
- Took second dose of remedy.

Day 4
- Wonderful feelings on waking. Serenity during the day.

Day 5
- On waking, pain in right hip joint.
- During the day episodes of empty memory.
- Itching inguinal region.

Day 6
- Much irritability. Intolerant of others.

From the 8th to the 19th day:
- Diffused irritability, always cross, intolerant with people.
- Felt well when in quiet places with few people.
- In the last days, alteration of taste for beer and cheese. (Usually I like them a lot and they don't have a sour taste.)

Ideas about the substance proved:
- A flower or flowering plant, yellow flower like a sunflower, without thorns.

Prover #10 • Male • 48 years old

Day 0
- Taken first dose of the remedy in the evening. I had a good deep sleep, no dreams.

Day 1
- Tired in the morning with low energy, also traveling was tiring anyway. More hunger after the first dose.

Day 2
- More energy, good appetite but always better for light meals, still > cold, moving about. I had a good sleep. Less tired.

Day 3
♦ I took a second dose in the evening before going to bed. As soon as I took the remedy, I experienced slight cramps in the stomach for a few seconds, as if it were contracted, cramped, which disappeared when I went to bed. I had a good sleep.

Day 4
♦ In the morning, I felt a bit tired and sleepy. During the day also tired. Tiredness, a bit more difficulties in digestion. Desire for fruits and a light meal without milk and dairy product, > moving, walking, > open air.

Day 5
♦ Tired and sleepy in the morning, hunger and > after a good breakfast. Desire to lie down and sleep during the day. Hunger in the evening, I had a rich meal but after, I had sensation of fullness and long digestion... Sleep was good with no particular dreams.

Day 6
♦ Great energy during the day. Hunger at lunch. I had a light lunch with sleepiness soon after the meal, better for rest (as usual), > open air (as usual). I took the last dose of remedy in the evening, before going to bed. Again I experienced cramps in the stomach as if the stomach were narrow. Stronger for 30 minutes (a bit stronger than the previous time). The cramps disappeared when I went to bed. I had a good sleep.

Day 7
♦ Tired in the morning with low energy, also traveling was tiring anyway. Desire for rest, which makes you feel better. This time I was a bit more tired then the last time I took the remedy. Also my wife noticed that I was tired with desire for rest. Still feeling hot, better for open and cool air.

Day 8
♦ Again tired in the morning with low energy, also traveling was tiring. Desire for rest, which makes me feel better. Anyway I felt better than the day before. During the next few days the sensation of tiredness gradually went away. I felt more energy, more active, more desire to do things, and optimism, as noticed also by my wife.
♦ More vivid dreams, usually about holiday, (the theme about holidays was present also before the proving).

General comments:
♦ 3 days after the last dose: more energy, more organized. I woke up in the morning before the usual time, with more energy.
♦ More vivid dreams.
♦ More disposed to love others, to do something helpful for others.
♦ Two episodes about forgetfulness: I forgot my camera; forgot the keys of the house where we had to meet. Forgetful about things I had just done.
♦ In general, I felt more relaxed.

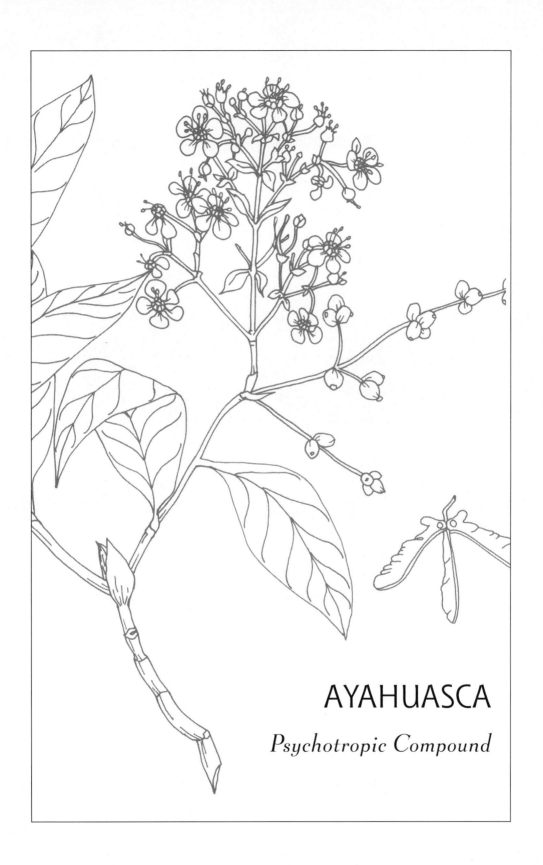

AYAHUASCA [AYAH.]
Psychotropic Compound

Banisteriopsis caapi and Psychotria viridis
Family: *Malpighiacea and Rubiaceae*
Miasm: *Syphilitic*

Ayahuasca or *yagé*, as it is commonly called, is a powerful medicine originating from the Amazonian rain forests. Believed to be primeval in use, Ayahuasca's influence on the culture and ethos of indigenous peoples throughout South America is pervasive. Once a tool of Amazonian Indians for diagnosis and treatment of disease, spiritual guidance, divination, rites of passage, and strength in battle, the vision-inducing power of yagé is now experiencing a great resurgence in shamanic healing practices all over the world.

Although there are numerous admixtures, two plants indigenous to the Amazonian rain forest, *Banisteriopsis caapi* (vine) and *Psychotria viridis* (bush), most often make up this psychoactive, synergistic compound. With small pink flowers much like apple blossoms, the *Banisteriopsis* vine climbs up adjacent tropical forest trees until its flowers find direct sunlight. It is so hungry for light that over time, it kills the very trees that support it. Known by Amazonians as the "vine of the spirits," *B. caapi* grows to half a foot thick with a rosette pattern inside composed of "hearts." The bark is essential to any *yagé* concoction. Belonging to the coffee family, *P. viridis*, a glabrous shrub up to fifteen feet in height, with glossy foliage, pale green to white flowers and red berries containing small brown seeds, thrives best in the rich, moist, soil under the forest canopy. Although studied most for its part in the Ayahuasca mixture, it is highly regarded as a medicinal plant in its native area, one of its uses being eye drops for migraines.

The major psychoactive ingredient in *B. caapi* is a three-ringed cluster of compound chemicals, referred to as the harmala alkaloids, the most powerful of which is harmaline. These alkaloids appear throughout the plant kingdom, and are even present in tobacco and the human pineal gland, reportedly more so in the pineal glands of highly advanced yogis (*Stafford, 344*). Despite its prevalence in nature, this compound's use as a mind-altering substance has been documented in only two regions of the world, Syria and northwestern South America (*333*). In the case of the Amazonian brew, the *P. viridis* plant introduces another intensely psychoactive alkaloid, DMT [dimethyltryptamine], which expands the length and vividness of the extraordinary *yagé* visions. DMT is not normally absorbed when taken by mouth because the enzyme MAO [monoamine oxidase] breaks down DMT while it is still in the stomach. However, in the *yagé* mixture the natural chemicals in the *Banisteriopsis* vine block MAO, thus allowing DMT to be absorbed. Richard Evans Schultes says of this compound: "One wonders how peoples in primitive societies, with no knowledge of chemistry or physiology, ever hit upon a solution to the activation of an alkaloid by a monoamine oxidase inhibitor" (*333*). Ralph Metzner, Ph.D. states: "We now know that it is this synergistic action between the two rainforest plants that makes Ayahuasca one of the most powerful and widespread shamanic hallucinogens in South America" (*Metzner, 17*).

Gathering these plants proves to be a difficult and delicate operation. Harvesters clamber to the top of very tall trees at a specifically determined time and place to find the *B. caapi* vine. At these precarious heights, chopping of the sturdy vine commences and once lowered, (**HIGH/LOW**) the scraping of the tough bark begins. The rare *P. viridis* bush provides the leaves that are mashed and mixed with the vine's bark. The concoction, carefully boiled and stirred in a large pot for up to twenty-four hours, is now finally ready. The potent brew tastes extremely foul bringing on immediate and powerful nausea which, apparently increases the more one is out of touch with his inner world.

The reward for all this effort, believers claim, is eminently worth the pain because with the experience comes profound revelatory visions. What do they reveal? According to practitioners, they reveal one's inner spiritual life and true relationship to the outer world, serving as a guideline, a powerful trajectory of information that changes one's life forever. (**FLOW/EXPANSION/POWER**)

Peter Stafford, in *Psychedelics Encyclopedia,* describes a study using harmaline conducted by Chilean psychiatrist, Claudio Naranjo: (In *Hallucinogens and Shamanism* Michael Harner and Naranjo independent of one another underscore the "constancy" of both *yagé* and harmaline visions.)

> Of the group of thirty subjects who were our volunteers, fifteen experienced some therapeutic benefit from their harmaline session, and ten showed remarkable improvement of symptomatic change comparable only to that which might be expected from intensive psychotherapy.... Such improvements usually occurred spontaneously, without necessarily entailing insight into the particulars of the patient's life and conflicts. As in all cases of successful deep therapeutics, it did involve greater acceptance by the patients of their feelings and impulses and a sense of proximity to their self. (*366*)

Stafford summarizes Marlene Dobkin de Rios' findings in her book *Visionary Vine*:

> Many of the patients go to jungle Ayahuasca sessions (in the language of Western medicine) "for psychiatric help." She calls "drug healing in the Peruvian jungle . . . a very old and honored tradition of dealing with psychological problems that predates Freudian analysis by centuries." Much of the treatment is non-verbal. In some places, natives refer to Banisteriopsis as "the vine of death"— meaning that it causes one to "die," and then be "born anew." (*354*) (**DEATH**)

The disciples of Ayahuasca, from all levels of society in Ecuador, Peru, Bolivia, and Brazil, as well as Asia, Africa, and most recently, the United States, drink *yagé* for just this depth of spiritual transformation and healing. A new religion with Ayahuasca as the central sacrament is active in Brazil having "several thousand . . . members . . . and . . . satellite centers in North America and Europe" (*Metzner, 19*). These congregations are always under the guidance of a *curandero* or shamanic teacher and are now a large and important force in mainstream South American spiritual life. The church ceremony, which uses some Christian motifs, involves singing hymns with a rhythmic beat, sitting in circles and taking the drink in a formal communion, quietly undergoing the effects, and then sharing experiences and descriptions of how lives are altered. Much of the ceremony occurs in very dim light or darkness which helps elicit the visions and dreams. Stafford notes: "To minimize distractions, urban users generally gather in the jungle at night, from about 8:00 p.m. to 2:00 a.m. rather than in someone's home" (*351*). Metzner concurs: "Minimizing external vision makes it easier to pay attention to the subtler visual phenomena coming from within" (*19*). (**BLACKNESS**) Reportedly, much of what comes from these church experiences is a heightened awareness of world ecology and an intense desire to save threatened plants and animals.

This spiritual relationship with the natural world is at the heart of shamanism. Understanding this is key to understanding the Ayahuasca experience. Shamanism, simply put, is the world-view that all things are living and all living things have an interconnection. In addition, plants, animals, and even rocks are believed to hold profound wisdom for anyone open and willing to hear their message. The shaman, one with extensive personal experience of the natural world, provides guidance for those seeking communication with this spirit world. In the introduction to *Ayahuasca: Human Consciousness and the Spirits of Nature,* Metzner describes the shamanistic understanding of the herbs used to facilitate this journey:

> In the tribal societies where these plants and plant preparations are used, they are regarded as embodiments of conscious intelligent beings that only become visible in

special states of consciousness, and that can function as spiritual teachers and sources of healing power and knowledge. The plants are referred to as "medicines," a term that means more than a drug: something like a healing power or energy that can be associated with a plant, a person, an animal, even a place. They are also referred to as "plant teachers" and there are still extant traditions of many years, long initiations, and trainings in the use of these medicines.

Michael Harner, an anthropologist studying for many years the Jivaros of the Ecuadorian Amazon, originally doubted reports of experiences under the influence of Ayahuasca until he experienced it himself; de Rios describes Harner's experience:

> For several hours after drinking the brew, Harner found himself, although awake, in a world literally beyond his wildest dreams. He met bird-headed people as well as dragon-like creatures who explained that they were the true gods of this world. He enlisted the services of other spirit helpers in attempting to fly through the far reaches of the galaxy. (**FLYING/BIRDS**) He found himself transported into a trance where the supernatural (**SUPERNATURAL**) seemed natural and realized that anthropologists, including himself, had profoundly underestimated the importance of the drug in affecting native ideology.... (*Stafford, 350*)

Stafford also concludes that, "Flying and long-distance perceptions seem to be characteristic of the telepathic element of Ayahuasca" (*353*). He quotes Villavicencio, who wrote the first published report about *yagé* use:

> As for myself, I can say for a fact when I've taken *ayahuasca* I've experienced dizziness, then an aerial journey in which I recall perceiving the most gorgeous views, great cities, lofty towers, beautiful parks, and other extremely attractive objects. Many natives claim not only to see, but to travel great distances under the influence of *yagé*. (*353*)

Koch-Grünberg describes the *yagé* experiences of the Tukano Indians, indigenous to the western Amazon region of Columbia, in Furst's *Flesh of the Gods*:

> According to what the Indians tell me, everything appears to be larger and more beautiful than it is in reality. The house appears immense and splendorous. A host of people is seen, especially women. The erotic appears to play a major role in this intoxication. Huge, multicolored snakes wind themselves around the house posts. All colors are very brilliant. (87)

The *yagé* experience includes another side, Furst recounts:

> Generally, the ingestion of an infusion or maceration of Banisteriopsis is said to cause vertigo, nausea, and vomiting, followed by more or less clearly defined states of euphoria or even aggressive excitation. Suddenly, brilliantly colored hallucinations appear, which may be of sublime beauty but which may also involve anxiety, or even stark terror. Animals sometimes appear in these visions—usually felines or even reptiles. Sometimes the individual finds himself flying on the winds, visiting far off places, or communicating with divinities, demons, or tribal ancestors. (86)

The physical effects of Ayahuasca are also significant. Indians have long drawn on the aggressive power that comes with the use of *yagé* before going into battle. (**ENERGIZED/STIMULATED**) In addition, *ayahuasqueros,* or shamans, according to many who have observed them, are remarkably nimble, energetic, and have unusually smooth skin. Andrew Weil, in *The Natural Mind,* describes Luis, an old *curandero* shaman:

> He would dance out the door and we would hear him chanting and singing off into the jungle, circling the house, disappearing into the night. Then he would burst through the doorway in an explosion of feathers and palm leaves, growling like a jaguar. (*Stafford, 347*)

Some of our most important remedies, such as *Cannabis indica* and *Anhelonium* include reports of poisonings and material dose experiences in our materia medicas. In keeping with this practice the following excerpts, published in *Ayahuasca* by Dr. Metzner, are contemporary accounts of the essence of the *yagé* experience in the participants' own words:

> **Death and Rebirth in Santo Daime** by Madalena Fonseca. *This is an account by a Brazilian copywriter in her thirties of a powerful experience in the context of a Santo Daime ritual....*
>
> ...When the fire reached my throat, I became aware of restraining cords pulling from the back of my neck. I focused my attention on the cords and followed them to their source. I saw a man looking at me with a very mean expression on his face. It was a very intense and frightening moment, because I realized I was looking the enemy right in the face. His features changed to those of other men, consecutively. Some of them I recognized as brothers, uncles, cousins, grandfathers, ex-lovers, and my own father. I had very intense and painful talks and experiences with each one, and all of them ended with faces falling off like masks to reveal the face of the Devil. In these

moments I felt the presence of God and heard him say, "This is all an illusion!"

This was a pattern that lasted throughout the whole episode. It was a history of crimes, ambition, betrayal, violence, and pain. (**AGGRESSION/COMPRESSION**) I experienced both sides of sadomasochistic relationships. I was victim and tyrant at the same time. Soon the experience took on a wider aspect, and I actually felt everything every criminal and every victim had ever felt at any point in time and space. It gave me deep understanding of human pain. I cried rivers. All my resentments, shame, and guilt dissolved. I forgave humanity. I forgave myself. . . . Since this experience there's been a general sense of lightness in my life, more humor, forgiveness, acceptance, compassion, and responsibility, not only for my actions, but also for whatever happens to me. I have no doubt that work was done within the deep unconscious and that it reflects in my ordinary life. . . . (*21-22*)

Nature Has Embraced Me, Blown the Breath of Life into Me by Stefan C. . . . *in the context of the União do Vegetal, this physician in his forties relates various visions*. . .

Shortly before leaving for an expedition to South America to participate in some sessions with the União do Vegetal, I was told that a new female acquaintance, R., would be joining us. I was not pleased to hear this news. R. was recently unattached and alluring. I was encountering ambivalence about my marriage, but not to the point of wanting to leave my family. R. had apparently decided one week before our departure that she wanted to accompany me on the journey. Before informing me of this, she had purchased her ticket. The day to leave came. We traveled together to South America, to the distant Amazon. Culture shock, sleep deprivation, the excitement of our mission. Opportunities to join in ceremonies employing ayahuasca, freshly prepared from local rainforest flora. R., filled with enthusiasm, embracing our vision, bonding with our hearts.

. . . For the night of Saint John the Baptist, a special outdoors session of ayahuasca is planned. I sit adjacent to R., in a reclining chair. I settle back and close my eyes. Visions come to me, beautiful, enchanting, soft, subtle reds, blues, and greens. My body starts to gently vibrate. In my reverie, I "see" R. and myself slowly begin to elevate out of our chairs, rising, until we are suspended above the congregation, bathed in beautiful and shimmering lights of divine hue. In this celestial palace, among the union of the assembled faithful, R. and I are being joined, married. I am enraptured, overwhelmed with ecstasy. But, from the distant periphery of my consciousness, comes a sound, a question, quiet at first, then rapidly building in intensity. I listen intently and finally decipher the words. It is asking me: But what about N.? N., my wife! N., with whom I have shared the past sixteen years. N., the mother of my child. I wake from the trance. The vision of R. explodes; I suddenly fall hurtling back to earth. (**HIGH/LOW**) I am in my chair again but stunned, desperate, terrified. My world implodes, and I am cast into the darkness (**BLACKNESS**), losing all orientation. Meaning loses its thread. The knowledge accrued over a lifetime vanishes, leaving only vague outlines of what had once been an identity, a life. Language loses its coherence. I know that such a phenomenon as language exists, but I have lost all capacity to use productions of sound symbolically. I know that there is such a word as "chair" but for the life of me, I have no idea what a "chair" is. Disjointed, fragmented images swirl through my nightmarish vision. I lie there, for all eternity, trapped in this whirlwind of anguish and grief. Finally, I slowly emerge, shaken. I turn to R. She, too, has been overwhelmed and exposed. She tells me she has "seen" all of the hurtful and cruel things she has ever done to others. She has suffered the unrelenting torment of the damned. She, too, is humbled.

Years later, as I look back on this episode, the meaning is finally clear. Ayahuasca had spoken to me, yet I could not immediately acknowledge the message. Over a longer period of time than prudence or good sense should have allowed, I failed to consistently act on the teaching, and paid the price. In spite of my misguided insistence that R. and I were fated for one another, the spirit of the vine had discerned only sorrow could grow from such a union. From its ethical core, ayahuasca spoke to me that night, and revealed to me that only action based on truth and integrity can prevail. My self-delusion was laid bare, a hard yet invaluable lesson.... (*22*)

The Plant Spirits Help Me to Heal Myself and Others by Eugenia G. . . . *a pharmacist in her forties* . . .

. . . Like most of those who experienced ayahuasca, I, too, experienced the breathtaking brilliant visions of nature's plants, animals, birds, and river scenes. However, to my amazement, what happened during the ayahuasca experience was not as dramatic as what happened afterwards. . . . I realized the plant kingdom was talking to me. Plants, berries, flowers, and trees were telling me of their medicinal properties and how to use them. . . . The plant kingdom had suddenly come alive to me. . . . For months, I was haunted by dreams of plants, and how to use some of them medicinally. . . I tried to shake them off, saying herbs were folk remedies and that I represented modern science. . . . The plant kingdom continued to direct me. I experienced a spontaneous healing from an herb in my garden. . . . It's been about four years since that life-changing experience. . . . Plants and herbs have become my passion, a private and holy experience. They take me to the deepest parts of my being, my soul. After my first ayahuasca experience, all kinds of plants began to speak to me directly of their medicine and how to use them. Wherever I went I seemed to merge with plants from the fields and gardens, houseplants, and even weeds. Ayahuasca opened me up to the experience of the plant kingdom as a "way in"—a deep connection with the divine. . . . I have come to realize my life's work: I am to follow the path of a shaman-healer,

> who does visionary journeying to help others. . . . I now have a focus, a technique, and a purpose that seem to be answering questions raised by the spiritual emergence. . . . The transformative powers of ayahuasca profoundly changed my life. . . . *(25)*

In Ayahuasca, we have a formidable combination of at least two plants that produce an emotional as well as physical effect on large numbers of people who use it for spiritual experiences. Acknowledged by anthropologists throughout the world as being the most powerful and most widespread shamanic hallucinogen, research on Ayahuasca's influence is growing (*Metzner*). Recent attempts to prohibit its use have resulted in several large studies done by the Brazilian government revealing that there is no evidence of social or physical disruption in those who use it. An international team of research scientists has begun the Hoasca Project to study the long-term effects of Ayahuasca on church members. As a result, there is a growing body of research amongst anthropologists in an attempt to learn how this entheogen is used to heal illness on both the mental and physical plane. Given this level of interest, it is apparent that Ayahuasca, little known in the United States and Europe, warrants further study as a homeopathic remedy.

Ayahuasca Themes

Banisteriopsis caapi and Psychotria viridis

- *Death/Suicide*
- *Aggression/Compression*
- *Blackness*
- *Supernatural*
- *Flow/Expansion/Power*
- *Energized/Stimulated*
- *Flying/Birds*
- *High/Low*

Death/Suicide

#1 . . . The feeling of horror could be described "as if my parents were shot in front of me, or if my best friend died in front of me.". . .

#3 Later in the evening I felt total despair, suicidal. I knew I didn't really feel this way but I thought about slitting my wrists or shooting myself in the head with a gun. This was a totally new feeling for me. I knew I wouldn't kill myself. I was a witness to this emotional state. I witnessed myself feeling completely desolate. It felt like a release of something unexpressed from within me. Couldn't feel any reason to be crying, but I kept crying. I couldn't feel any reason for wanting to die, but also felt there was no reason to live. The sadness was very deep. If I was going to kill myself, I would do it quickly, with a revolver. I wouldn't write a suicide note, I just would do it quickly. . . .

#5 Dream: People dying, and the feeling was poignant, a transition. The group house was at first well populated, then everyone seemed to be dropping like flies.

#11 . . . Urge to leap out of a third floor window.

#8 . . . "Why do people have children? What is the point of life? How many people can offer things that are indispensable?" I had nihilistic feelings.

#10 I was intensely suicidal. Imagining ways of killing myself, by taking too much aspirin or slicing my wrists.

#11 Dream: About Yama, the god of death, coming toward me with large, red, fiery nostrils. I opened, and he melted into me, then peace. This is a recurrent dream I've had, but this time I felt open and fearless, and death seems irrelevant.

#5 Dream: I stopped dreaming about the past and started dreaming about death, but it wasn't disturbing at all. . . . [I dreamt that] a woman at the group house died of cancer.

#11 Dream: . . . Sense of death and destruction is just another expression of universal energy.

(de Rios, ref. Stafford) In some places, natives refer to Banisteriopsis as "the vine of death"—meaning that it causes one to "die," and then be "born anew."

Aggression/Compression

#4 During that vacation week I felt very put upon. I felt boxed in, that there were expectations of me, that I had to act a certain way, and it was driving me crazy. I didn't want to be told how to act. I didn't want any kind of regimented behavior, and I felt very agitated by that. . . .

#1 . . . I feel aggressive towards others and don't feel like taking shit from anyone. This hyper-aggressiveness is unusual for me.

#2 I felt a sense of compression. . . .

#8 Dream: Driving my motorcycle off the road onto the shoulder, but then got the bike back onto the road. I consciously woke up when I saw a cop in my rear view mirror.

#2 I was confrontational, aggressive, not wanting to take any shit from anybody, a bit impulsive. . . .

#10 I felt angry, distrustful and closed.

#8 Felt physically tired, uptight and alienated. . . .

#7 Dream: I lost my temper when someone tried to take my toast. I was making lunch for the next day, preparing it the way I like it, and someone salted it for me, and I lost my temper and stormed away.

#1 I feel horrible, very aggressive and irritable. I only want to stop it. It is outside of the parameters of what I expected from the remedy. It feels like I am coming down from a bad acid trip, and there is nothing to be done about it. I still feel in touch with reality, but I am not coalesced in one spot. Feel a little mentally unbalanced and also feel stoned.

#7 Dream: Confrontational dream of a stranger walking around the house, and friend made sure the man had reason for being there. (Usually he doesn't confront people.)

#8 Dream: An innocuous pill that was actually a bomb that made a huge hole in someone's front yard. I avoided the authorities.

Blackness

#1 ... By 2 a.m. I was very agitated, as if Pandora's box was opened in my chest and in my head, with blackness, and unnamable horror coming out of me. It was very uncomfortable. It went on and on. I couldn't put a name on any of it. It was blackness.

#10 Dream: Black gulls circled off the ocean over a castle, they landed on the ramparts and were called to fight. . . .

#1 ... It came as an unbroken river of black emotion, grief, sorrow, weight, thickness. . . .

#3 ... I wondered about what the remedy was and felt it was like a black widow spider would feel, busy, shiny and black and alone. Felt self-destructive.

#10 Dream: . . . There were enemies of the crow in the shadows, in the dark, which came over to attack the crow. . . . Of imprisonment and black birds. . . . The dark side was more prevalent.

(Stefan C., ref. Metzner) I am in my chair again but stunned, desperate, terrified. My world implodes, and I am cast into the darkness, losing all orientation.

Supernatural

#5 I would often have fear of ghosts in the past, and when I took this remedy, I had intensification of that fear. Had the feeling that there was something in my room, but it didn't bother me as much.

#4 Had first feeling of some force moving on a different level—like ghosts. I was working late at night . . . when I had a creepy feeling that something was coming down the hallway to get me. I felt afraid of ghosts, and kept feeling that something was watching me. . .

#5 Dream: I was entering a dark room, and seeing a red and blue, foot high, elf-like marionette man. The next day I was thinking about it, and realized as a child that kind of dream would have terrified me. The issue was seeing something in the room that wasn't supposed to be there. It wasn't a monster, but it wasn't right.

#4 . . . I was convinced that the upstairs of the house we were staying in was haunted. There was a closed up room behind the main upstairs bedroom, and the door was covered with an old blanket. It felt like something was wrong up there. The last night I put up my teachers' pictures and lit some incense, thinking that if they (the ghosts) were going to do something, this was their last chance.

#1 . . . During the first five or six nights, I had incredible meditations. I had increased ability to see things as the big picture. Able to get quiet and focused quickly. Had more psychic ability to see into things. Some of the best meditation I've ever had. Able to keep my mind very quiet. . . .

#1 . . . Felt like I was on drugs, like reality could shift.

#6 Dream: About M. who died. There was a big Ganesh statue, and M. was there. M. took me to other planes [of existence.—Ed.]

(Eugenia G., ref. Metzner) After my first ayahuasca experience, all kinds of plants began to speak to me directly of their medicine and how to use them. Wherever I went I seemed to merge with plants from the fields and gardens, houseplants, and even weeds. Ayahuasca opened me up to the experience of the plant kingdom as a "way in"—a deep connection with the divine. . .

Flow/Expansion/Power

#11 . . . I had a sense of calmness, shoulders relaxing, expansiveness of breath, everything was floating up to my head and expanding outward. . . . a feeling of relaxation through my whole body. . . . My right sacroiliac pain lessened significantly. . . . Lungs and chest felt fuller, able to take in more air, sense of lightness and fluidity. I had easier meditation. . . . Aware of keenness of sight and hearing. Increase of peripheral vision.

#1 . . . There was a flowing out from my chest and head. Every bad experience I ever had was flowing out of me. All the compacted emotional energy, all the grief and sadness within me was coming out, like a river. It seemed infinite, and I wasn't sure how long I could go through it. It came as an unbroken river of black emotion, grief, sorrow, weight, thickness. It wasn't fearful. The horror was that it kept coming out like a flood. I started out hating the remedy, but ended up loving it, as I ended up having a feeling of power and confidence. . . .

#1 Mental state now in steady rhythm. Sense of expansiveness, sense of power, assertiveness, capability. Ability to reach quiet mental state quickly and stay focused longer.

#4 I was doing some hatha yoga exercises, and I made a discovery. When I sat in a certain way, and shifted my weight back into my pelvis, there was a feeling of release through my whole lower body for the first time. Every little tiny muscle released. There was a feeling of a flow through the pelvis and down through my legs. Was able to actually isolate and feel a flow into aching area of left hip area. I had the feeling that something had shifted and that the problem was going to go away at some point.

#11 Feeling a sense of expansion and breath. Awareness of connectedness of everything and lack of distinct boundaries. . . .

#3 Woke happy and refreshed, felt euphoric. . . . This euphoria is one of extreme happiness. It is consistent and long lasting. This is a state of being awake, energetic and grounded, not spacey. It's a very free feeling. It is just great to have all these things happening at once.

#1 I felt a sense of being strong in myself, of moving from my own center, with an increased sense of power. Physical energy good. . . .

#10 Feeling expansive, open, relaxed, sexual, opposite of the previous days.

Energized/Stimulated

#3 . . . After the remedy, I was wide awake right away. This was a big change. I liked that, as I could wake up and do things right away. It was like caffeine, without the nervousness, almost like amphetamines, at times. . . . What I liked most about the remedy is that my energy was even and consistent from the time I woke up to the time I went to bed, even if I stayed up late. It wasn't fast or speedy, I just never got tired. Normally I get tired from 3–7 p.m., but on the proving I never felt fatigued. . . .

#4 For the next few days I felt even, a lot of energy, felt great, almost like I had too much energy, didn't know what to do with it. I felt great overall.

#2 . . . Energy high. Impatience. Awoke tired. It felt like too much caffeine.

#3 My thoughts felt very clear, clearer than normal. Normally my thoughts are fuzzy and dull, and my thinking is difficult. It's like wading through something. On this remedy I thought so clearly, it reminded me of how my thoughts were in the past. . . . On the remedy I got lots of work done, good mental capabilities. . . . I lost my craving for caffeine and sweets, right from the first day of the remedy.

#2 I felt agitation, excitement, tense energy, like taking amphetamines. . . .

#10 . . . Body felt energized from exercise of the previous day.

#3 . . . Felt so much energy in my body. It was an odd combination of tension and despair. . . .

Flying/Birds

#10 Dream: Black gulls circled off the ocean over a castle, they landed on the ramparts, and were called to fight. I was a bird, flying down to the ground. . . . I also felt like a bird in temperament, looking out over her shoulder, constantly watching for danger. A three-foot tall crow with a neck chain. . . .

#11 Saw a jay outside and thought it would be easy to fly. . . . Feeling close to birds and having an urge for flying. . . . Picking cherries, and had an urge to jump out of the cherry picker and fly. I had the feeling that I could fly and had to restrain myself.

#6 . . . Had quick images of a bee on a flower, fly wings and a feather.

#9 Dream: Flying in a forest. At first it was fun, then I lost the ability to fly and became fearful, hanging onto a branch high up in a tree, and felt scared of falling, and not knowing how to get down from the tree. I lost my previous feeling of confidence in flying.

#11 Ran up the mountain, with an urge to leap out into space at the top of the mountain, as if I am so light that the wind could carry me. . . . Urge to fly whenever I am at any height. Urge to leap out of a third floor window.

#6 Dream: . . . Swinging on a swing, trying to get high enough so that I could flip off of it.

(Furst) Sometimes the individual finds himself flying on the winds, visiting far off places, or communicating with divinities, demons, or tribal ancestors.

(Villavicencio, ref. Stafford) As for myself, I can say for a fact when I've taken ayahuasca I've experienced dizziness, then an aerial journey in which I recall perceiving the most gorgeous views, great cities, lofty towers, beautiful parks . . .

(de Rios, ref. Stafford) . . . Harner found himself, although awake, in a world literally beyond his wildest dreams. He met bird-headed people as well as dragon-like creatures who explained that they were the true gods of this world. He enlisted the services of other spirit helpers in attempting to fly through the far reaches of the galaxy.

High/Low

#4 . . . As I was going up over the bridge, it felt like I was leaving my body, starting at the feet. I started to come up and out of my body. I quickly suppressed that feeling because I hated it.

#6 . . . Swinging on a swing, trying to get high enough so that I could flip off of it.

#9 Dream: . . . hanging onto a branch high up in a tree, and felt scared of falling, and not knowing how to get down from the tree. . . .

#11 Ran up the mountain, with an urge to leap out into space at the top of the mountain, as if I am so light that the wind could carry me. Had the desire to feel my body falling and striking the earth. . . .

(Stefan C., ref. Metzner) My body starts to gently vibrate. In my reverie, I "see" R. and myself slowly begin to elevate out of our chairs, rising, until we are suspended above the congregation, bathed in beautiful and shimmering lights of divine hue. . . . The vision of R. explodes; I suddenly fall hurtling back to earth. I am in my chair again but stunned, desperate, terrified.

AYAHUASCA RUBRICS *Banisteriopsis caapi & Psychotria viridis*

MIND
    ACTIVITY; clairvoyant, like that of a
      increased excessively
      morning
      waking on
    AGITATION; with any kind of regimented behavior
      waking on
    AGGRESSION
      oppressive
    ALTERNATING STATES
      talkative and wanting to be alone
    ANGER, irascibility
    ANXIETY
      food would not be there if she didn't eat it right away
      speaking, when; talk in company, on attempting to
    AVERSION; interference
      being told how to act
      people asking stupid questions
    AWARENESS heightened
      connectedness of everything
      of body
    CALM
    CALMNESS
    CHEERFUL
    CLAIRVOYANT
    CLARITY OF THOUGHTS
    COMPANY; aversion to
      solitude, fond of
    CONFIDENCE; increased
    CONFRONTATIONAL
    DANCING (Weil)
    DELUSIONS
      act; a certain way, she had to
      animals, of
        birds; he is a
          fly, and it would be easy to
        spiders;
          feeling as a black widow would
      blackness
        unnamable horror flowing out from his chest and head, unable to stop it, with
      body; leaving her body, she was
        expanded, is
        chest and head
      boundaries are not distinct between objects
      boxed in, she felt
      colors, brilliant (Koch-Grünberg)
      compression
      demons, communicating with (Furst)

    dragon like creatures, bird-headed people (Harner)
    drug trip; as if coming down from, bad
    dying;
       his best friend died in front of him
    emotional energy was coming out of him like a river, like a flood
    enemy; surrounded by
    expansion; of self
       of breath
    fly, it would be easy to
    flying; far reaches of galaxy (Harner)
    ghosts; coming to get her
       are watching her
         pursued; he was; ghosts, by
    God, the divine, communicating with (Fonseca)
    grief and sadness flowing out of him like a flood
    house;
       haunted, is
         upstairs of the house is
    heads; off, he could take people's
    horror; as if his parents were shot in front of him
    light; incorporeal, he is
       lightness and fluidity, of
    nature, embraced me, blew breath of life into me (Stefan C., ref. Metzner)
    Pandora's box is opening in his chest and unnamable horror is coming out of him
    reality, not in touch with
    snakes, brilliant colored, huge (Koch-Grünberg)
    tribal ancestors, communicating with (Furst)
    unbroken river of black emotion, grief, sorrow, weight, thickness
    visions, animals, felines, reptiles (Furst)
       beauty, sublime (Furst)
       cities, great, towers, lofty, aerial views (Furst)
       devil, revealed the face of the (Fonseca, ref. Metzner)
       light, beautiful, shimmering, divine hue, bathed in (Stefan C., ref. Metzner)
       palace, celestial, saw (Stefan C., ref. Metzner)
    watched; that she is being
DESIRES; leap out into space, to
DESPAIR
    releasing something unexpressed within her
    witnessing herself feeling desolate
DETACHED
    as if the experience of living is about a sense of herself, not about what she does
DISCONNECTED, people from
DREAM, as if in
DREAMS
    affair, mother confessed to having
    amorous
    anger
    animals, of
      birds, of
        black
        black gulls circling off the ocean
        fighting birds
        she is a bird
        three foot tall crow with sharp teeth was her pet

fights, of
   between a bear, who could not contain his contempt, and the enemy
flying, of
   she is a bird
lion, that he was a
mice, doing dissection on, saw pain and felt horrible
rat, experiments on and almost bite her
rats
salamanders with cucumber like sections of seed pods
snakes
   being naked with snakes of different size in the forest
spiders; Brown Recluse
apartment, brother and parents moving in, no room
anxious
avoiding authorities
   powerful and controlling
beach with lots of people but no one to play with
beautiful, things were more
birdfeeders too costly to maintain by government
birthday cake, making, but sister ate half of the dough
body; parts of
   foot, someone shot my
   hacked up and gruesome
bomb, an innocuous pill that was a bomb
brother, wanting to be with him but can't
buildings, high rise
children, about; babies
chocolate bars
cleaning with vacuum cleaner
coition; of, with a classmate, professor says "have fun"
colorful
condoms, cleaning up, one broke and sprayed on her
country; Central America
crossing a bridge with a limp, push self on rails, didn't want to be in anyone's way
darkness
death, of; dying, of
   destruction as an expression of universal energy
   fearless; death is irrelevant
   people, feeling it was a poignant transition
   woman of, by cancer
   Yama, God of Death
distorted, face is, thick and swollen
driving a car
   holding a baby
   in New York City, with his brother
driving his motorcycle off the road
dying, people are, feels poignant
elf-like man, foot high and red and blue
enemies
errand boy, he was
escape, of
falling; high places, from
family, own
father holding a baby like he used to hold her

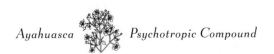

fetus, she is the size of a, lying in her teacher's chair
food
   messenger girl delivering food to her
   rendering his guru's food inedible
   waiting a long time for food to be prepared
friends
   meeting, of
   old, of
   seeing, of
frightening, fear of falling from a tree
Ganesh statue
girl, of, and her benefactor
graduating, everybody she knows is
head
   a bloody wound to the back of a man's head; masonry fell under him to cradle
     his head, taking care of him
house, old, that she grew up in
houses, of
   doing carpentry on a house
humiliation
imprisonment
job, he had not done the job right
judgmental about an irresponsible person
magic
man in black leather doing a lip synch
mansion, exploring a big, empty
marionette
meditating with big rocks as cushions
men
   Chinese, watching her
   gay, having relations with women for politics
   tap dancing
mentally retarded kid in a marching band being trained in right and wrong
movie, watching it and in it at same time
museum, going with father to
musical instruments, a room full of
nightmare
Nityananda's hand on her forehead
outhouse
past, of the
peeling signs and surfaces, like scabs
penis infected with worms
places, Central America
planes
plants, wanting to buy
professor, who made sexual innuendo
realistic
sexual abuse
singing messenger girl
smell, old and musty
snow, catching buses in a storm, of
socks, colorful
something in room which isn't supposed to be there
strangers, of
   confronting, walking around the house

   strip tease dance
   supernatural things
   taking orders from customers
   threats
   tornado happening
   town, that she grew up in
   train, going somewhere
   treasure, hidden, like a secret gold mine
   tree, hanging onto a high branch
   tricks, of
   vacation
   vertigo
     on a bridge looking down the grid
   vivid
   walking, of
     in the mountains
   war
   war; American Revolution
   wedding
     two friends in the tropics, of
     women wore red silk dresses
ENERGY, as if on amphetamines
  as if on caffeine
EUPHORIA
EXCITEMENT, excitable
FASTIDIOUS
FEAR, bridges, crossing
  ghosts, of
  ghosts, of; night
  narrow place, in, claustrophobia
  pursuit, of
FEARLESSNESS
  of death or change
FLOWING feeling during yoga class through her muscles
FLY, desire to
FORGIVENESS; forgave humanity (Fonseca, ref. Metzner)
  forgave myself (Fonseca, ref. Metzner)
FORSAKEN, feeling
  isolation, sensation of
  peace with his loneliness, at
FREEDOM remarkable, in doing what he had to do
GRATITUDE
  nurtured feeling
HOME; desires to, go
HOMESICKNESS, nostalgia
HURRY, haste
  occupation, in
IMPATIENCE
IMPULSE, morbid
  to leap into space at mountaintop
  to feel body falling and striking the earth
  to swing so high I could flip off of the swing
IMPULSIVE
INDIFFERENCE

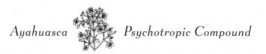

        apathy
        starting a new job
INDUSTRIOUS; mania for work
INQUISITIVE; supernatural or spiritual matters, about
IRRITABLE; from being cold
JOY
JUMP, impulse to
MEDITATION; deep, profound
    during with acrid tears
MOOD; oppressive
NIHILISTIC
POWER; increased sense of
RELAXED feeling, letting go
SADNESS, despondency, dejection, mental depression, gloom, melancholy
SELF-CONTROL
SENSES; acute
SENSITIVE, oversensitive; everything, to
    noise, to
SINGING (Weil)
STARTING, startled; easily
STRENGTH increased, mental
SUICIDAL disposition
    despair, from
    delusions, from
    self-destructive
    shooting, by
    slicing her wrists, by
    taking too much aspirin, by
    weeping
    would not write a note, just do it quickly
SUSPICIOUS, mistrustful
    self-destructive
THOUGHTS; clearness of
    creative
    morbid
TRANCE-LIKE states (Harner)
TRANQUILITY
    calmness
    serenity, waiting, while
WEEPING, tearful mood
    causeless; knowing why, without
    easily
    inconsolable
    sad news, to
    sensitive, being teased, to
WEEPY

HEAD   HAIR; affections of
        falling out; offensive
        greasy

EYE   DISCOLORATION; conjunctiva, red
    LACHRYMATION; left
    REDNESS; left

VISION	ACUTE	
NOSE	SNEEZING	
	morning	
HEARING	ACUTE	
FACE	BURNT; marks down her, by acrid tears	

VISION ACUTE

NOSE SNEEZING
　morning

HEARING ACUTE

FACE BURNT; marks down her, by acrid tears
DISCOLORATION; eyes, under
ERUPTIONS; acne
　herpes
　lips; upper
PAIN; jaws
　drawing; jaws, right
　spasm; jaws, right

STOMACH NAUSEA; alcohol, from
THIRST; afternoon
　four p.m.

RECTUM CONSTIPATION; difficult stool
　flatulence, with
　painful
　strain, must
　urging; ineffectual
PAIN; general; stool, after

FEMALE MENSES; clotted, coagulated
　frequent, too early, too soon
　mucous
　painful, dysmenorrhea

CHEST PAIN; burning
　burning; sides; inspiration, during
　sides; pressure agg.
　sides; right
PALPITATION heart; lying, while; side, right; amel.

BACK TENSION; cervical region; sleep, during, causing insomnia and frustration

EXTREMITIES CRACKED skin; feet; soles
ERUPTION; general; itching
　general; rash
　upper limbs; itching
　lower limbs
　lower limbs; rash; itching
　rash; itching
ITCHING; upper limbs
　upper limbs; afternoon

EXTREMITY PAIN
GENERAL; waking, on
ACHING; upper limbs
　wrist

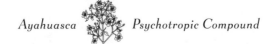

                              BURNING, foot, sole, left
                                  upper limbs
                                  upper limbs; afternoon
                                  lower limbs; foot; walking, while
                                  inflamed cracks
                              PULSATING; hand; right
                              SORE, bruised
                                  upper limbs, as if doing too much massage, but hadn't done any
                                  foot, sole
                              STIFFNESS; hip
                              STINGING, foot, sole, left
                                  upper limbs; shoulder; right

PERSPIRATION   ODOR; chocolate
                                  metallic

SLEEP   POSITION; abdomen, on
                                  hands under thighs
                                  side, on; left
                              SLEEPLESSNESS; fear, fright, from
                                  from of ghosts
                              UNREFRESHING
                              WAKING, happy
                                  refreshed

GENERALITIES   ACTIVITY; increased
                              FOOD and drinks;
                                ailments from
                                alcohol; agg.
                                aversion
                                mustard, desires
                                sweets; desires
                              SENSATION as if flowing while doing yoga
                              WEAKNESS, enervation
                              WEARINESS; afternoon

JOURNALS..*Ayahuasca*

EDITOR'S NOTE: *Punctuation, abbreviations, and individual stylistic nuances of the original journal entries have been preserved wherever possible.*

> **Prover #1 • Male • 37 years old**

Day 1
◆ Took first dose about 10:00 a.m. Immediately felt a little "stoned" and also felt a sense of expansion in my head and chest, a kind of a high, a good feeling. By 9 p.m. that night I felt more intense symptoms, was agitated, uncomfortable in myself, like coming down off a bad drug trip, where you don't quite have touch with reality, where you can't touch the markers of where you are. By 2 a.m. I was very agitated, as if Pandora's box was opened in my chest and in my head, with blackness, and unnamable horror coming out of me. It was very uncomfortable. It went on and on. I couldn't put a name on any of it. It was blackness.
◆ I didn't sleep much.
◆ I felt I was in a bad place in myself. I wanted to antidote the remedy. I went over to Starbucks and had a cup of decaf coffee, in attempt to antidote the remedy.

Day 2
◆ I feel horrible, very aggressive and irritable. I only want to stop it. It is outside of the parameters of what I expected from the remedy. It feels like I am coming down from a bad acid trip, and there is nothing to be done about it. I still feel in touch with reality, but I am not coalesced in one spot. Feel a little mentally unbalanced and also feel stoned.
◆ My eyes are very glassy.
◆ Tried to antidote remedy with a cup of decaf coffee because I felt like I was in a terrible place in myself. A place where I would never EVER be by choice. The coffee didn't antidote it though.
◆ There was still a sense of expansion associated with the feelings of dread but I couldn't get past all the blackness coming out of me to enjoy it or go with the expansion.

Day 3
◆ It has come down a notch. Still feel aggressive, not happy with myself. I feel an expansion in my head and center of my chest, but it's not filled with darkness anymore. I feel aggressive towards others and don't feel like taking shit from anyone. This hyper-aggressiveness is unusual for me.
◆ Got in touch with supervisor at noon and she told me not to try to antidote it anymore. She said to ride it out.
◆ Rest of the day was agitated, didn't feel like being around anyone. Felt like I was on drugs, like reality could shift.

- Went to sleep early, exhausted at 10:00 p.m.
- Skin felt warm, tingling, but seemed to feel porous as if I couldn't really tell where skin ended.

Day 4
- Woke up feeling a little more balanced but still agitated. Sense of dread emanating from head and chest almost gone. Still feel sense of expansion beyond my mind and physical body. Took a long nap today, kind of tired and emotionally worn out.
- Eating normal, all physical aspects normal.
- Felt kind of angry, pissed off and a little agitated. Feelings of imbalance gone.
- Still feel a sense of expansiveness coming from center of head and chest. Also general feeling of being a little pissed off, but not agitated.
- Psychic abilities improved as if I can see internal or external things from above—as a whole—a sense of greater perspective.
- Had one of my best meditation classes ever. Was able to get very quiet and still and keep out of my head for entire period.

Day 5
- Continued sense of expansiveness, but today combined with a lot of agitation. Also sense of power—physical and something more. Feeling very aggressive, like I'm not going to take shit from anyone.

Day 6
- Feel kind of fuzzy and stoned; a little out of it today. Mental energy very fuzzy, hard to tune into things. It was a lot of work to get through the day.
- I felt a sense of being strong in myself, of moving from my own center, with an increased sense of power. Physical energy good. Eating stayed the same. The only real change was the emotional things.
- Went out for a few drinks at night. Usually never drink. Usually after one or two drinks I have a three-day hangover. Drank four drinks with little hangover effect.

Day 7
- It's easier for me to quiet my mind during morning meditation. And easier for me to get quieter during my day.
- Still have sense of aggressiveness, although it's not like I'm looking for a fight.
- More ready to stand my ground in any confrontation.
- Hearing is more sensitive and sharper.
- Eating a lot more carbohydrates this week. Examples are pizza, spaghetti, etc. Feel more of a sense of grounded determination, too, over last week.

Day 8
- Same sorts of mental feelings. Head clear, sense of confidence, determination.
- Meditation sessions continue to be better—quieter, deeper.
- Physical things—appetite, digestion, elimination—no real change over normal state.

Day 11
- Mental state now in steady rhythm. Sense of expansiveness, sense of power, assertiveness, capability. Ability to reach quiet mental state quickly and stay focused longer.
- General well state of feeling and being.
- Eating more cheese and carbos. Poops regular, one time a day—well formed.

Day 12
- After this the remedy seems to have worn off. Back to "normal."

Comments:
The aggression died down by the sixth or seventh day. By the twelfth day, I was back to my regular state, almost without my noticing it. During the first five or six nights, I had incredible meditations. I had increased ability to see things as the big picture. Able to get quiet and focused quickly. Had more psychic ability to see into things. Some of the best meditation I've ever had. Able to keep my mind very quiet. That was a great thing about the remedy. Since the remedy has worn off, this has dissipated. On day six I felt stoned, out of it. Dreams were not out of the ordinary, just situational dreams, just bits and pieces of things.

The feeling of horror could be described "as if my parents were shot in front of me, or if my best friend died in front of me." There was a sense of not being able to stop it. There was a flowing out from my chest and head. Every bad experience I ever had was flowing out of me. All the compacted emotional energy, all the grief and sadness within me was coming out, like a river. It seemed infinite, and I wasn't sure how long I could go through it. It came as an unbroken river of black emotion, grief, sorrow, weight, thickness. It wasn't fearful. The horror was that it kept coming out like a flood. I started out hating the remedy, but ended up loving it, as I ended up having a feeling of power and confidence, and had great meditations while on it. The anger was a product of me being overly agitated for too long, and that got me pissed off.

Prover #2 • Male • 46 years old

Day 1
- I felt a sense of compression. Concentration good, mind a bit worried.
- Energy throughout was mid to high.
- Frequent urination at night, which is unusual for me.
- Deep sleep, woke up rested.
- I was supervising service day at the house, and I felt some aggression. People weren't moving fast enough for me, people were acting stupid, asking stupid questions that were irritating to me. Felt I could take people's heads off. There was a feeling of agitation. I felt agitated while being videotaped to provide instruction about the masonry project.
- As the day went on, I felt more centered, my emotions settled down, and I felt a feeling of joy.

Day 2
- I felt agitation, excitement, tense energy, like taking amphetamines. Felt sense of compression—concentration good and mind worried. Energy level mid to high. It wasn't a nervous energy.
- Urinated three times between 11:30 p.m. and 5:30 a.m.
- Shoulders tight—little pain.
- Woke early, 4–5 a.m. Deep sleep, woke up rested. Low tolerance for others. Feeling tired.

Day 3
- I was confrontational, aggressive, not wanting to take any shit from anybody, a bit impulsive. Irritated, agitated—felt people I worked with were not moving fast enough—impatient.
- Felt alienation from close friend even.
- Head tight.
- Energy level high. As day went on became more centered—mind clearer—emotion settled. Feeling of joy. No significant sex drive.

Day 4
- Agitation, excitement, intense energy (like I had taken amphetamine). Energy level high.
- Low tolerance with others.
- Cough light.
- Sleep restless, awoke feeling tired—5:00 a.m.
- I had to go high up on scaffolding, and felt a little nervous going up, but once up on top felt fearless.
- Concentration was very sharp. Felt strong, fearless, it was a good feeling. The agitation was going down.

Day 5
◆ Agitation—confrontational—little patience, impulsive. Energy high. Impatience. Awoke tired. It felt like too much caffeine.
◆ Mind wasn't quiet, it was noisy.

Day 6
◆ Strong, fearless—work on a building 30 ft. off ground—calm, strong, clear—no fear.
◆ Woke 4:30 a.m.
◆ From there on it was fading. My energy stayed high, but I became more calm. No significant dreams, no physical symptoms.
◆ Impatience, irritability and agitation were the key feelings.

Day 7
◆ Like too much caffeine. Excitable—not quiet, noisy mind. Energy level high. Sleep restful.

Day 8
◆ Calm, enthusiastic. Energy level high. Legs, back stiff. Pain in knees.

Day 9
◆ Calm, enthusiastic. Energy level high. Sleep deep.

Day 10
◆ Relaxed, calm. Upbeat. Energy level high.

Day 11
◆ Quiet, calm, happy. Energy level high. After hiking—got chilled. Felt dizzy, chest—right side hurt—face flushed.

Day 12
◆ Calm, relaxed. Energy level high.

Day 13
◆ Relaxed, happy. Energy level mid. Cough—mild.

Day 14
◆ Worried—happy—calm. Energy level mid to high. Cough—mild.

Day 15
◆ Calm, relaxed. Energy level tired to mid. Sleep deep. Woke up tired.

Day 16
◆ Agitated—somewhat—got calm as day went on. Energy level tired—mid. Thirsty.

Day 17
◆ Agitated. Energy level mid. Woke up tired. Druggy.

Day 18
◆ Agitation. Energy level mid. Woke up tired.

Day 19
◆ Energy level high.

Day 20
◆ Relaxed, calm—happy. Energy level high. Blister on throat.

Day 21
◆ Relaxed, calm—happy. Blisters on throat.

Day 22
◆ Relaxed, calm, happy.

Prover #3 • Female • 38 years old

I loved the remedy.

Day 1
◆ The first morning I woke up very refreshed, which is unusual for me. I normally wake up feeling fuzzy in the head, partly in a dream state. After the remedy, I was wide awake right away. This was a big change. I liked that, as I could wake up and do things right away. It was like caffeine, without the nervousness, almost like amphetamines, at times.
◆ What I liked most about the remedy is that my energy was even and consistent from the time I woke up to the time I went to bed, even if I stayed up late. It wasn't fast or speedy, I just never got tired. Normally I get tired from 3–7 p.m., but on the proving I never felt fatigued. Sometimes a little impatient.
◆ My thoughts felt very clear, clearer than normal. Normally my thoughts are fuzzy and dull, and my thinking is difficult. It's like wading through something. On this remedy I thought so clearly, it reminded me of how my thoughts were in the past.
◆ On the remedy I got lots of work done, good mental capabilities.
◆ I lost my craving for caffeine and sweets, right from the first day of the remedy.
◆ Appetite was average, thirst was average.
◆ No stool—very unusual for me. I did not feel constipated.
◆ Slept very deeply. Knew I had a lot of dreams, but woke up so fast that I couldn't recall them—a purple bird is about all I could remember.
◆ Felt very cheerful and energetic overall.

Day 2
- Woke happy and refreshed, felt euphoric.
- Also noticed that before the remedy I had lots of mucous in my nose, and that went away.
- An old symptom came up, I developed deep cracks in the heels, so painful I couldn't walk on my heels, with some bleeding—especially right heel. Very inflamed and painful. I am unable to step down on it. Heels usually only worse from caffeine but I'm not having caffeine and my heels reacted.
- Red blotches on my face after shower. Unusual.
- This euphoria is one of extreme happiness. It is consistent and long lasting. This is a state of being awake, energetic and grounded, not spacey. It's a very free feeling. It is just great to have all these things happening at once.

Day 3
- I woke cheerful and relaxed, and this persisted, even though I spent the day with my parents, with whom I am usually impatient. I was more able to relax, not just work all the time. For the first time in months just sat around a bit. Usually I work/do things around the house all the time. Had good level of energy all day.
- Started sleeping on my left side, usually sleep on right side.
- Got my period—only 15 days after last period ended. Normal for me is about 21 days apart although there was a time last year that I got my period every two weeks for about four months.
- Cracks in feet became extremely inflamed and painful to walk. Soaked in Epsom salts and hot water—at first didn't help. Later feet felt less inflamed.
- Dream: B. and M. (a couple who are friends) got married. Their house was in the tropics. The wedding rings were made out of tropical wood. Two women were embroidering a special gown. Our teacher called to see how things were going. The women wore red silk dresses. The dream felt like the future, like something that really happened. It was very realistic, as if these things could really happen. The feeling was happy.

Day 4
- Energy level was good, although a little lower than previous days—but probably due to my period.
- Less mucous in nose and throat than usual.
- Soft stool.
- Cracked feet getting better—bathed with oil and used lots of moisturizer—helped as well.
- I had been warm, but I felt chilly. But also the weather had gotten a little colder. Got irritable from being cold, was wearing more clothes. Better from a hot bath.
- Slept on left side.
- Dreams: Could not remember my dreams. Notice that since remedy it is easier for me to get up in the morning—feel more refreshed and more mentally alert upon waking. Far less desire for caffeine or sweets.

Day 5
- I woke up feeling happy. Had energy all day.
- Started to feel very emotional in the late afternoon—five- or six-ish, teary eyed. I cried during meditation, which isn't so unusual for me. What was unusual was that the tears were acrid, and they left burn marks down my face. I was in a happy mood afterwards.
- On remedy I have a much harder time remembering my dreams. There is a greater distinction between my sleep and my wake states—meaning when I wake up I feel more awake immediately, as if I sharply left the dream state and then can't remember dreams. I previously would feel very dreamy waking up and have a harder time thinking, talking or functioning upon waking but I would more easily remember dreams.

Day 6
- I woke up feeling irritated. Good energy level but felt very tense and irritable all day. Felt strong energy moving through my body. Felt very emotional in late afternoon. Had uncontrollable tears, even though nothing had happened to upset me.
- Later in the evening I felt total despair, suicidal. I knew I didn't really feel this way but I thought about slitting my wrists or shooting myself in the head with a gun. This was a totally new feeling for me. I knew I wouldn't kill myself. I was a witness to this emotional state. I witnessed myself feeling completely desolate. It felt like a release of something unexpressed from within me. Couldn't feel any reason to be crying, but I kept crying. I couldn't feel any reason for wanting to die, but also felt there was no reason to live. The sadness was very deep. If I was going to kill myself, I would do it quickly, with a revolver. I wouldn't write a suicide note, I just would do it quickly. Wanted to be alone, and was averse to company. Consolation would have pissed me off. Couldn't sleep, muscles in neck very tight. Felt unsettled and tense. Felt frustrated from not being able to sleep. Felt so much energy in my body. It was an odd combination of tension and despair. I wondered about what the remedy was and felt it was like a black widow spider would feel, busy, shiny and black and alone. Felt self-destructive.
- I wanted to be alone. I felt self-destructive, not violent toward anyone else. It was an internal experience.

Day 7
- I woke up very sad, despairing. All day long I had easy tears. Someone was joking with me, and I said, "Don't kid with me, because I'll start crying." I was very sensitive to any kidding or sad news. Extremely sensitive. Would cry for no reason at all. Better in the afternoon and evening.
- Still had consistent good energy, not tired. Went between being talkative and wanting to be alone, moody. When feeling up I was talkative, and when down, I wanted to be alone. I felt better alone during the despair. Worked until 11 p.m., and wasn't even tired.
- Tears were no longer burning, but they weren't salty either.
- Still on period! Long time for me.

Day 8
- I was happy, energetic, back to the euphoric state. Open, happy, even, and stable! Still on period!

Day 9
- Felt remedy was wearing off. Energy was lower overall, thinking less clear.
- Period ended.
- Sleeping on left side.
- Everything was reverting back to my old state, felt fuzzy in the head.
- I'm still sleeping on the left side, but everything else is gone.
- Bothersome back pain in the upper back, then in the lower back, then on the left side, then the right side.
- I felt impatient that the group didn't meet last week as planned, because I wanted to get more of the remedy, and couldn't get more of the remedy.

Prover #4 • Female • 42 years old

Day 1
- When I first took the remedy I got very tired.
- Dream: I went with friends to a plant nursery, and I looked at plants I wanted to buy. Then I went to a big, empty mansion at the end of a lot that I explored; it was completely empty.

Day 2
- For the next few days I felt even, a lot of energy, felt great, almost like I had too much energy, didn't know what to do with it. I felt great overall.

Day 3
- After a few days my energy went back down to normal, even, but not like it had been before.
- Had some symptoms in my legs and feet. At bottom of the left foot, there was a feeling that a blood vessel had burst, hot and stinging, and a bruise in the center of my foot. Deep aches and cramping in the legs, not better from propping them up. It felt like varicose veins, like little blood vessels were breaking inside my legs. This is something that I had felt in the past.

Day 4
- Dream: A group of people were cleaning my teacher's apartment, and he left for the airport.

Day 5
- I had aching in my left sacroiliac joint, which is a chronic complaint that flared up. In the past my legs would give out from under me while walking, but that didn't happen, it was just aching. I got nervous, because I was about to go on vacation the following week, and didn't want to have trouble with my back again. I was careful about my activities. I was looking forward to my vacation.

- My energy level was even, just less than it had been at the beginning of the proving.
- I took the remedy again.

Day 6
- I was doing some hatha yoga exercises, and I made a discovery. When I sat in a certain way, and shifted my weight back into my pelvis, there was a feeling of release through my whole lower body for the first time. Every little tiny muscle released. There was a feeling of a flow through the pelvis and down through my legs. Was able to actually isolate and feel a flow into aching area of left hip area. I had the feeling that something had shifted and that the problem was going to go away at some point.

Day 7
- Really looking forward to vacation.
- Cramping sensations in calves, as if veins ached.

Day 8
- I had recurrence of my fear of driving over bridges. As I was going up over the bridge, it felt like I was leaving my body, starting at the feet. I started to come up and out of my body. I quickly suppressed that feeling because I hated it.

Day 9
- Had first feeling of some force moving on a different level—like ghosts. I was working late at night, to finish things up before my vacation, when I had a creepy feeling that something was coming down the hallway to get me. I felt afraid of ghosts, and kept feeling that something was watching me. I couldn't get to sleep. I turned on the TV for awhile to help me to get to sleep.
- The next day I went on vacation.
- That night I was convinced that the upstairs of the house we were staying in was haunted. There was a closed up room behind the main upstairs bedroom, and the door was covered with an old blanket. It felt like something was wrong up there. The last night I put up my teachers' pictures and lit some incense, thinking that if they (the ghosts) were going to do something, this was their last chance.
- I continued to have the pain in my left side, but during the week, as I was doing my hatha yoga exercise, I noted I could fine tune my postures so that they weren't painful anymore.
- During that vacation week I felt very put upon. I felt boxed in, that there were expectations of me, that I had to act a certain way, and it was driving me crazy. I didn't want to be told how to act. I didn't want any kind of regimented behavior, and I felt very agitated by that. I finally spoke up about that and cleared the air, and everything was better.
- One night I felt heart palpitations, better lying on the right side.
- Dream: A room full of music instruments. Everyone took the instruments I wanted, and I ended up with an oboe which I didn't want.
- I got recurrence of painful pimples on my face, which resolved after three days.

- Dream: Making a birthday cake, but my sister ate half of the dough, and I was worried that I wouldn't be able to make the cake.
- Had craving for mustard.
- Couldn't tolerate any alcohol, even a sip of red wine. I normally can drink a beer or two or a glass or two of wine before reaching my limit. Even thinking about drinking any alcohol gave me a nauseous feeling. It was a normal thing intensified. Then everything went away, and there weren't any further symptoms.

Prover #5 • Female • 25 years old

Day 1
- I would often have fear of ghosts in the past, and when I took this remedy, I had intensification of that fear. Had the feeling that there was something in my room, but it didn't bother me as much.
- I took the remedy three times, because I didn't feel I had a reaction right away. The strongest reaction was in my dreams. Normally I have vivid dreams, but during this period, the dreams were particularly intense. Every dream was a blast from the past.
- Dream: The old house I grew up in, of old friends.
- Dream: I was with my brother back in Cincinnati where we grew up. Felt an intense nostalgia, a wanting to be back there, a kind of homesickness, paired with a feeling of loneliness.
- I had strong heart palpitations that frightened me. I had them in the past, but they had never frightened me. They would go on for ten seconds or more.
- I didn't want to go to bed, even though I was sleepy. I kept finding things to do. Slept well overall, but woke up several times during the night.
- Dream: I was entering a dark room, and seeing a red and blue, foot high, elf-like marionette man. The next day I was thinking about it, and realized as a child that kind of dream would have terrified me. The issue was seeing something in the room that wasn't supposed to be there. It wasn't a monster, but it wasn't right.
- Dream: My father and my teacher got into a big argument. There were obvious psychological meanings, in this case about me wanting to be close to both of them.
- Dream: I was at the beach, and I didn't have any friends, no one to play with, even though there were lots of people around. I was looking for someone, but there was no one there.

Day 2
- I would get thirsty in the afternoon. Not usually aware of my thirst. Around 4 p.m. I'd get very thirsty.
- Stiffness in the hips, like they were still asleep and never woke up.
- Dream: My mother confessed to me about having an affair. I was very upset, but in my dream I was still trying to be nice to her, because I could sense she regretted telling me.

♦ Dream: Of first coming to the house, of the feelings I had early on, the displacement of moving 3,000 miles.

Day 3
♦ I suspected that I had a strong body odor, and was embarrassed about it. It was a stronger smell than I usually have. My hair and skin were oilier than usual. My face and hair seemed greasy, and my hair was hard to comb.
♦ Dream: About fear when crossing a bridge. I was walking on a long, high approach to a bridge, and had a limp in my left leg in the dream. I felt scared, but couldn't stop because there were people behind me, and I didn't want to be in their way. I had to push myself along with the handrails. I found some of my personal articles in the water, a hairbrush and a comb.
♦ In general I noticed more color in my dreams.
♦ Dream: Of my family house.
♦ Almost every dream was about something from my past.
♦ Dream: Of visiting my home town. Things were more beautiful than they actually were. Every hotel was glass.

Day 4
♦ Noticed a metallic smell from my left upper arm. I would sniff an odor and decide that it was coming from me. It was hard to localize the odors.
♦ Dream: Of a party, where my father held a baby in one arm, like he used to hold me when I was a baby.
♦ Dream: Of being in my old house and wanting to take a nap.
♦ Dream: Of watching a movie, but being in it at the same time. Saw a movie poster, and I was in it.
♦ Tonight I smelled like a full vacuum cleaner.

Day 5
♦ My energy has been generally even and I have been quite happy, even though I have just started a new job.
♦ Dream: Of being back east with my brother, and he was going to take an apartment, but I was confused what I was doing, as half of my stuff was back in Portland, and my parents were moving into the same apartment, and there wasn't enough room. Everything there was old and smelled musty. The dream was upsetting, and the next day it stayed with me.

Day 6
♦ Someone was asking impertinent questions about my brother, and it made me intensely mad. He moved back in with our parents, and I felt unhinged about the whole thing. I started crying, and felt emotional. I helped him move, and started crying again.
♦ Dream: With my brother. I wanted to ride in the car with him, but they had to drive two separate cars, so I couldn't be with him, and this was frustrating.

Day 7

◆ The next day I smelled like chocolate.
◆ Dream: I stopped dreaming about the past and started dreaming about death, but it wasn't disturbing at all.
◆ Dream: We were having meditation class outside in the parking lot, and the biggest rocks were the cushions to sit on.
◆ Dream: A woman at the group house died of cancer.
◆ Dream: People dying, and the feeling was poignant, a transition. The group house was at first well populated, then everyone seemed to be dropping like flies.
◆ Dream: Of an old friend that had moved away.
◆ Dream: A graduation, where everyone I knew or had ever known were graduating.

Day 16

◆ On day sixteen I was very depressed.

Prover #6 • Female • 38 years old

I took the remedy 3 times. Felt I didn't have strong reactions.

Day 1

◆ When I first took the remedy, I was doing Chi Gung, and felt a quick, sharp pain on the back of my right hand. Felt that my hand was pulsating. Had quick images of a bee on a flower, fly wings and a feather.
◆ I usually don't wake refreshed, but the first morning I was more foggy than usual. I had lots of dreams.
◆ Dream: Of driving in a car, holding a baby. I was in a room at school, having sex with a classmate, and a professor came in and got a condom out of a file cabinet and threw it at us, and said have fun. It was all matter of fact.
◆ I went into the bathroom and looked in a mirror, and my face was very distorted. My internal feeling was sweet and pleasant, but my face was thick and swollen, especially around the nose and lips.

Day 2

◆ The next day, woke unrefreshed.
◆ My stool was darker than usual.
◆ My actions were more hurried than usual when performing tasks, not a mental agitation, but a physical agitation.
◆ I woke unrefreshed. Got tired in late afternoon, especially from 5:30 to 6:30 p.m.
◆ Dream: Back in Boston, and forgot that it was Christmas. Was afraid that I messed up the family gathering by forgetting about it.

- Dream: About a friend who was buying a new home. The dream was about relationship issues.
- Dream fragment: About a friend being very organized.
- Dream: Of a friend who had a big orange pupil, and the pupil had feathered edges.
- Desire for sweets stronger than usual.
- Constipation with ineffectual urging. Bloating with gas, but no odor. Pain after straining for stool. Some sharp pain with straining. Pain in my back, in the quadratus area.
- Dream: About people in the house, a woman was crying.

Day 3
- Took the remedy again.
- Dream: About a sudden shift in the atmosphere, like a tornado happening.

Day 4
Recorded four dream fragments.
- Dream: Was outside near parked cars, with elements of sexual abuse.
- Dream: About being at my teacher's home for dinner, with lots of other people. He left a message for me on my message machine, and I played it back and it said I was hanging out with the wrong people.
- Dream: Hanging out with an oriental sailor.
- Dream: Of going to a movie with some people.

Day 5
- Dream: Of a basketball game, and one person was taller than he actually is, and people holding chocolate bars.
- Dream: About M. who died. There was a big Ganesh statue, and M. was there. M. took me to other planes [of existence.—Ed.]
- Dream: About old friends from college who now live in Hollywood. There was a theme of friends and relationships and connection.
- Started feeling burning and itching in both upper arms, starting in the afternoon. Soreness and aching in the hands and wrists, as if from doing too much massage, but I hadn't been doing any.
- Sensitive to objects in my peripheral vision.
- I was more direct in my communication, less diplomatic than usual. Felt more self-conscious.
- Felt fastidious, especially at school.

Day 6
- Dream: About watching my mother's TV, and how I would never pick the type of TV cabinet my mother had. A man on the TV was lying, and some curtain fell away, revealing the truth of what he was talking about.
- Felt foggy on waking, was staring into space.
- Felt a dull aching in the wrists, with a sharp pain in the right wrist. Pain in upper trapezius.

♦ Went to visit friends in Seattle and felt claustrophobic when getting on the train, a new sensation for me. I felt disconnected from my friends, who I am usually close to.
♦ Very tired in late afternoon.

Day 7
♦ Dream: Doing a dissection at school, and injecting something into the eyes of mice, and saw lines of pain in the mouse's body, and felt horrible. The only humane thing to do was to cut the mouse's head off.
♦ Slept on stomach with hands under my thighs, which is unusual for me.
♦ Felt my nerves were raw in the hypothenar area.
♦ I was having fun with my friends, but I wanted to be alone and do nothing.
♦ I had allergies on waking, much stronger than normal. My left eye was red and watery, with lots of sneezing.

Day 8
♦ Dream: Of a professor who made an improper sexual innuendo, which I ignored.
♦ Dream: Of a girl that hurt my sacrum, and I was treating it, not caring what people would think as I sat with her in class, with my arm across the girl.
♦ Dream: Of being irritated at my friend for my friend's lack of direction.
♦ Dream: Of sagittal sections of penises that were infected with worms.
♦ Dream: Of a high-rise building.
♦ Dream: Of colorful socks with McDonald's logos.
♦ Dream: Of a gay man who was having relationships with women for political purposes.
♦ Developed cold sores on my upper lip that stayed for a week. They were painful and stinging.
♦ Got some large itchy bumps on my left hand and wrist, like poison ivy bumps.

Day 9
♦ Dream: Of friend helping two gay men from stopping their fights.
♦ Dream: About my two brothers fighting.
♦ Dream: Of having to go somewhere by train.
♦ Dream: About school, having to do a dance to music, a schoolmate did a strip tease down to her underwear. A man in a black leather jacket did a lip-synch and magic tricks.
♦ Dream: A man friend who was crying, related to discovering history of previous sexual abuse.

Day 10
♦ The cold sores were still painful.
♦ Dream: On vacation with some friends. I was cleaning the house. Had to clean up some used condoms, and one broke and sprayed on me. I was wearing chain mail.
♦ Dream: An older man tap dancing, and I followed him.
♦ I developed a rash on my upper thighs, and my upper lip was swollen around the cold sores.

Day 11
♦ Dream: Of traveling from Boston to New York, trying to find the airport. I was in the wrong building at an airport. I can see the planes in a hangar next door. Everything seems old. Next door is a train station.
♦ Dream: Doing experiments with a pet rat, and almost got bitten by it as the rat tried to escape, and I was fearful and agitated.
♦ Dream: About my father falling off a bicycle every time he turned left.
♦ Dream: Of starting the American Revolution, which started because I started shooting, including shooting someone in the face.
♦ Dream: Of cleaning with a fancy Saab vacuum cleaner.

Day 12
♦ Menses were a week early, in conjunction with the full moon, with clots, mucous and cramping, which was unusual for me.
♦ Dream: Of being in an outhouse with large glass windows, and Chinese men were watching me.
♦ Dream: Of lifting a girl over a fence.
♦ I developed dark circles under my eyes.

Day 13
♦ Dream: About a brown recluse spider.
♦ Dream: Of my cousins being in a joint wedding. Swinging on a swing, trying to get high enough so that I could flip off of it.
♦ Had lots of sneezing and coryza with hay fever.

Day 14
♦ This week I have had pain in right upper chest, with burning, < pressure and < inspiration, and I took some Arnica.

Day 15
♦ Dreamed of being in Central America, and someone shot me in the foot.
♦ Having spasmodic jaw pain on the right side.

Prover #7 • Male • 40 years old

I took the remedy 3 times. Didn't have much of a reaction.

Day 1
- Had stabbing pinprick sensation in the right thumbnail.
- Had a knot in the upper neck, lasting several days.
- Dream: Of working on a house, doing carpentry.

Day 2
- Had vertex headache.
- Dryness of upper lip, chapped, unusual for me.
- Dream: I lost my temper when someone tried to take my toast. I was making it for lunch for the next day, preparing it the way I like it, and someone salted it for me, and I lost my temper and stormed away.
- Dream: Of a salamander, with cucumber-like sections of seed pods.

Day 3
- I started a new job recently, and felt quite blasè about it.
- Dreamed of catching buses in a snowstorm, like where I grew up in Ohio. Signs and surfaces were peeling, being pulled back like duct tape or scabs.

Day 4
- Tick in the right temple, feeling like an insect on the skin.
- Dream: Of having vertigo on a bridge and looking down the grid.
- Dream: Confrontational dream of a stranger walking around the house, and friend made sure the man had reason for being there. (Usually he doesn't confront people.)
- Dream: Driving around New York City with my brother, and going to a museum with my father.

Day 5
- Aching in the right thigh to the anus, subcutaneous, like an intense flu ache. It was impossible to localize it by touch.

Prover #8 • Male • 40 years old

Day 1
♦ I did have a recurrent thought, a dark one: "Why do people have children? What is the point of life? How many people can offer things that are indispensable?" I had nihilistic feelings.
♦ I had a strong sugar craving, stronger than usual for me.
♦ Felt tired, and a little tense after only sleeping three hours.
♦ I was at peace with my loneliness for the first time.
♦ I felt a bit more at ease with people. Was irritated with certain people as usual, but they didn't bother me as much.

Day 2
♦ Lots of dreams.

Day 3
♦ Dream: Of being in the foothills around Los Angeles. There were huge bird feeders that had been filled by the government, and they were to be discontinued, as it was too costly to keep them maintained.
♦ Dream: Hiking in the mountains.
♦ Felt physically tired, uptight and alienated, especially during chanting and meditation.

Day 4
♦ Dream: Customer service, taking orders.

Day 5
♦ Felt a feeling of pressure on the right side of my abdomen (which has persisted).
♦ My boss commented that I should try to get some sleep, that I looked tired.
♦ I usually stay up too late at night.

Day 6
♦ Had a moody, teary day. Thinking about a person who represented failure to make a connection. Had strong emotions in meditation class.
♦ Went to dentist, and found it enjoyable to have two fillings filled.
♦ Started practicing French horn again, after taking a month off.
♦ I could stop dreams at will if they got too weird or violent.
♦ Dream: With my teacher and I rendered his rice inedible by emptying it too soon.
♦ Dream: An innocuous pill that was actually a bomb that made a huge hole in someone's front yard. I avoided the authorities.
♦ Dream: Driving my motorcycle off the road onto the shoulder, but then got the bike back onto the road. I consciously woke up when I saw a cop in my rear view mirror.
♦ Dream: Had a strong dream on my birthday, in which I was in a marching band. There was a mentally retarded kid in the band, who was being trained in right and

wrong. They discovered some hacked up body parts, it was gruesome. I consciously woke myself up during this dream as well.

Day 7
- Dream: A girl and her benefactor. I was an errand boy. Everyone in the dream was dressed nicely, except I was in my pajamas.
- I have recently stopped working on my computer at night and am doing much more reading.

Prover #9 • Male • 44 years old

Day 1
- Dream: Flying in a forest. At first it was fun, then I lost the ability to fly and became fearful, hanging onto a branch high up in a tree, and felt scared of falling, and not knowing how to get down from the tree. I lost my previous feeling of confidence in flying.

Day 2
- Dream: Waiting for a long time for a meal to be prepared. The feeling was unusually peaceful. Waiting like this would usually cause impatience in real life.

Day 9
- Had burning and stabbing pain in stomach, feeling like shards of glass, starting around 9 p.m.

Day 10
- Fine until 9 p.m. when there was recurrence of the same stomach pain.

Day 12
- Dream: Having a patient at the clinic who didn't show up for his appointment. I rescheduled it for another day, but he showed up late that day, and was rescheduled again. Felt judgmental about person being irresponsible about the appointment. I later felt guilty as the patient was an important illustrative case of a remedy that I was supposed to have seen and reported to the class. I felt guilty as I had not done the job right, and was embarrassed.

Day 13
- Dream: Bookshelf with sliding door and a hidden treasure, which was a fabulous homeopathic library with full descriptions of lesser-known remedies. This was like a secret gold mine and the feeling was very happy.

Prover #10 • Female • 41 years old

Day 1
- When I took the remedy I had a strange physical sensation in the legs. Felt a sudden rush of relaxation moving downwards. Then extreme feeling of heaviness of the legs, which stopped abruptly.
- Dream: A messenger girl (who looked like Jessica Lange), and I was delivering food to her.
- Dream: Black gulls circled off the ocean over a castle, they landed on the ramparts and were called to fight. I was a bird, flying down to the ground. The enemy was powerful and controlling, and they called out their commands in a forced town gathering. I advised my two male companions (a man and a bear) to smile, clap and cheer as the others were doing, so as to not be discovered as the opposition. There was a confrontation between the bear, who could not contain his contempt, and the enemy. Fighting ensued. The man fell with a bloody wound to the back of his head. As he fell, the masonry fell under him, to cradle his head, as if the masonry was taking care of him. I kept waking to the messenger girl singing. I heard laughter and singing. I fell in and out of sleep in the dream and woke some time later, and went upstairs to eat. My boisterous aunt said, "Oh dear, you must be famished. It's too bad we didn't save you much!"
- I was hungry the whole time of the proving, feeling like a bird, eating all the time. I also felt like a bird in temperament, looking out over her shoulder, constantly watching for danger.

Day 2
- Dream: Had a sexual dream, of being naked with snakes of different sizes in a forest. There was a man and some other people there.
- Dream: Of trying to escape from an area which was being held by the enemy. There was mistrust for artwork in the dream.
- Dream: A three-foot tall crow with a neck chain that was my pet, who had sharp pointed teeth. There were enemies of the crow in the shadows, in the dark, which came over to attack the crow. The feeling was anxious, being on edge.
- I felt anxious, buzzing and nervous right after taking the remedy.

Day 3
- I was irritable and impatient. General energy level varied from lightness to lethargy and heaviness. Felt heaviness in muscles. Irritable.
- Sleep not restful at all.
- Slight headache moving like a wave from front to back, covering the whole skull. I never get headaches normally. Awoke at 2 a.m., couldn't get back to sleep until 4:15.
- Dream: Of imprisonment and black birds.

Day 4
- Another headache along the midline to the vertex.
- Feeling expansive, open, relaxed, sexual, opposite of the previous days.
- Sensual dreams that night.

Day 5
- I felt angry, distrustful and closed.

Day 6
- I was eating whatever I could. Anxious that the food was not going to be there if I didn't eat it right away. Felt depressed, suicidal, angry and distrustful. Energy very low. Forced myself to go do a heavy workout.

Day 7
- I was intensely suicidal. Imagining ways of killing myself, by taking too much aspirin or slicing my wrists.

Day 8
- I was still depressed, but not suicidal.

Day 9
- I felt flat, on the edge of feeling positive. Body felt energized from exercise of the previous day.
- During the proving I noticed that my usual discomfort from uterine fibroids during sex had cleared up, and I was hoping that relief might last.

Day 10
- Dream: Recurrent dream images: Birds, fighting, feeling of constant threat, which was countered by feeling safe, open, sexual and expansive. The dark side was more prevalent.
- I felt mistrustful, that I needed to watch my back. The unknown enemy was everywhere. Everyone was suspect, even my husband. It was an oppressive mood overall.

Prover #11 • Female • 39 years old

I took the remedy right after the rat blood proving, and had to antidote that one to start this one.

Day 1
- On holding the remedy in my hand before taking it, I had a sense of calmness, shoulders relaxing, expansiveness of breath, everything was floating up to my head and expanding outward. I took the remedy and noted a feeling of relaxation through my whole body.
- My right sacroiliac pain lessened significantly.
- Lungs and chest felt fuller, able to take in more air, sense of lightness and fluidity. I had easier meditation.
- Aware of keenness of sight and hearing. Increase of peripheral vision.

- Saw a jay outside and thought it would be easy to fly.
- Posterior vertex headache, lasting most of the evening, disappearing around 9 p.m.
- Energy level full throughout the proving.
- Appetite good, digestion settling down after the last proving. I was averse to sweets, unusual for me.
- Premenstrual cramps before the remedy that disappeared by the next morning.
- Not heat tolerant at all. Had to get out of the hot tub. Chilly in the early morning, which is unusual for me.

Day 2
- I had a craving for raw greens or salad.
- Had ribbony soft stool, which was unusual for me.
- Sweating on forehead with menstrual flow.

Day 3
- Ligaments relaxing, and much flexibility in my body.
- Still had increased sensitivity of sight and hearing.

Day 4
- Took another dose.
- Got high posterior vertex headache, which was gone by evening.
- Feeling close to birds and having an urge for flying.
- Feeling fearless, doubts are minimal, and feeling a fine, light clarity.
- Sensitive to loud sharp noises, and increased startle reflex.

Day 5
- Averse sweets, but desire for nuts.

Day 11
- Picking cherries, and had an urge to jump out of the cherry picker and fly. I had the feeling that I could fly and had to restrain myself.
- Woke up at 4:30 a.m., with the first light.
- My brother had a dream that I was at a wedding, a man with a radio cut off my head with a samurai sword when I asked him to turn off his radio. They wouldn't arrest him because I didn't need stitches.

Day 12
- Had difficulty sleeping, waking at 4:30.
- Deep burning in my forehead and vertex headache.
- Continued sense of lung expansion.
- Ovulation starting with more mucous than usual.
- Dream: Nityananda's hand on my forehead.
- Dream: I was lying in Rudi's chair, in fetal position. I was the size of a fetus. My

teacher is laughing and won't let me leave the chair. I feel deeply nurtured, and feel gratitude on waking.

Day 14
◆ Thoughts are soft, more creative than analytical. Can't sense distinct boundaries between objects.
◆ Ran up the mountain, with an urge to leap out into space at the top of the mountain, as if I am so light that the wind could carry me. Had the desire to feel my body falling and striking the earth. No judgment or fear, every act seemed equal. Felt a sense of detachment, as if the experience of living is about a sense of myself, not about what I do.
◆ Waking and sleeping seem similar, sense that dreamtime and this dimension are only slightly different.

Day 15
◆ Soft edges again.
◆ Noticing a sweet smell to my sweat.
◆ Craving cold drinks in large quantities.
◆ Stool smells like strawberries.

Day 16
◆ Dream: About Yama, the god of death, coming toward me with large, red, fiery nostrils. I opened, and he melted into me, then peace. This is a recurrent dream I've had, but this time I felt open and fearless, and death seems irrelevant.

Day 18
◆ Urge to fly whenever I am at any height. Urge to leap out of a third floor window.

Day 19
◆ Sense of clarity and softness.
◆ Continued expansion in the chest.
◆ Still have posterior high headache.

Day 20
◆ Amazing lack of urge for sweets or chocolate.
◆ Dream: Another dream of Yama, breathing into my left ear, hot and erotic. Sense of death and destruction is just another expression of universal energy.

Summary:
Feeling a sense of expansion and breath. Awareness of connectedness of everything and lack of distinct boundaries. Fearlessness about death or change. Sense of muscular strength. Overall relaxation of muscles and ligaments. Posterior vertex headache. Increased visual acuity and peripheral vision. Desire for nut meats and cold drinks. Sweat smells sweet. Increased nasal mucous and cervical mucous at ovulation. Averse to sweets and heavy foods.

ANHALONIUM

Peyote

ANHALONIUM [ANH.]
Peyote

Lophophora williamsi
Family: Cactaceae
Miasm: Cancer

Anhalonium, also known as Peyote, Mescal button, or simply "Mescalito," is a modest little blue-green spineless cactus about two inches tall that grows only in southern Texas and northern Mexico. It is found in clusters with the roots of several individual plants connected at the base. Its humble appearance belies the power held within the soft green knobs. It is hard to imagine that this, the smallest of all cacti, has been a major religious and spiritual influence for indigenous Meso-American culture since pre-Columbian times, with current adepts reaching over 225,000 in the Native-American Church.

Listed by the Drug Enforcement Agency in the same category as heroine and LSD, possession in the United States is a felony and can result in imprisonment. Only those individuals with a minimum of one-quarter Native-American blood and belonging to the Native-American church may legally use the cactus. Why is it outlawed by the DEA yet revered for centuries by Native-Americans? Research may provide part of the answer. A study conducted in 1953 revealed that the peyote plant has eleven different psychoactive alkaloids, the only cactus with alkaloids in such significant amounts. Mescaline is the simplest of these and it strongly affects the central nervous system producing extraordinary visions and powerful spiritual experiences. The state produced by Anhalonium is described by Aldous Huxley in *The Doors of Perception*:

> The glory and wonder of pure existence, beyond the power of even the highest art to express . . . it had delivered me for the moment from the world of selves, of time, of moral judgments, of utilitarian considerations, the world of self-assertion, of cocksureness, of overvalued words and idolatrously worshipped notions . . . without question the most extra-ordinary and significant experience. . . . (*12-13*)

These words express a unique experience that is far beyond what most of us encounter in daily living. Another, more prosaic description, based on extensive

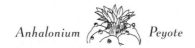

research by Havelock Ellis, Weir Mitchell, M.D., and Alexander Rouhier, is found in *Peyote* by David Flattery, Ph.D.:

> . . . . most subjects became aware of a sensation that is described in numerous ways, but which generally expresses a feeling of contentment, well being and relaxation. For some, this is the central component of the entire experience; yet it is almost thoroughly lacking for a few. The common denominator of the feeling seems to be a certain lack of hostility, of anger, and along with this a decrease in the tendency to attribute hostility toward others. One subject described a feeling that a great weight had been lifted, which he had carried since his earliest memories, and, on considering the matter, he was able to say that this burden had consisted of nothing more than fear and anger. Perhaps related to this freedom is the loss of many of the usual drives. During the experience there seems to be nothing that the subject wants badly enough to take from the others. The appetites are diminished and the mental phenomena are such that external realities become less important. There is thus no threat posed to another, and no threat is felt by the subject. In reference to these feelings, many psychiatric workers use the term "depersonalization," usually in a manner implying that such a feeling is uncomfortable at best and at worst damaging to mental health. Many takers of the drug make a specific point of rejecting this word, stressing instead that there is a greater personal feeling or sense of identity. Others note that they experience something related to a loss of personality, but the feeling is pleasant, leaving them with a realization that much of their "social" activity in the world would be seen (by them) as absurd and useless. (*39*)

Since ancient times, the Native-American has understood Peyote to be a divine force providing spiritual knowledge and guidance. As with many spiritual traditions, the journey toward knowledge includes challenges. The first challenge is finding the little button in the largely dry and brown desert earth. Often a great ceremony is made of the event. Weston La Barre in *The Peyote Cult* writes:

> An early Comanche party going for Peyote in the Apache region had much the character of a war journey. It involved a clairvoyant discovery of the enemy, prophecy of the outcome, and a horse raid. The Lipan tribe says: Peyote is pretty hard to find when you are looking for it. . . . a person who is not used to it doesn't recognize it though he is in the middle of a whole clump of Peyote. Once he sees one, another appears and so on until they all come out just like stars. If you are having a hard time finding them you do this: when you find just one by itself you eat it. When it takes effect, when you get a little dizzy, you will hear a noise like the wind from a certain direction. Go over there . . . from the place where the noise is coming you will get many peyote plants. (*57*)

After the buttons are collected the ceremony begins in the evening and lasts all night. The people gather around a crescent-shaped earthen altar in a teepee or around a sacred fire in a simple building. There is an assortment of ceremonial paraphernalia in place, including gourd, rattle, drum, drum stick, staff, feathers, eagle wing, bone whistle, corn shucks, loose tobacco, bags for Peyote, cedar incense, altar cloth, sage, water bucket, and ritual breakfast containers. These things are passed around in a ritualized manner. Then the chief leads a prayer. This may be very long-lasting up to an hour. La Barre reports, "The speaker's voice becomes louder as he proceeds, earnest and quavering as he sways with the fullness of his emotions and stretches out his hands toward the Peyote and the fire. Sometimes his speech is wholly interrupted by uninhibited broken sobbing as he cries out for the pity of the supernatural." John Rave, the Winnebago teacher said, "Only if you weep and repent will you be able to attain knowledge" (81). During the whole time the group is instructed to gaze at the Peyote plant placed atop a crescent in the center of the room. Peyote buttons are passed to each member and they may take as much as they wish. No conversation occurs about what one is experiencing or the effects of the meeting.

> The rules regarding use by the Indians are brief and simple. In the legendary account of how Father Peyote made himself known to the Indian, he is made to say: "There are several different ways that you can use me, but unless you use me in only one way, the right way, I may harm you. Use me the right way and I will help you.". . . It must be approached in a reverent, contemplative frame of mind and accepted as a great power through which one may reach the great spirit. Perhaps the only real rule is that one must surrender himself completely and unreservedly to Peyote if he is to use it at all. (*Flattery, 18*)

The tenets of the church are these: brotherly love, family care, self-support through steady work and the avoidance of alcohol (these last two are no doubt modern). These are the very essence of the teachings of "Mescalito." In *The Yaqui Way of Knowledge*, Carlos Castenada reports the words of the shaman, Don Juan, "The devil's weed (Stramonium) has never protected anyone. It only serves to give power. Mescalito, on the other hand is gentle like a baby. It . . . has constant qualities of being a protector and a teacher. . . ." Peyote is related to the acquisition of wisdom or the knowledge of good and evil.

In the beautiful book, *Huichol Indian Sacred Rituals*, Susana Eger Valadez reveals the power of the Peyote culture:

> Under the proper ritual circumstances, the Peyote brings enlightenment to the shamans and their apprentices; the Peyote illuminates their consciousness and attunes

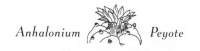

them to the life forces of Nature. One of the abilities they master is psychic communication with plant, animal and spirit entities, who grant them healing powers. . . . The *mara akame* is the shamanic healer who protects the health of his family and community. While some herbal remedies are employed, most of the healing is done through ritual. The shamans and the patients work together to contact the spirit entities responsible for causing the illness and, once the proper rituals are performed, sending the healing white light energy that effects the cure. (*Valadez, 75*)

Peyote as also used by the Huichol and many other Native-American tribes as a topical and herbal medicine especially for the curing of wounds, snakebite and rheumatism. But some tribes, notably the Kiowa and the Shawnee, eat Peyote as a panacea medicine or tonic to heal all conditions. They give it to all members of the tribe including infants and very young children. In days long past, Peyote was given to anyone in the tribe who was injured, very old, or a mother and child who could not keep up with the tribal movement and had to be left behind. The Peyote was said to aid their transmigration from this life into the next. There is a legend that a Wichita, held captive in a prisoner of war camp, successfully escaped using his Peyote plant as a shamanic trickster (*LaBarre, 28*).

The Huichol Indians are currently gaining worldwide notoriety for their powerful and provocatively colorful artwork depicting visions seen during the Peyote ceremonies. Like the celebratory colors and hallucinogenic images seen in the Huichol artwork the themes of the proving suggest an otherworldly sense of spiritual elevation and sensory exultation. But like all of the drug remedies in which there exists an often dangerous "split" between its high and low points, Anhalonium presents a dark side as well. This powerful dichotomy suggests that this remedy may be especially useful in the treatment of schizophrenia.

In spite of the fact that Anhalonium is so well known homeopathically and is thoroughly represented in the repertory, most of the symptoms come from material doses or one small proving. I felt it might be useful to get another look at this valuable remedy from a homeopathic perspective. So, in October of 1994 I undertook the task of proving Anhalonium homeopathically. As with every other proving in this book, the provers took a (legal) homeopathic dose of Anhalonium 30C, one to three times, carefully recording over a three week period any and all physical symptoms, dreams, emotions or unusual experiences they may have encountered.

I have chosen to include it in this book. First, because it so closely relates to the other provings of sacred plants and second, because a great deal of interesting new material surfaced in the course of the proving. However, due to the availability of extensive material on Anhalonium, I have chosen to include only those themes, rubrics and journal entries that shed new light on this substance. May it serve as a guide to deeper understanding of this sacred plant's essence.

Conducted by Nancy Herrick with ten provers
Collated by Claire Green N.D.

It has been my experience that the sacred plants or "drug remedies" in their provings have a peculiar characteristic of manifesting both sides of many symptoms. Although each side may not be equally expressed in the proving, we do often see these polarities. Anhalonium is a good representative of this, having quite clear opposite poles which are outlined below.

POLARITIES

Calm, Quiet	Quarrelsome
Selflessness	Selfishness
Thoughts quiet	Thoughts vanishing
Increased insight	Confusion
Involvement	Withdrawal

Editor's note: The following material is all that is available from the original proving. Wherever a prover's number is known it is indicated. Mental states, which were not expressive of a common theme, are listed under the heading: Random Entries. Following the themes, entries regarding physical states are listed according to body systems. They are not in rubric form.

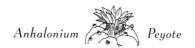

Anhalonium **Themes**

Peyote

- *Calm/Quiet*
- *Energetic/Productive*
- *Well-Being*
- *Dullness*
- *Sadness/Compassion*
- *Anxiety/For children*
- *Danger/Violence/Explosions*
- *Escape*
- *Surreal*
- *Old Things/Ancient*
- *Sensual impressions/Smells–Sight–Taste*
- *Water/Tropical*
- *Sexuality*
- *Animals*

Calm/Quiet

#2 Before proving, was overwhelmed. Now handles everything with ease, no judgment, no anger, when usually would be. Amazingly calm.

#2 No anxiety about situations that usually made one anxious. Confident—centered. Clarity. New insights. Alert. I knew it would be fine. No fear in fearful situations.

#1 Calm in the eye of the storm.

#2 Right away felt calm, not anxious though was very busy, not bothered. Centered. Confident.

#1 Quiet reflective, as though a deep trust that everything will work out all right, no need for agitation. Not very social, not needing people but glad to speak to or see them. Introspective, connected to self.

#2 All problems at work easy to take care of. Before remedy was overwhelmed. Real marked difference after remedy. Felt fine, not tired.

#2 She felt happy, centered all day. Workshop led by medicine woman went well. No judgment about children who were up all night. Would usually feel that parents who bring kids to late night events are abusing their kids. She cared for kids, but was not irritated. Not worrying about things—unusual for her. Got insights about what she was doing wrong: she needed to be gentler. Shook man and he collapsed; realized he is delicate. New ways to deal with him.

#3 Stressful time, but very calm without problems. Life very busy but not bummed out.

#1 Goes swimming, feels very playful. While in hot tub realizes she has been liking to go underwater and open her eyes, an impression of being womb-like. Weightlessness, warmth, and seeing her limbs faintly. So the calmness I have been feeling is the same sort of watery warm sense of safety and comfort. Uncomplicated. At peace with myself.

#5 . . . felt good . . . calm.

#1 Still feels very calm in spite of external situation, lots of work, would usually be in a spin at this point, but still feel very connected and in myself.

#1 (With) Children; anger is easily averted. Good feelings.

#1 Peaceful, introverted self-contained mood. Felt very happy in the water, diving, especially good underwater. Good to stretch and feel weightless.

#3 Dream: Driving car. Stopped at a bridge with a lot of people waiting. Had to wait 35 minutes but felt patient.

#1 Still feeling very quiet and wishes could curl up in chair and sort of dream.

Anxiety/For Children

#6 Dream: Anxiety, panic, hurry, going to wedding. Dress unraveling, wrong shoes, no flowers. Hurry.

#1 Feeling slightly anxious about son who has not been heard from in a month during his travels.

#9 Anxiety in chest.

#7 Felt like couldn't keep life together. Big struggle. Overwhelmed by responsibilities. Too much. Fretting.

#6 Dream: Driving into the outskirts of a town. People on the street are running, panicking. Sound of sirens, smell of smoke. Got to a neighborhood where my sister lived. Father and brother there saying that my sister and her children were missing. We tried to find them but police restrained us. Feeling of helplessness, grief, shock.

#1 Dream: In building that is about to explode because a flaming jeep has crashed through the wall. Running down lots of steps. . . . Wake feeling disturbed, anxious about son.

#4 Dream: Motorcycle chase, children in danger. I observed children were fine. I woke with the feeling of anxiety about the children.

#5 Dream: In ruins with a friend. Odd feelings. We should not be here. Very ancient wall, crumbling. Ominous feelings. Daytime, alone. Felt anxious. Need to leave.

Energetic/Productive

#? First night had PMS—usually a difficult time, foggy but instead felt great—clear—on track, dynamic. Even better the next day. Energetic; really like it. Got a lot done. Handled a lot. Very busy but no problem.

#5 Full of energy felt good. . .

#? Alert. "Amped up" energy like an animal. Ever ready, Alert. Aware.

#? Cautious. Steady and alert. Higher vibration.

#9 Feel great, lots of energy, happy, excited for the day. Enjoying things, worked out at gym, feeling great.

#? After taking the remedy felt light bubbly, uplifting sensation. Aware of breathe with a need to sigh.

Well-Being

#1 Spontaneous, open to expressing happiness, fatigue, within myself in a very true way. Not feeling so self-conscious while in conversation with others. Wonders if she sounds silly but does not mind. Feels freeing.

#5 Full of energy felt good, felt well-being. . . .

#9 I'm strong, steady, able to take care of the world. Felt comfortable. Feet and arms could move. I could roam. Open and centered. I'm in my world and well taken care of.

#1 Deep sense of well-being continues, related to self-connectedness. This feeling of connectedness to self and a higher place continues to be joy.

#2 Before proving, was overwhelmed. Now handles everything with ease, no judgment, no anger, when usually would be.

#1 Flowing with life and work. Feeling there is plenty of time to do everything.

#1 Attitude of self-care towards myself, using nice smelling bath salts and moisturizers after shower. Wearing clothes that feel good. Almost a sensuality, a pleasure in caring for myself.

Dullness

#9 During the day, read things over and over; forget things; difficult organizing things; didn't know word "heart."

#? Dull, slow mentally.

#9 Thickheaded and mental dullness. Small range. Like a little kid in front of TV all day. Narrow expression. Dull. Resignation. In a waking free association.

#9 Difficult to do a puzzle.

#5 Irritable, impatient. Dullness in afternoon. Impatient with child during headache.

Sadness/Compassion

#1 Feels sad, as if have forgotten something or have done something hurtful to someone or been dishonest. Sort of guilty but can think of nothing specific. Compassionate feelings for anybody's hurt. I notice I am feeling others feelings more clearly.

#9 Saying good-bye to someone I would not see again, wanted to savor the moment.

#1 A dog patient died, and although I had only been given the case minutes before he died, I felt sad and cried. Felt remorse that if I had not been so selfish and considered their urgency the dog might have lived.

#5 Sadness while watching news and reading newspaper about the state of the world.

#1 Walk through a shop and smells a perfume my mother used to wear. Keep walking back and forth sniffing it, makes me feel a little sad, missing her.

#5 Feeling of missing being closer to family.

#8 Dream: Buying property from Russians, then watched a parade. Someone was called the town drunk in local newspaper and I wrote to demand a retraction. . . .

Sensual Impressions/Smells–Sight–Taste

#1 Attitude of self-care towards myself, using nice smelling bath salts and moisturizers after shower. Wearing clothes that feel good. Almost a sensuality, a pleasure in caring for myself.

#5 Sensitivity to odors—very unusual; ginger odor seems so strong. Nobody else noticed it. I felt I would choke.

#1 Walk through a shop and smell a perfume my mother used to wear. Keep walking back and forth sniffing it, makes me feel a little sad, missing her.

#6 Dream: Driving into the outskirts of a town. . . . Sound of sirens, smell of smoke.

#1 . . . Feel particularity drawn to rocks while taking walk in the hills. Lie down next to a moss covered rock that feels very friendly, leaves a warm impression for the remainder of day.

#9 Liked sensation of coolness and air on my body.

#? After taking the remedy felt light bubbly, uplifting sensation. Aware of breathe with a need to sigh.

#9 Wanted to go outside to feel coolness on face. Deep but narrow range of experience.

#1 Goes swimming in the sea which is unusual because usually dislike the cold water, feels very good.

#9 Touch, aversion to being.

#2 Dream: Desires stuffed grape leaves.

#4 Dream: Food theme: very unusual, walk through restaurant. All dressed in black. People at tables, smells of food.

#6 Dream: Sales people at Macy's passing out cinnamon rolls in shape of cats. Feeling of pleasure, especially because they are whole wheat.

#4 Dream: Children waiting for huge pot of colorful food to cook. Multiple colors. Was not hungry.

#6 Dream: At very elegant restaurant with friends. Food is very clean, organic, beautiful, nouvelle cuisine—"frou-frou." Everyone took turns going around describing how their food tastes. "I have a bean terrene layered with veggies, garlic." Savory, herbal, floral. Very creative dream, exquisite and beautiful.

#1 Dream: As I fell asleep saw images of African/Aztec colorful designs: zigzags and arrows. Dreamt of an unknown dark skinned or black man who was a guide. Swimming through warm tropical rivers. Silky smooth very sensual feeling water that had gentle waves washing me along. Under tropical foliage in a jungle.

#6 Dream: Shopping for shoes at department store. Old schoolmate is the salesman and tries to sell me a pair of ugly deck shoes. I want navy blue shoes, and see a pair of strappy navy blue sandals, very beautiful and impractical. Leave without buying anything.

#6 Dream: We are under the space shuttle, watching it take off with fire raining down all around. Noise, smoke. Then we are in the shuttle looking down at the earth dropping away below us. Cool! Then driving in a car along the ocean, but it is not the earth, on another planet. The ocean and foliage are unearthly colors. Surrealistic.

Danger/Violence/Explosions

#4 Dream: Motorcycle chase, children in danger. . . .

#7 Dream: In house with no security. Impervious to robbers who were coming through walls. Impotent. Felt like killing them by strangling.

#8 Dream: Bad guys shooting at me. . . .

#10 Dream: Violence; imprisoned with wife and another couple against our will. Managed to send for help to rescue us. Bicycling on a farm, rebelled. Got farm implements to use as weapons. A man took a rake and hit another in the head. I took a pitchfork and stabbed him in the chest. I thought, "He has a tension pneumothorax and he is going to die." A feeling of: either we kill or we will be killed. No remorse. Unusually vivid dream.

#7 Dream: Car left in parking structure. Broken into. Pissed off, "not again." Four gangsters on motorcycles. I was very neutral. No fear, no anger. I ask, "What do you suggest to me?"

#1 Dream: Prophetic dream: In a house with ten young women and a guru figure who is male. He tells us planet is about to explode. . . .

#1 Dream: In building that is about to explode because a flaming jeep has crashed through the wall. Running down lots of steps. See pool of water, which I am about to go into, until I see that it is filled with disgusting toads and fish half-buried in mud. Yucky. Wake feeling disturbed, anxious about son.

#2 Dream: Strange hospital. Dark hall, no fear; he was friendly and nice. Offered wine, surrealistic. Long dark corridors with candle. I felt OK. He was a wizard of Oz. Mysterious, powerful, dangerous person. I knew it would be OK.

#6 Dream: Victorian house turned into a shop. Party being held there, lots of seductive women in period costumes late 1800's. Spooky man who wanted a very expensive piece of jewelry. I said, no he could not take it; he had to pay for it. Who do you think you are?

#6 Dream: Driving into the outskirts of a town. People on the street are running, panicking. Sound of sirens, smell of smoke. Got to a neighborhood where my sister lived. Father and brother there saying that my sister and her children were missing. We tried to find them but police restrained us. Feeling of helplessness, grief, shock.

#2 Dream: Dead bodies, unusual but [ed: had recently] read about bodies in newspaper. Surrealistic. Stack of decomposing bodies. Wanted to avoid it. Malevolant spirits. . . .

Animals

#? "Amped up" energy like an animal. Ever ready, Alert. Aware.

#4 Dream: Large group of animals in a forest, I lead some kangaroos and dogs to safety. I had to protect them. "Got to care." Two giant, friendly dogs. Whatever is chasing will get hurt.

#9 Dream: Leading a horse to corral. It needed further training. Stubborn, and yet resigned. Didn't want to do it.

#8 Dream: Driving somewhere with my Airedales (who died several years ago and I dream about them once a month). Thinking about going to medical school and that I was too old to do so, but was pleased nonetheless.

#8 Dream: Two Dobermans, one pregnant, bought a large amount of meat for them, was concerned it might be dog meat.

#1 Dream: . . . Sea lions come swimming towards me—I feel very happy.

#7 Dream: Tropical place. Friend fishing, caught it. In water a huge fish swam at my feet. He caught a big fish.

#8 Dream: Buying property from Russians. . . . Property purchase fell through because of fire ants.

#1 Dream: . . . See pool of water, which I am about to go into, until I see that it is filled with disgusting toads and fish half-buried in mud. Yucky.

#? Dream: Examining a patient's foot: Looking at a dark area, a spider came out of hole. Felt surrealistic. Weird. Strange. Not upsetting. It was supposed to be that way. Large dark spider.

Old Things/Ancient

#1 When holding the remedy had impression of something very ancient, powerful and hard.

#5 Dream: In ruins with a friend. Odd feelings. We should not be here. Very ancient wall, crumbling. Ominous feelings. Daytime, alone. Felt anxious. Need to leave.

#6 Dream: Victorian house turned into a shop. Party being held there, lots of seductive women in period costumes late 1800's. . . .

Escape

#5 Dream: In ruins with a friend. Odd feelings. We should not be here. Very ancient wall, crumbling. Ominous feelings. Daytime, alone. Felt anxious. Need to leave.

#6 Dream: Riding bikes at Hanford Nuclear Reservation, like a Department of Energy theme park. Husband wanted to ride his bike off road, I said, "No, there is plutonium all around, we should not be here, we don't belong here."

#9 Lots of physical sensations; feelings of roaming, more needing the space and not wanting to be enclosed.

#1 Dream: Awareness of escaping some sort of situation, not really scary; can't remember the details; fleeting impression on waking but seems to include water.

#1 Dream: Prophetic dream: In a house with ten young women and a guru figure who is male. He tells us planet is about to explode. We must kill ourselves before it does. We must sit in a lotus posture and hold our arms up in a particular mudra: just surrender up our spirits to death. I realize it is quite easy to do, but then realize: Hey, I don't want to do this! I ask another girl if she really wants to do this and she says no, so we escape and I feel very relieved.

#8 Dream: Bad guys shooting at me, I fell into a pond, they disappear. I go to the store.

Water/Tropical

#1 Dream: Ocean: not clearly remembered but seems to have ocean or water in it.

#1 Dream: As I fell asleep saw images of African/Aztec colorful designs: zigzags and arrows. Dreamt of an unknown dark skinned or black man who was a guide. Swimming through warm tropical rivers. Silky smooth very sensual feeling water that had gentle waves washing me along. Under tropical foliage in a jungle.

#1 Dream: We run and come to a section of sea with ice melting. I jump as far as I can, trying to reach an iceberg, but fall into the water. It is unexpectedly warm and really pleasant. I grab onto a pole to pull myself up and that is too warm. Even the iceberg is warm. Sea lions come swimming towards me—I feel very happy.

#7 Dream: Tropical place. Friend fishing, caught it. In water a huge fish swam at my feet. He caught a big fish. Use current situation to accomplish task. Pleasant. Warm water.

#10 Dream: Driving in a bucolic setting, Very impressionistic, rolling hills, picturesque. At one point the road was washed out and all around were tremendously eroded fields with tufts of land sticking up like reefs. Road impassable. We marveled at the power of the water. I wanted to get back home; no sure sign of were we were. No emotions.

#1 Dream: In building that is about to explode because a flaming jeep has crashed through the wall. Running down lots of steps. See pool of water, which I am about to go into, until I see that it is filled with disgusting toads and fish half-buried in mud. Yucky. Wake feeling disturbed, anxious about son.

#1 Goes swimming, feels very playful. While in hot tub realizes she has been liking to go underwater and open her eyes, an impression of being womb-like. Weightlessness, warmth, and seeing her limbs faintly. So the calmness I have been feeling is the same sort of watery warm sense of safety and comfort.

Surreal

#? With eyes closed saw: colorful images moving rapidly. Bubbling feeling. Surreal, rapid-fire montage of images. Like Peter Max art or Yellow Submarine/Beatles movie. Flowers.

#6 Dream: We are under the space shuttle, watching it take off with fire raining down all around. Noise, smoke. Then we are in the shuttle looking down at the earth dropping away below us. Cool! Then driving in a car along the ocean, but it is not the earth, on another planet. The ocean and foliage are unearthly colors. Surrealistic.

#10 Dream: Wife and I had lost our clothes, had sandwiched ourselves between blankets and were going to ride the subway home. Lost in the middle of nowhere. Suddenly thought, "I can't ride on subway like this!" and we put clothes on. Shoes looked like fire trucks. Then a fire truck came up and was selling ice cream.

#2 Dream: Dead bodies, unusual but [ed: had recently] read about bodies in newspaper. Surrealistic. Stack of decomposing dead bodies. Wanted to avoid it. Malevolent spirits. Not afraid but felt disgust. Felt centered and happy all the next day.

#1 Wanting to be near rocks and trees, feel drawn to them as if they had a message, which they usually do. Notice colors, shades, trees against the sky, sudden flowers in the sidewalk.

#? Dream: Examining a patient's foot: looking at a dark area, a spider came out of hole. Felt surrealistic. Weird. Strange. Not upsetting. It was supposed to be that way. Large dark spider.

#2 Dream: Strange hospital. Dark hall, no fear; he was friendly and nice. Offered wine, surrealistic. Long dark corridors with candle. I felt OK. He was a wizard of Oz. Mysterious, powerful, dangerous person. I knew it would be OK.

#9 Sensation of face elongated, nose elongated.

Sexuality

#? Amorous.

#8 Dream: Very bizarre, sexual dream: butter, dildos and earthquakes.

#6 Dream: Flirtatious. Composite dream of people from college days. Scenes of classrooms, parties, friend's apartments. Meeting people, pleasant, no particular point to the dream.

#6 Dream: Victorian house turned into a shop. Party being held there, lots of seductive women in period costumes late 1800's. . . .

RANDOM ENTRIES

#9 Aloof, alone quality.

#5 Got in argument with parents. Not good.

#2 Dream: Usual stuff: work, people, children.

#2 Dream: New clinic, too much furniture; abrasive unpleasant people. I was abrasive back to them.

#7 Dream: Sister getting married. Secret wedding. Family is angry and feeling left out.

#6 Dream: Big party with Barbara Mandrell as hostess. The idea of the party was to bring the black sheep of the family back into the fold. Theme of forgiveness, but it was actually just for show.

#4 Dream: In public place, had to have a bowel movement. Went to closet with clothes. Spots of stool all over the room. Had to clean it up. Felt humiliated. No control.

#8 Dream: On a country estate with wife and some friends. Behind farm was a field filled with potted plants, all dead. A woman was gathering the plants saying she did not want to take all the dried mustard. Barrel of carved staves, rakes, tools, one was made into a musical instrument. They were rushes or reeds, five feet long, with cattails at the end. A woman and a friendly bald man came up and I asked the woman how she was. She smiled shyly and walked away without talking, no real emotions.

PREDOMINANT PHYSICAL STATES

Energetic.
Groggy—tired. Unusual fatigue. Sleepy.
Headache—frontal and occipital.
Sensitive to noise.
Gas, diarrhea, spluttering stool.
Nausea. Cutting pain in stomach.
Tingling sensation on buttocks on sitting—herpes sores.
Increased sexuality.

Editor's note: The following are not in rubric form. They are direct quotes from the proving journals (followed by the prover's number in parenthesis wherever possible) and organized under body systems.

HEAD

- Pain: dull frontal lasted 1–2 hours. (3)

- Pain: cramping, irritable dull frontal headache in evening; premenstrual worse. loud noise, and impatient with child. (5)

- Pain: aching in occiput. Bones wanted to move. Throbbing. Bursting open. (9)

- Pain: sensation of wire cutter bisecting head, started afternoon 3 PM and built as the day went on. Worse noise, eating. Nausea. Vision blurred better warm bathing, lying. (6)

EYES

- Difficult to read small print. (1) Pain, throbbing. (9) Ptosis. (9)

- Photophobia. (7) Needed sunglasses. (9)

VISION

- Blurred during headache better warm bathing. With eyes closed saw: colorful images moving rapidly. Bubbling feeling. Surreal, rapid-fire montage of images. Like Peter Max art or Yellow Submarine/Beatles movie. Flowers. (6)

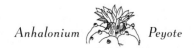

FACE

- Sensation of face elongated, nose elongated. (9)
- Energy concentrated in face, head. (9)

THROAT

- Pain: felt swollen and burning, dry, constricting. (9)
- Swollen and hot. (9)

STOMACH

- Anorexia and nausea: late afternoon and early evening. (5)
- Desires: garlic (1), spaghetti (1), rice cakes (1), spicy hot, salsa. (1)
- Distention: feels bloated after eating a little, in morning on waking. (1)
- Hunger: but knows not what for (1), and thirst for something I cannot see or buy, frustrating!!(1)
- Nausea: on waking lasting into midmorning. (6) Nausea brief, for five minutes. (7)
- Pain: gnawing in stomach, felt warm, wanted nothing in body and felt sensitive, confinement if anything on her body. (9)
- Pain: severe cutting pains Waking from sleep 1 a.m. better passing stool. (1)
- Sensation of pressure and fullness extending to small of back on waking. (1)

ABDOMEN

- Distention. (7)

RECTUM

- BM spluttering and loose (1), BM still looser than usual, less gas. (1)
- Flatus ameliorates (1), flatulence (1), flatulence with BM, sputtering, looser stool than normal. (1) Flatulence. (7)

BLADDER

- Drank lots of water but no need to urinate. (2)

FEMALE

- Menses: started day took remedy and finished next day, very short. (1)
- Menses: no cramps. Tired, weighted-down feeling. (5)
- Sex drive returned dramatically at 1 p.m. Nipples sensitive. Had been low. (2)

CHEST

- Pain: stitching in the right outer breast. (6)
- Pain: soreness, tenderness in left breast. (5)

BACK

- Neck stiff on waking. (1) Pain: stitching sacroiliac joint left. (6)
- Pain: shooting extending from kidney area to top of back of leg. (1)
- Pain: sore. Drove 2.5 hours and usually her hips would be sore but this time not, although back sore. (2) Pain: Lower backache. (5)
- Numbness: Buttocks numb sitting in meditation. Tingling, painful. (2)
- Right-sided sciatica. (2)

EXTREMITIES

- Pain: stitching Finger joint. (6) Pain: stitching knee right. (6) Restless – moving feet while lying in bed. (6)

SLEEP

- Waking: 1 a.m. with severe cutting pains in stomach. Felt like diarrhea. Gas distress like when pregnant. Could not pass. Felt urge. Then relaxed and passed huge stool. Felt>> deeply cleansed. Slept well rest of night. (2)

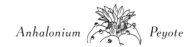

GENERALS

- Fatigue: Very groggy in the morning. Unusual. (Daughter woke me 3x/night.) (5)
- Fatigue: afternoon 3:30 PM (5), fatigue: noon. (5)
- Fatigue: Feels tired in the evening especially if around other people, easily tired by others. (1)
- Fatigue: Difficult waking in a.m. (1) Fatigue: Sleepy after lunch. (?)
- Fatigue: Extreme, did not want to do anything, napped. (3)
- Feels like doing things in slow motion, like mind and body moving through thick molasses. (1)
- Pain, slight, achy with flu like symptoms. (5)
- Pain, on waking: feeling tired, with under the weather blah feeling, muscles aching, weak lower back. (5)
- Aversion to direct sun. (1) Felt chilled. (5)

BIBLIOGRAPHY

Adams, George, and Olive Whicher. *The Plant Between Sun and Earth*. Boulder, Colorado: Shambhala, 1982.

Allen, Jane E. "Researcher Germinates 1,288-Year-Old Seed" [online]. *Gainesville Sun*. 14 November 1995. [cited 24 June 2002]. Available from: <http://aquat1.ifas.ufl.edu/pick1.html>

Apostolos-Cappadona. *The Dictionary of Christian Art*. New York: Continuum, 1994.

Beales, Peter. *Classic Rose*. New York: Henry Holt and Company, 1985.

Bown, Deni. *Encyclopedia of Herbs and Their Uses*. New York: Dorling Kindersley, 1995.

"A Brief History of Ginseng" [online]. In *Red Cloud Ginseng*. South Yarra, Australia: 1997. [cited on 12 Dec. 2001]. Available from: <http://www.jarvis.com.au/ginseng/Rchist1.htm>

Brill, "Wildman" Steve, and Evelyn Dean. *Identifying and Harvesting Edible and Medicinal Plants: In Wild (and Not So Wild) Places*. New York: Hearst Books, 1994.

Brother Thomas of Celano. *The Life of St. Francis of Assisi* and *The Treatise of Miracles*. Translated by Catherine Bolton. Assisi, Italy: Editrici Minerva Assisi, D.p.

Brun, Charles A. *Online Guide to Ginseng Production in the Pacific Northwest* [online]. 12 Dec. 2001. [cited on 28 Mar. 2002]. Available from: <http://clark.wsu.edu/horticulture/Ginseng/Cover/cover.html>

Cameron, Marilyn. "Aphrodite's Favorite Blossom: The Rose" [online]. In *Chamomile Times* [cited on 25 Mar. 2002]. Available from <http://www.chamomiletimes.com>

Carroll, Lewis. *Through the Looking Glass*. In *The Complete Works of Lewis Carroll*. New York: The Modern Library, 1936.

___. *The Path of Roses*. In *Complete Works*.

Castaneda, Carlos. *The Teachings of Don Juan: A Yaqui Way of Knowledge*. Berkeley: Univ. of California Press, 1968.

Chang, Chin-ju. "Lotus, Flower of Paradise" [online]. Translated by Jonathon Barnard. *Sinorama*, 22, no. 7 (July 1997). [cited on 24 June 2002]. Available from: <http://www.sinorama.com.tw/en/8607/607038e1.html>

Clarkson, Rosetta E. "Chinese Red Ginseng" from *Herbs: Their Culture and Uses*. New York: Collier Books, 1990.

Collura, Jennie O. "Ginseng: prince of tonics. (The Herbalist)" [online]. In *Vegetarian Times* (March, 1997) [cited on 12 Dec. 2001]. Available from: <http://www.findarticles.com/cf_1/m0820/n235/19173888/p1/article.jhtml>

Coulter, Merle C., and Howard J. Dittmer. *The Story of the Plant Kingdom*. Chicago: The Univ. of Chicago Press, 1964.

Dewan, Asheesh. "Ginseng: Delving into the Myth and Lore." *Resonance Homeopathy* 18 (Nov./Dec. 1996).

Dharmananda, Subhuti. "Safety Issues Affecting Chinese Herbs: The Case of Ginseng" [online]. In *Institute for Traditional Medicine*. Portland, Oregon: Institute for Traditional Medicine, 2000. [cited on 2 Dec. 2001]. Available from: <http://www.itmonline.org/arts/ginseng.htm>

Dobkin De Rios, Marlene. *Hallucinogens: Cross-Cultural Perspectives*. Great Britain: Prism Press, 1990.

Duke, James A. *Herbs of the Bible: 2000 Years of Plant Medicine*. Loveland, Colorado: Interweave Press, 1997.

Durrani, Anayat. "A Rose By Any Other Name" [online]. In *Arabia On Line*. 6 June 2001. [cited on 25 Mar. 2002]. Available from: <http://www.arabia.com/life/article/english/0,11827,48582,00.html>

Emboden, William. *Narcotic Plants: Revised and Enlarged*. New York: Macmillan Publishing Company, 1979.

___. "The sacred journey in dynastic Egypt: shamanistic trance in the context of the narcotic water lily and the mandrake" [online]. *Journal of Psychoactive Drugs* 21 (1) (Jan-Mar 1989): 61-75. Abstract. *The Vaults of Erowid*, 2000. [cited on 27 May 2001]. Available from: <http://www.erowid.org/plants/bluelotus/bluelotus_journal1.shtml>

Essick, Robert N. *William Blake at the Huntington: an Introduction to the William Blake Collection in the Henry E. Huntington Library and Art Gallery*. New York: Harry N. Abrams, 1994.

Flattery, David S., and J. M. Pierce. *Peyote*. Berkeley: The Berkeley Press, 1965.

Furst, Peter. *Flesh of the Gods: The ritual use of hallucinogens*. Prospect Heights, Ill.: Waveland Press, 1972.

Gasnick, Roy M., OFM, ed. *The Francis Book*. New York: Macmillan Publishing, 1980.

Grieve, Maud. "Mandrake" [online]. *A Modern Herbal*. In *Botanical*. New York: Dover Publications, 1971. (unabridged and corrected republication of *A Modern Herbal*. Harcourt, Brace … Company, 1931). [cited on 6 May 2001]. Available from: <http://www.botanical.com/botanical/mgmh/m/mandra10.html>

____. "Ginseng" [online]. *A Modern Herbal*. [cited on 12 Dec. 2001]. Available from: <http://www.botanical.com/botanical/mgmh/g/ginsen15.html>

____. "Roses" [online]. *A Modern Herbal*. [cited on 25 Mar. 2002]. Available from: <http://www.botanical.com/botanical/mgmh/r/roses-18.html>

Grohmann, Gerbert. *The Plant*. Vol. 2. Kimberton, Penn.: Bio-Dynamic Farming and Gardening Association, 1989.

Harriman, Sarah. *The Book of Ginseng*. New York: Pyramid Books, 1975.

Harris, Marvin. *Cows, Pigs, Wars, and Witches: The Riddles of Culture* [online]. In *The Witching Hours*. New York: Vintage Books, 1989. [cited on 05 July 2002]. Available from: <http://shanmonster.lilsproutz.com/witch/flying.html>

Heinerman, John. *Heinerman's Encyclopedia of Fruits, Vegetables and Herbs*. West Nyack, N.Y.: Parker Publishing, 1988.

Heiser, Charles B., Jr. *The Fascinating World of the Nightshades: Tobacco, Mandrake, Potato, Tomato, Pepper, Eggplant, etc*. New York: Dover Publications, 1987. (unabridged and corrected republication of *Nightshades: The Paradoxical Plants*. San Francisco: W.H. Freeman and Company, 1969).

Hobbs, Christopher. *The Ginsengs: A User's Guide*. Santa Cruz, Ca.: Botanica Press, 1996.

____. "Adaptogens — Herbal Gems to Help Us Adapt" [online]. In *HealthWorld Online*. Santa Monica, Ca.: D.p. [cited on 12 Dec. 2001]. Available from: <http://www.healthy.net/asp/templates/article.asp?PageType=Article&ID=934>

____. "Drugs with Adaptogenic Effects for Strengthening the Powers of Resistance" [online]. In *HealthWorldOnline*. [cited on 28 Mar. 2002]. Available from: <http://www.healthy.net/scr/Article.asp?Id=962>

Hufford, Mary. "American Ginseng and the Idea of the Commons" [online]. In *American Folklife Center*, Library of Congress. Reprinted from *Folklife Center News* 19 (nos. 1 and 2) (Winter-Spring 1997). [cited on 28 Mar. 2002]. Available from: <http://memory.loc.gov/ammem/cmnshtml/essay1/index.html>

___. Audio excerpts, "Stress Rings and the Value of Ginseng" [online]. *American Folklife Center's* Coal River Folklife Project (1992-99), Library of Congress. *Randy Halstead* access to audio interview. [cited on 28 Mar. 2002]. Available from: <http://memory.loc.gov/ammem/cmnshtml/essay1/essay1b.html>

Huson, Paul. *Mastering Herbalism: A Practical Guide.* New York: Stein and Day, 1975.

Huxley, Aldous. *The Doors of Perception* [online]. In *The Psychedelic Library.* First published in Great Britain: Chatto & Windus Ltd., 1954. [cited on 26 Jan. 2003] Available from: <http://www.druglibrary.org/schaffer/lsd/doors.htm>

Hyam, R., and R. Pankhurst. *Plants and Their Names: A Concise Dictionary.* Royal Botanic Garden, Edinburgh, Oxford: Oxford University Press, 1995.

Ikeda, President, Katsuji, Saito, Takamori, Endo, and Haruo, Suda. "Wisdom of the Lotus Sutra" [online]. Panel Discussion Series. In *Etherbods. Soka Gakkai International Newsletter*, 1995-2000. [cited on 24 June 2002]. Available from: <http://etherbods.com/sutra/wisdom/index.shtml>

"Images of Korean Culture: Korean Ginseng" [online]. In *Korea.net: Korean Government Homepage.* [cited 12 Dec. 2001]. Available from: <http://www.korea.net/koreanculture/imagesofkorean/imagesofkorean_07.html>

Jacobson, David. "Want a Love Potion? Alternatives to Viagra" [online]. In *WebMDHealth* [cited 12 dec. 2001]. Available from: <http://my.webmd.com/content/article/11/1668_50389>

Joh, Dr. Jason Namsik, trans. "The Young Man and the Wild Ginseng" [online]. In *Homepage of Korean Folktales.* [cited on 12 Dec. 2001]. Available from: <http://www.csun.edu/~hcedu004/ginseng.html>

Johnson, Timothy. *CRC Ethnobotany Desk Reference.* Boca Raton, Florida: CRC Press, 1999.

Kavanaugh. "The Apothecary's Rose" [online]. In *Herbal Health Plants.* [cited on 25 Mar. 2002]. Available from: <http://www.herbalhealthplants.com/article1011.html>

Khuda-Bukhsh, Anisur Rahman and Sharmisthat Banik. "Assessment of Cytogenetic Damage in X-irradiated Mice and Its Alteration by Oral Administration of a Potentized Homeopathic Drug, Ginseng D200." Paper presented at the VIIth All India Congress of Cytology and Genetics, Kalyani University, W.B., 22-26 Dec. 1990.

Krüssmann, Gerd. *The Complete Book of Roses.* Portland, Oregon: Timber Press, 1981.

La Barre, Weston. *The Peyote Cult.* Hamden, Connecticut: The Shoe String Press, 1969.

Lewis, Mark. "U.S. History Shaped By China Dreams" [online]. In *Forbes*. (6 Nov. 2001). [cited on 12 Dec. 2001]. Available from: <http://www.forbes.com/2001/11/06/1106chinamarket.html>

Lewis, Walter H., P. R. Elvin-Lewis, and Memory Elvin-Lewis. *Medical Botany: Plants affecting man's health*. New York: John Wiley and Sons, 1977.

Lowndes, Florin. *Enlivening the Chakra of the Heart*. London: Sophia Books, Rudolf Steiner Press, 1998.

Luciano Canonici. *Francis of Assisi*. Translated by Catherine Bolton Magrini. N.p.

"Lycanthropy" [online]. *The Columbia Encyclopedia*, 6th ed. New York: Columbia University Press, 2002. [cited on 6 May 2001]. Available from: <http://www.bartleby.com/65/ly/lycanthr.html>

Markoe, Karen. "200 Years of the China Trade" [online]. *Scholastic Search* (Nov. 14, 1980) [cited on 12 Dec. 2001]. Available from: <http://www.columbia.edu/itc/eacp/webcourse/chinaworkbook/for_pol/ch_trade.htm>

McKeon, Judith C. *The Encyclopedia of Roses*. Emmaus, Penn.: Rodale Press, 1995.

Metzner, Ralph. "Ayahuasca and the Greening of Human Consciousness." *Shaman's Drum*, no. 53 (1999).

Miller, Richard Alan. *The Magical and Ritual Use of Herbs*. Rochester, Vermont: Destiny Books, 1993.

Mooney, James. "The Snake Tribe" [online]. *Myths of the Cherokee*. In *Sacred Texts*. Nineteenth Annual Report of the Bureau of American Ethnology 1897-98, Part I. [1900] [cited on 12 Dec. 2001]. Available from: <http://www.sacred-texts.com/nam/cher/motc/motc049.htm>

"Panex Ginseng" [online]. In *Herbal Remedies*. [cited on 12 Dec 2001]. Available from: <http://www.herbalremedies.com/panginkorhis.html>

PDR for Herbal Medicines, 2nd ed. Montvale, NJ: Medical Economics Company, 2000. [Most references are in German].

Pelikan, Wilhelm. *Healing Plants: Insights through Spiritual Science*. Vol. 1. Spring Valley, New York: Mercury Press, 1997.

Pettit, Jeremy L. "Alternative Medicine." *Clinician Reviews* 10 (August 2000).

Pickles, Sheila. *The Language of Flower* [online]. New York: Harmony Books, 1989. [cited on 25 Mar. 2002]. Available from: <http://www.allrosesrosesroses.com/history.shtml>

Rätsch, Christian. *Plants of Love: Aphrodisiacs in history and a guide to their identification.* Berkeley, California: Ten Speed Press, 1997.

___. *The Dictionary of Sacred and Magical Plants.* Dorset: Prism Press, 1992.

"Ren Shen: panex ginseng" [online]. In *Herbal Hall: Professional Herbalists Discussion List.* [cited on 12 December, 2001]. Available from: <http://www.herb.com/files/ginseng.html>

"Rose." *Flower History* [online]. [cited on 25 Mar. 2002]. Available from: <http://www.flowermonthclub.com/history.htm>

Rudgley, Richard. *The Encyclopedia of Psychoactive Substances.* New York: St. Martin's Press, 1999.

Rumi. Mathnawi. (Mesnevi), II, 278. D.p.

Schaefer, Stacy B. "The Crossing of the Souls: Huichol Perceptions of Peyote." *Shaman's Drum* (Spring 1996).

Shen-Miller, J., Mary Beth Mudgett, J. William Schopf, Steven Clarke, and Rainer Berger. "Exceptional Seed Longevity and Robust Growth: Ancient Sacred Lotus from China." *American Journal of Botany*, Vol. 82 Issue 11 (Nov., 1995).

Slotte, Anita. "Chakras: Tools for Transformation" [online]. In *Alternative Culture.* [cited on 24 June 2002]. Available from: <http://www.alternativeculture.com/spirit/chakra.htm>

St. Clair, Richard. "The Wonderful Law of the Lotus Sutra" [online]. In *Pure Land Buddhism,* October 1998. [cited on 24 June 02]. Available from: <http://web.mit.edu/stclair/www/lotus.html>

Stafford, Peter. *Psychedelics Encyclopedia.* Berkeley, California: Ronin Press, 1978.

Sullivan, Dorothy. *Cherokee Heritage Calendar.* Norman, Oklahoma, 1996.

Ullman, Robert. "Ginseng (*Panax quinquefolium*)." *Resonance Homeopathy* 18 (Nov./Dec. 1996).

Valadez, Susana Eger. *Huichol Indian Sacred Rituals.* Oakland, California: Dharma Publishing, 1992.

Vento, Marie. "One Thousand Years of Chinese Footbinding: It's Origins, Popularity and Demise" [online]. In *University of Memphis.* 7 Mar 1988. [cited on 24 June 2002]. Available from: <http://www.people.memphis.edu/~kenichls/1301ChineseFootBinding.html>

Walsh, James J. "Anaesthesia" [online]. *Catholic Encyclopedia.* Vol. 1. New York: Robert Appleton, 1907. [cited on 6 Nov. 2001]. Available from: <http://www.newadvent.org/cathen/01447b.htm>

Waters, Jack. "The History of American Ginseng" [online]. *Tellico Plains Mountain Press.* [cited on 12 Dec. 2001]. Available from: <http://www.telliquah.com/Ginseng/Ginseng.htm>

Weidner, Marsha, ed. *Latter Days of the Law: Images of Chinese Buddhism 850 to 1850.* Spencer Museum of Art, University of Kansas: University of Hawaii Press, 1994.

Weiner, Michael A., and Janet Weiner. *Herbs That Heal: Prescriptions for Herbal Healing.* Mill Valley, California: Quantum Books, 1994.

Willard, Terry. "Herbs for your Health – Ginseng" [online]. *Alberta Agricultural Food and Rural Development.* [cited on 12 Dec. 2001]. Paper presented at Prairie Medicinal and Aromatic Plants Conference, Olds, Alberta. March 3-5, 1996. Available from: <http://www.agric.gov.ab.ca/crops/special/medconf/willardb.html>

Williams, Cheryll. *Wellbeing Magazine*, No. 69 (September 1997).

Williams, Joseph J., S.J. "Applied Magic" [online]. *Psychic Phenomena of Jamaica.* In *Sacred Texts.* New York: Dial Press, 1934. [cited on 05 July 2002]. Available from: <http://www.sacred-texts.com/afr/ppj/ppj002.htm>

Zimmer, Heinrich. *Myths and Symbols in Indian Art and Civilization.* Edited by Joseph Campbell. Vol. 6 of Bollingen Series. Princeton, New Jersey: Princeton Univ. Press, 1974.

RESOURCES

There are two pharmacies which carry the remedies made as a result of the provings in this book, as well as other remedies newly proven by Nancy Herrick.

From **Deutsche Homöopathie Union** in Germany, the following remedies are available:

Lac delphinum (Milk of the Dolphin)
Lac equinum (Milk of the Horse)
Lac leoninum (Milk of the Lion)
Lac lupinum (Milk of the Wolf)
Buteo jam (Red Tail Hawk)
Rosa gallica (Yellow Rose)

These are available to all homeopaths in 12c, 30c, 200c, 1M, and 10M potencies. Practitioners should request that their remedy vials be labeled "for research" when ordering.

Orders should be sent to:

DHU - ARZNEIMITTEL
GMBH & CO. KG
Ottostrasse 24
D-76227 Karlsruhe-Germany

Phone 011 49 721 4093-230
Fax 011 49 721 4093-244

From Hahnemann Pharmacy:
Sanguis soricis (Blood of the Rat)
Limenitis bredowii (Butterfly)
Maiasaura lapidea (Dinosaur)
Lac loxodonta (Milk of the Elephant)
Lac delphinum (Milk of the Dolphin)
Lac equinum (Milk of the Horse)
Lac leoninum (Milk of the Lion)
Lac lupinum (Milk of the Wolf)
Buteo jam (Red Tail Hawk)
Rosa gallica (Yellow Rose)
Ginseng (American and Korean)
Ayahuasca
Nilumbo nucifera (Lotus)
Anhalonium (Peyote Cactus)
Mandragora (Mandrake Root)
Rosa St. Francis (Rose of St. Francis)

Call Pharmacy for available potencies and prices. **1-888-4ARNICA** (1-888-427-6422)

ORDERING INFORMATION

To order copies of Nancy Herrick's books:

Sacred Plants, Human Voices
Animal Mind, Human Voices

Send check or money order, payable to Hahnemann Clinic Publishing.

Enclose $ 39.95 for each book
Tax (CA only) @ $3.30
US Shipping and Handling @ $6.00
Foreign S/H @ $20.00

Allow two weeks for US delivery.
Foreign air: twelve days.

MAIL TO:
Hahnemann Clinic Publishing
13974 Glenn Pines Rd.
Grass Valley, California 95945
Telephone and facsimile: 530–477–7397
jaffemarks@yahoo.com

Other material by Nancy Herrick:

Foundations of Homeopathy: Home Study Video Course is a comprehensive introduction to classical homeopathy. The program consists of live video taped lectures from the Hahnemann College of Homeopathy a four year course of study for medical professionals, featuring the world renown faculty: Nancy Herrick, PA, Roger Morrison, MD, and Jonathan Shore, MD, plus guest lecturers Deborah Gordon, MD, Todd Rowe, MD, and Anna Shore, PA. At this printing the series includes:

Foundations of Acute Prescribing
12 Tapes / 14 hours

Introduction to Acutes – Trauma and Injury – Otitis – Cystitis – Fever & Exanthem – Coryza – Allergy – Sinusitis – Cough – Pneumonia – Pharyngitis – Nausea & Vomiting – Stomach Pain – Abdominal Pain – Diarrhea

Includes *Desktop Companion to Physical Pathology* by Roger Morrison, MD.

Foundations of Homeopathic Theory Vol. I
8 Tapes / 8 hours

Overview of Homeopathy – Introduction to the Organon – Research in Homeopathy – Law of Similars – Evolution of a RX – Essence vs. Central Delusion – Introduction to Books – Introduction to Repertory: Generals – Introduction to Repertory: Mentals – Acute Case Taking

Foundations of Homeopathic Theory Vol. II
9 Tapes / 9 hours

The Kingdoms – History I & II – Antidotes – Aggravations – Remedy Reaction – Miasms – Provings – Potency – Acutes During Chronic – Chronic Case Taking for Essence – Chronic Case Taking for Data

Includes *Desktop Guide to Keynotes and Confirmatory Symptoms* by Roger Morrison, MD.

Foundations of Materia Medica Vol. I
12 Tapes / 14 hours

Introduction to Materia Medica – Pulsatilla – Natrum Muriaticum – Calcarea Carbonica – Phosphorous – Sulphur – Staphysagria – Lachesis – Sepia – Graphites – Nux Vomica – Aurum – Apis – Lac Caninum – Barytas – Ignatia – Lycopodium – Magnesias – Thuja – Psorinum – Arsenicum

Includes Nancy Herrick's *Animal Mind, Human Voices*.

Foundations of Materia Medica I Vol. II
12 Tapes / 14 hours

Acids – Cations – Anions – Cannabis – Chamomilla – Silica – Calcarea Salts – Argentum – Anacardium – Carcinosin – Tuberculinum – Lyssinum – Syphilinum – Hydrophobinum – Kali Salts & Carbonicum – Causticum – Aurum Salts – Ferrum – Halogens

To order *Foundations of Homeopathy: Home Study Video Course*
visit our website at
www.hahnemanncollege.com

The lectures are offered in five series which may be purchased individually or as a complete set. A comprehensive exam and certificate of completion is available from Hahnemann College which qualifies toward the CHC exam. For more information contact:

Hahnemann College of Homeopathy
80 Nicholl Avenue
Point Richmond, CA 94801
Telephone: 510-232-2079
Email: hahnemann@igc.org